# Nutritional Management of the Surgical Patient

# Nutritional Management of the Surgical Patient

Edited by

## Mary E. Phillips
### OStJ BSc (Hons) RD DipADP

Advanced Clinical Practitioner and Senior Specialist Dietitian
(Hepato-Pancreatico-Biliary Surgery)
Royal Surrey NHS Foundation Trust
Guildford, UK

**WILEY** Blackwell

*Registered Offices*
John Wiley & Sons, Inc., 111 River Street, Hoboken, NJ 07030, USA
John Wiley & Sons Ltd, The Atrium, Southern Gate, Chichester, West Sussex, PO19 8SQ, UK

For details of our global editorial offices, customer services, and more information about Wiley products visit us at www.wiley.com.

Wiley also publishes its books in a variety of electronic formats and by print-on-demand. Some content that appears in standard print versions of this book may not be available in other formats.

Trademarks: Wiley and the Wiley logo are trademarks or registered trademarks of John Wiley & Sons, Inc. and/or its affiliates in the United States and other countries and may not be used without written permission. All other trademarks are the property of their respective owners. John Wiley & Sons, Inc. is not associated with any product or vendor mentioned in this book.

*Limit of Liability/Disclaimer of Warranty*
While the publisher and authors have used their best efforts in preparing this work, they make no representations or warranties with respect to the accuracy or completeness of the contents of this work and specifically disclaim all warranties, including without limitation any implied warranties of merchantability or fitness for a particular purpose. No warranty may be created or extended by sales representatives, written sales materials or promotional statements for this work. This work is sold with the understanding that the publisher is not engaged in rendering professional services. The advice and strategies contained herein may not be suitable for your situation. You should consult with a specialist where appropriate. The fact that an organization, website, or product is referred to in this work as a citation and/or potential source of further information does not mean that the publisher and authors endorse the information or services the organization, website, or product may provide or recommendations it may make. Further, readers should be aware that websites listed in this work may have changed or disappeared between when this work was written and when it is read. Neither the publisher nor authors shall be liable for any loss of profit or any other commercial damages, including but not limited to special, incidental, consequential, or other damages.

*Library of Congress Cataloging-in-Publication Data*
Names: Phillips, Mary E. (Mary Elizabeth), editor.
Title: Nutritional management of the surgical patient / [edited by] Mary E.
    Phillips.
Description: Hoboken, NJ : Wiley-Blackwell, 2023. | Includes index. |
    Summary: "Nutrition in the surgical patient explains the role of
    clinical nutrition in patients undergoing surgery to their
    gastro-intestinal tract and within the thoracic and abdominal cavities.
    This book will provide an overview of assessment, current practice and
    considerations in the management of the surgical patient for clinicians
    working in clinical nutrition"– Provided by publisher.
Identifiers: LCCN 2023003632 (print) | LCCN 2023003633 (ebook) | ISBN
    9781119809098 (paperback) | ISBN 9781119809104 (adobe pdf) | ISBN
    9781119809111 (epub) | ISBN 9781119809128 (obook)
Subjects: MESH: Nutrition Therapy | Perioperative Care | Nutrition
    Assessment | Nutritional Status
Classification: LCC RM217 (print) | LCC RM217 (ebook) | NLM WB 400 | DDC
    615.8/54–dc23/eng/20230317
LC record available at https://lccn.loc.gov/2023003632
LC ebook record available at https://lccn.loc.gov/2023003633

Cover Design: Wiley
Cover Images: © David Malan/Getty Images; DIGICOMPHOTO/Getty Images

Set in 10.5/13 STIX Two Text by Straive, Pondicherry, India

SKY10052221_073123

# Contents

# Contributors

**Lindsey Allan**
Department of Nutrition and Dietetics
Royal Surrey NHS Foundation Trust
Guildford, UK

**Maria Ashworth**
Academic Department of Gynae-oncology
Royal Surrey NHS Foundation Trust
Guildford, UK

**Neil Bibby**
Department of Nutrition and Dietetics
Manchester University Hospitals NHS
Foundation Trust
Manchester, UK

**Jayanta Chatterjee**
Academic Department of Gynae-oncology
Royal Surrey NHS Foundation Trust
Guildford, UK

**Wissam Abou Chedid**
Department of Urology
Royal Surrey NHS Foundation Trust
Guildford, UK

**Alison Culkin**
Department of Nutrition and Dietetics
St Mark's Hospital
London Northwest Healthcare University Trust
London, UK

**Nárbhla Donnelly**
Department of Nutrition and Dietetics
Guy's and St Thomas' NHS Foundation Trust;
Department of Nutrition and Dietetics
The Royal London Hospital
Barts Health NHS Trust
London, UK

**Adam Frampton**
Department of HPB Surgery
Royal Surrey NHS Foundation Trust
Guildford, UK

**Oonagh Griffin**
Department of Nutrition and Dietetics
St Vincent's University Hospital;
School of Physiotherapy, Public Health
and Sports Science
University College Dublin
Dublin, Ireland

**Fiona Huddy**
Department of Nutrition and Dietetics
Royal Surrey NHS Foundation Trust
Guildford, UK

**Jeremy R. Huddy**
Department of Surgery
Frimley Health NHS Trust
Camberley, UK

**Chris Jones**
Department of Anaesthetics
Royal Surrey NHS Foundation Trust
Guildford, UK

**Rajiv Lahiri**
Department of HPB Surgery
Royal Surrey NHS Foundation Trust
Guildford, UK

**Anne Langan**
Department of Nutrition and Dietetics
Guy's and St Thomas' NHS Foundation Trust;
Department of Nutrition and Dietetics
The Royal London Hospital
Barts Health NHS Trust
London, UK

**Evanna Leavy**
Intestinal Failure & Gastrointestinal Surgery
St George's University Hospitals NHS
Foundation Trust
London, UK

**John S. Leeds**
HPB Unit
Freeman Hospital;
Population Health Sciences Institute
Newcastle University
Newcastle upon Tyne, UK

**Callum Livingstone**
Clinical Biochemistry Department
Royal Surrey NHS Foundation Trust
Guildford, UK

**Rebekah Lord**
Department of Nutrition and Dietetics
Manchester University Hospitals NHS
Foundation Trust
Manchester, UK

**Thanuya Mahendran**
Academic Department of Gynae-oncology
Royal Surrey NHS Foundation Trust
Guildford, UK

**Ashleigh Maske**
Department of Nutrition and Dietetics
Manchester University Hospitals NHS
Foundation Trust
Manchester, UK

**Helen McNamara**
Department of Occupational Therapy
Royal Surrey NHS Foundation Trust
Guildford, UK

**Nabeel Merali**
Department of HPB Surgery
Royal Surrey NHS Foundation Trust
Guildford, UK

**Gregory J Nason**
Department of Urology
Royal Surrey NHS Foundation Trust
Guildford, UK

**Ann-Marie Nixon**
Department of Nutrition and Dietetics
Wythenshawe Hospital
Manchester University NHS Foundation Trust
Manchester, UK

**Katy O'Rourke**
Department of Anaesthetics
Royal Surrey NHS Foundation Trust
Guildford, UK

**Alessandro Parente**
Department of Hepatopancreatobiliary
Surgery and Liver Transplantation
University Hospitals Birmingham
NHS Foundation Trust
Birmingham, UK;
Institute of Immunology and Immunotherapy
University of Birmingham
Birmingham, UK

**Rupal Patel**
Department of Nutrition and Dietetics
Royal Brompton and Harefield Hospitals
Guy's and St Thomas' NHS Foundation Trust
London, UK

**Krishna Patil**
Department of Urology
Royal Surrey NHS Foundation Trust
Guildford, UK

**Matthew J.A. Perry**
Department of Urology
Royal Surrey NHS Foundation Trust
Guildford, UK

**Mary E. Phillips**
Department of Nutrition and Dietetics
Royal Surrey NHS Foundation Trust
Guildford, UK

**Sarah Powell-Brett**
Department of Hepatopancreatobiliary Surgery
and Liver Transplantation
University Hospitals Birmingham NHS
Foundation Trust
Birmingham, UK

**Charles Rayner**
Department of Surgery
Royal Surrey NHS Foundation Trust
Guildford, UK

**Keith J. Roberts**
Department of Hepatopancreatobiliary Surgery
and Liver Transplantation, University Hospitals
Birmingham NHS Foundation Trust
Birmingham, UK;
Institute of Immunology and Immunotherapy
University of Birmingham
Birmingham, UK

**Cathy Skea**
Clinical Lead Dietitian
Department of Nutrition and Dietetics
Royal Victoria Hospital, Belfast
Belfast Health and Social Care Trust
Belfast, Northern Ireland

**Sara Smith**
School of Health Sciences
Queen Margaret University
Edinburgh, UK

**Naomi Westran**
Department of Nutrition and Dietetics
Royal Surrey NHS Foundation Trust
Guildford, UK

**Jennifer Wetherden**
Major Trauma & Critical Care
St George's University Hospitals NHS
Foundation Trust
London, UK

# INTRODUCTION

# CHAPTER 1

# Introduction

Welcome to this book exploring the nutritional management of the surgical patient.

An understanding of anatomy and surgical procedures is vital to ensure that nutritional management meets the needs of the surgical patient. This book is designed to give all surgical dietitians, surgical trainees, and gastroenterology trainees specialising in nutrition an overview of the impact of surgery on nutritional status and an insight into the nutritional management of complex conditions.

My first experience of the impact of surgery on nutrition came early in my career. As a junior dietitian I was referred a patient (Mr A) who had lost 50% of his body weight in three years.

Mr A came to my clinic in a wheelchair, very frail, weighing barely 40 kg. A detailed dietary history demonstrated that he consumed more than enough energy and protein to be gaining weight. Unfortunately, as he had continued to lose weight despite reporting compliance with nutritional advice and oral supplement drinks, it had been assumed that he was non-compliant. He had a good appetite, was not vomiting, but he did report he had rather frequent stools.

He was rather embarrassed to discuss this, but we eventually established that he was actually having his bowels open more than 10 times a day and was passing bright orange/yellow oily stool with visible food particles.

When I took a clinical history, he told me he had had an operation for a tumour on his pancreas four years ago, and a year after that an operation on his back. This wound had never healed and was still being dressed daily by district nurses.

I had never heard of a pancreatico-duodenectomy, so headed to the library (Google was not around back then!). Mr A was taking 10 000 units of enzymes with each meal, none with snacks, nor the supplement drinks he had been given. I had carried out my undergraduate dissertation in cystic fibrosis, so was familiar with pancreatic enzymes, and the much higher doses used there. After lengthy discussions with a very supportive GP (who had also never prescribed enzymes before) and Mr A's consultant surgeon, we escalated his enzyme dose. After several dose increases, we finally stopped the weight loss, restored normal bowel function, and the wound on his back started to heal, but we couldn't achieve

*Nutritional Management of the Surgical Patient*, First Edition. Edited by Mary E. Phillips.
© 2023 John Wiley & Sons Ltd. Published 2023 by John Wiley & Sons Ltd.

weight gain. Hence, we brought Mr A into hospital to establish nasogastric feeding. After six months of overnight tube feeding at home with a semi-elemental feed, Mr A walked into clinic at 65 kg having spent the weekend building a shed for his neighbour, and the wound on his back had healed.

Sadly, this story does not have an entirely happy ending, as nine months after, in his words, 'getting his life back' he developed liver metastases and quickly succumbed to his disease. We were able to give him nine months of good quality of life, but he lived for over five years after his cancer surgery. If we knew then what we know now, I suspect he could have had the full five years of good quality of life.

Roll forward more than 20 years and I am now privileged to work in a fully inclusive surgical multidisciplinary team, where collaborative working supports the early identification and management of the nutritional consequences of surgery, but I still see evidence of cases like Mr A's in clinical practice. So, this book is my attempt at filling what I see is still a gap in education in both dietetics and medicine.

Surgical procedures are becoming more complex and post-operative management is evolving to include more therapeutic nutritional management. The advent of immuno-nutrition, a greater understanding of the microbiome, the impact of sarcopenia, and continued improvements in survivorship following extensive cancer surgery mean we still have a lot to learn. I imagine the content of this book will change considerably in editions to come.

I would like to thank everyone who took the time to write chapters for this book, and the team at Wiley for their support, especially with all the stress of the global pandemic, which in hindsight was not the best time to undertake this project! I am delighted that we have been able to present a truly multiprofessional approach to nutrition.

So, this book is dedicated to Mr A, without whom I would not be in the job I am in now; to Professor Nariman Karanjia, who had the foresight to include a dietitian in the development of our tertiary hepato-pancreato-biliary centre 20 years ago, (and gave me the job!); and to Tanya Klopper, my manager, who has always supported me, however crazy some of my ideas may seem. Finally, thank you to my family, to whom I owe a massive debt of gratitude for putting up with the late nights and weekends of editing and listened to random sentences while I tried to get the wording right. As a consequence, I am the proud parent to teenagers who can pronounce encephalopathy and pancreatico-duodenectomy!

I hope this book is useful, and I welcome any suggestions for the next edition.

Happy reading
Mary E. Phillips
Advanced Clinical Practitioner/Senior Specialist
Dietitian (hepato-pancreatico-biliary surgery)

# BEFORE AND DURING SURGERY

# CHAPTER 2

# Nutrition Screening and Assessment

Sara Smith

*School of Health Sciences, Queen Margaret University, Edinburgh, UK*

---

**KEY POINTS**

- Nutrition screening and assessment are integral to effective multidisciplinary multimodal management of surgical patients.
- The loss of muscle mass and/or impaired function significantly increases peri-operative risks and delays post-operative recovery independently of body weight and body mass index (BMI).
- The screening of patients should ideally incorporate consideration of age, disease status, nutrition impact symptoms, changes in food intake/assimilation of food, signs of systemic inflammation, and losses in muscle mass and/or function.
- Those identified at risk on screening should be referred to a dietitian for a comprehensive assessment of nutrition status, including objective measures of muscle mass and function.

---

Early proactive screening and assessment of nutritional status are vital in identifying those at risk of malnutrition and other nutrition-related disorders to optimise readiness for surgery, minimise recognised peri-operative risks, and support enhanced post-operative recovery [1].

A globally agreed definition of malnutrition is lacking; most recently the European Society for Clinical Nutrition and Metabolism (ESPEN) has adopted a definition of malnutrition (synonym undernutrition) as 'a state resulting from a lack of intake or uptake of nutrition that leads to altered body composition (decreased lean tissue mass) and body cell mass leading to a diminished physical and mental function and impaired clinical outcome from disease', which can result from starvation, disease, or advanced ageing (>80 years), alone or in combination [2].

*Nutritional Management of the Surgical Patient*, First Edition. Edited by Mary E. Phillips.
© 2023 John Wiley & Sons Ltd. Published 2023 by John Wiley & Sons Ltd.

## OVERVIEW OF BODY COMPOSITION

Technological advancements in body composition assessment have allowed the identification of several distinct body tissue compartments (Table 2.1) variably affected by both deficiencies and excesses in nutrient intake, as well as the coexistence of metabolic derangements caused by certain conditions (e.g. infection, diabetes) and interventions (e.g. surgery).

The presence of an acute or chronic systemic inflammatory response because of underlying disease, trauma, or surgery has been shown to negatively impact on the preservation, utilisation, and function of the body's lean tissue stores [5]. Low levels of muscle mass and/or impaired function of existing muscle stores combined with the other metabolic effects of the systemic inflammatory response directly contribute to a significant increased perioperative risk, delayed recovery from surgery, and worse outcomes independent of body weight and body mass index (BMI) [3, 6].

## NUTRITION-RELATED SYNDROMES

Greater knowledge and understanding of body composition have in turn led to the recognition of other nutrition-related syndromes beyond malnutrition (Table 2.2). Presently the reported prevalence of these nutrition-related syndromes varies considerably due to differences in the diagnostic criteria utilised and the clinical population studied. Despite this, the published literature consistently reinforces the importance of nutrition screening and assessment in surgical patients to minimise the adverse impact of nutrition-related syndromes. Ongoing global work [7] to unify terminology and diagnostic criteria should support a better understanding of prevalence, as well as the earlier identification of those at risk and the most effective interventions.

As there is considerable overlap between the recognised nutrition-related syndromes with the coexistence of one or more syndromes possible [12, 13], further work is required to establish the significance of single versus concurrent syndrome occurrence, in relation to peri- and post-operative clinical outcomes and the development of targeted multimodal interventions [14].

## NUTRITION SCREENING

The process of nutrition screening is intended to provide a rapid, straightforward, cost-effective way of identifying those at risk of nutrition-related problems [15]. In doing so it aims to improve outcomes through the delivery of timely and targeted nutrition interventions. Screening should guide rather than replace clinical decision making and the

**TABLE 2.1** Body composition compartments.

| Body compartment | Description |
| --- | --- |
| Fat-free mass (FFM) | Lean tissue plus bone mineral content |
| Lean soft tissue mass (LSTM) | Sum of all lean tissues excluding bone. Includes protein, extracellular water (ECW) and intracellular water (ICW), carbohydrates, non-fat lipids, and soft tissue minerals |
| Skeletal muscle mass (SMM) | Primary component of lean tissue |
| Fat mass (FM) | Lipid content, forming 80% of adipose tissue |
| Adipose tissue (AT) | Connective tissues (adipocytes, collagenous, elastic fibres), fibroblasts, and capillaries |
| Intermuscular adipose tissue (IMAT) | Presence of lipids in adipocytes underneath the deep fascia of muscle. Includes the visible storage of lipids in adipocytes located between the muscle fibres and between muscle groups |

Source: Adapted from [3, 4].

**TABLE 2.2** Nutrition-related syndromes.

| Syndrome | Diagnostic criteria |
|---|---|
| Malnutrition | Global Leadership Initiative on Malnutrition (GLIM) proposes a diagnosis of malnutrition based on the presence of at least one phenotypic criterion *and* one aetiological criterion, with a further Stage 1/moderate or Stage 2/severe classification depending on severity [7]<br><br>*Phenotypical criteria:*<br>1. Weight loss >5% within past 6 mo, or >10% beyond 6 mo<br>2. Low BMI (kg/m [2]) <20 if <70 yr, or <22 if >70 yr. Asia: <18.5 if <70 yr, or <20 if >70 yr<br>3. Reduced muscle mass – determined using a validated body composition technique. When not available mid-arm muscle circumference or calf circumference can be used. Functional assessments like handgrip are considered as supportive measures<br><br>*Aetiological criteria:*<br>1. Reduced food intake or assimilation ≤50% of energy requirement >1 wk, or any reduction for >2 wk, or any chronic gastrointestinal condition that has adverse impacts on food absorption<br>2. Inflammation – acute disease/injury (e.g. major infection, burns, trauma, surgery, closed head injury) or chronic disease related (e.g. malignancy, chronic obstructive pulmonary disorder). C-reactive protein (CRP) can be used as a supportive laboratory measure |
| Sarcopenia | Progressive and generalised skeletal muscle mass disorder in older adults associated with increased likelihood of adverse outcomes including falls, frailty, physical disability, and increased mortality [8]<br><br>Primary sarcopenia: age-related loss of muscle mass with no other underlying cause identified [8]<br>Secondary sarcopenia: causal factors other than (or in addition to) ageing are evident, e.g. systemic disease, malnutrition, or physical inactivity and/or bed rest [8]<br><br>Proposed diagnostic criteria [8]:<br>• A probable diagnosis based on evidence of low muscle strength (handgrip, chair stand test); a confirmed diagnosis based on low muscle strength and quantity or quality of muscle stores determined via validated dual energy x-ray absorptiometry (DXA) or bio-electrical impedance analysis (BIA)<br>• Severe sarcopenia can be diagnosed based on these criteria plus evidence of low physical performance determined via validated test, e.g. gait speed |
| Sarcopenic obesity | Defined as the coexistence of obesity and sarcopenia. Considered a unique condition separate from obesity or sarcopenia alone, not confined to older adults [9]<br><br>Recommended screening should be based on [9]:<br>• A high body mass index (BMI) or waist circumference (WC), based on ethnic cut-points<br>*and*<br>• Surrogate parameters for sarcopenia, e.g. clinical symptoms/suspicion (e.g. age >70 yr, chronic disease diagnosis, recent acute disease, history of falls/fatigue/weakness/mobility limitations) or validated screening questionnaires (e.g. SARC-F for older adults) |

(Continued)

**TABLE 2.2**   (Continued)

| Syndrome | Diagnostic criteria |
| --- | --- |
| | Proposed diagnostic process/criteria [9]:<br>1. Stage 1: Altered skeletal muscle function, e.g. handgrip strength, sit to stand (chair rise). If stage 1 parameters are suggestive of sarcopenic obesity (SO), diagnosis should progress to stage 2<br>2. Stage 2: Altered body composition: increased fat mass (%FM) and reduced muscle mass as assessed by appendicular lean mass adjusted for weight (ALM/W) measured by DXA or skeletal muscle mass adjusted for weight (SSM/W) measured by BIA (If neither DXA nor BIA is available, calf circumference adjusted for BMI may provide a practical alternative)<br>For diagnosis **both** altered body composition and skeletal muscle function should be present. On confirmation of SO staging/severity can be determined as follows:<br>• Stage 1 SO: No complications<br>• Stage 2 SO: Presence of at least one complication attributable to SO, e.g. metabolic diseases, functional disabilities resulting from high FM and/or low muscle mass, cardiovascular and respiratory diseases |
| Cachexia | Complex metabolic syndrome associated with an underlying illness and characterised by loss of muscle with or without the loss of FM, which is associated with anorexia, inflammation, insulin resistance, and increased loss of lean tissue mass [10]<br>Proposed diagnostic criteria [10]:<br>• Weight loss of $\geq$5% (oedema/ascites free) in 12 mo or less (or BMI <20 kg/m$^2$ where weight loss cannot be determined) in the presence of underlying illness<br>*Plus three* of the following criteria:<br>• Decreased muscle strength (lowest tertile)<br>• Fatigue (defined as physical and/or mental weariness resulting from exertion; an inability to continue exercise at the same intensity with a resultant deterioration in performance)<br>• Limited food intake (total energy intake less than 20 kcal/kg body weight/day; <70% usual intake) or poor appetite<br>• Low fat free mass index/lean tissue depletion (mid-upper arm muscle circumference <10th percentile for age, sex)<br>• Increased inflammatory markers, e.g. CRP (>5.0 mg/l)<br>• Anaemia (haemoglobin <120 g/l)<br>• Low serum albumin (<32 g/l)<br>In making a diagnosis of cachexia, starvation, malabsorption, primary depression, hyperthyroidism, and age-related loss of muscle mass should be excluded |
| Frailty | Lack of universally accepted definition and criteria; can be defined as a multidimensional syndrome of decreased reserve and resistance to stressors, resulting from cumulative declines across multiple physiological systems, and causing vulnerability to adverse outcomes. Fried et al. [11] proposed phenotypical diagnostic criteria:<br>• Unintentional weight loss (>5% in last 12 mo)<br>• Self-reported exhaustion<br>• Weakness (grip strength in the lowest 20% baseline adjusted for age, sex, and BMI)<br>• Slow walking speed (slowest 20% of the population based on time to walk 15 ft (4.57 m), adjusted for sex and standing height)<br>• Low physical activity (male <383 kcal/week; female <270 kcal/week)<br>Positive for frailty phenotype when three or more criteria are present. Intermediate or pre-frail when one or two criteria are present |

identification of those at risk should be accompanied by a clear management plan.

The use of a validated and reliable screening process is vital to avoid the misclassification of patients. Multiple validated screening tools are available. Most malnutrition screening tools have been validated in adult patient settings and sarcopenia screening tools in healthy community-dwelling older adults [16].

Table 2.3 provides a summary of the recommended screening tools. In the UK, the Malnutrition Universal Screening Tool (MUST) has been commonly recommended for the purpose of routine malnutrition screening. While of proven value in identifying patients at risk of malnutrition [19], it does have limitations; for example, it does not specifically consider the presence of systemic inflammation, changes in muscle mass and function, or

**TABLE 2.3** Summary of commonly used nutrition screening tools.

| Screening tool | Description |
|---|---|
| Malnutrition Universal Screening Tool (MUST) | A five-step validated tool considered to provide a rapid and simple method of identifying adults at risk of malnutrition. Focuses on current and recent changes in tissue mass, e.g. body mass index (BMI); involuntary weight loss history and current dietary intake linked to the presence of acute disease<br>Patients are classified as low, medium, or high risk, and scores and immediate management guidelines based on risk category are provided [17]<br>A self-screening version is also available |
| Subjective Global Assessment (SGA) | A validated tool used to identify adults at risk of malnutrition [18]. Considered more of an assessment tool than a screening tool due to the inclusion of clinical history and physical examination [19]. As it is more complex, it is less suitable for rapid screening purposes [19]<br>Focuses on history of involuntary weight loss, reduced dietary intake, nutrition impact symptoms (e.g. early satiety, constipation, nausea, diarrhoea, vomiting), self-reported function, disease state in relation to the presence or absence of metabolic stress, a physical examination of fat/muscle stores, and the presence of ascites and oedema<br>Patients are classified as SGA-A (well nourished); SGA-B (mildly/moderately malnourished); or SGA-C (severely malnourished) |
| Patient Generated SGA (PG-SGA) | The PG-SGA was derived from the SGA for specific use within oncology populations [20]. The first four sections are designed to be completed by the patient and focus on current and previous weight history, changes in food intake/current type of intake, nutrition impact symptoms, and activities and function. Like the SGA it is a hybrid of screening and assessment and is more complex and time consuming to complete |
| Mini Nutrition Assessment (MNA) | MNA is validated for use with adults older than 65 yr [21]<br>The original full (18-item) version includes elements of screening and assessment including changes in body weight, dietary intake, mobility, psychological stress or acute disease, neuropsychological status, BMI, measurement of mid-arm and calf circumference, and presence/absence of pressure sores. Scores vary from 0 to 30, with ≤17.5–23.5 indicating risk<br>Due to the time required for completion of the 18-item version, a shorter screening version, MNA-SF, was developed [22]. Scores vary from 0 to 14, with ≤11 indicating risk. Subsequently a self-completion version has been developed [23] |

(Continued)

**TABLE 2.3**   (Continued)

| Screening tool | Description |
| --- | --- |
| Strength; Assistance with walking; Rising from a chair; Climbing stairs; and Falls (SARC-F) | Validated for use in older adults. Five-item self-reported questionnaire allowing the rapid identification of those at risk of sarcopenia and associated adverse outcomes. Focuses on perceptions of limitations in strength, walking ability, rising from the chair, stair climbing, and fall risk [24]. Due to its low-moderate sensitivity and high specificity, likely to primarily detect severe cases [8]. May also offer some utility as a screen for frailty [25]<br>Scores range from 0 to 10 points, with ≥4 being predictive of sarcopenia risk [24]<br>SARC-CalF combines the five items of SARC-F with a measurement of calf circumference (CC), which may provide improved sensitivity for screening [26]. CC is scored as 0 in the absence of a low muscle mass (<31 cm) and as 10 where low muscle mass is evident. A total score of ≥11 points indicates a risk of sarcopenia [27] |
| Clinical Frailty Scale (CFS) | Validated nine-point scale for use with older adults: based on medical history, cognitive status, and physical/activities of daily living history [28]. Increasingly recommended as a rapid, valid, and reliable screening tool for determining peri-operative frailty risk [29]<br><br>The CFS classifies patients as (1) very fit; (2) well; (3) well with treated comorbid disease; (4) apparently vulnerable; (5) mildly frail; (6) moderately frail; (7) severely frail; (8) very severely frail; or (9) terminally ill |

disease-specific nutrition impact symptoms that can increase risk. Additionally, the likelihood of at-risk overweight/obese patients not being identified was recognised some time ago [30]. Alternative screening tools have been recommended in a bid to address some of these limitations (see Table 2.2). However, currently there is no single validated screening tool that allows the simultaneous screening of malnutrition, sarcopenia, and cachexia [16]. Some nutrition screening tools allow for elements of patient self-reporting (e.g. MUST self-screening, Patient-Generated Subjective Global Assessment [PG-SGA]), which can result in lower specificity and reliability due to possible misinterpretation of the questions [31]. Therefore, use and interpretation of self-reported questions should be done with consideration of individual factors that can influence responses such as levels of health literacy, depression, anxiety, and impaired cognition [5]. The choice of screening tools in practice should be influenced by whether appropriate validation studies have been undertaken in the target population and have demonstrated sufficient sensitivity and specificity [32].

Where the use of a screening tool is not practically possible, more subjective criteria and visual signs can provide an indication of risk. For example, it has been suggested that a person who is visually thin; whose clothes and/or jewellery have become loose fitting; who has a history of decreased food intake, reduced appetite, or dysphagia over three to six months; and who has underlying disease or psychological /physical disabilities likely to cause weight loss should be deemed at risk of malnutrition [17].

## NUTRITION ASSESSMENT

When nutrition screening identifies individuals at high risk of nutrition-related problems, this should be followed by a comprehensive nutrition assessment by an appropriately qualified individual, for instance a dietitian, to determine the cause (diagnosis) and extent (severity) of the nutrition-related problems in order to guide anticipated outcomes and targeted interventions [15].

While it is possible to utilise computed tomography (CT), magnetic resonance imaging (MRI), dual-energy x-ray absorptiometry (DXA), or ultrasound scanning (USS) to quantify body tissues and functionality more accurately, these methods are not generally part of routine clinical care [5]. This is primarily due to practical reasons linked to local accessibility and experience, costs, and what could be considered unnecessary exposure to radiation (CT, DXA). However, in some clinical areas, such as oncology, the simultaneous use of abdominal and pelvic scans for diagnostic and nutrition purposes is increasing [5]. Further advances in the development of automated quantification technology may afford increased opportunities to utilise these types of scans on a more routine basis.

There are several validated methods that can be utilised to quantify fat, skeletal muscle mass, and function in day-to-day clinical practice. These are summarised in Table 2.4.

**TABLE 2.4** Summary of nutritional and functional markers/indices.

| | |
|---|---|
| Body Mass Index (BMI) | Considered to be a quick marker of chronic nutritional status linked to health risk |
| | At a population level, low or high BMI is consistently associated with increased morbidity and mortality. At an individual level, BMI has several limitations: it doesn't discriminate between fat and lean tissue stores; differences in fat distribution (e.g. visceral, subcutaneous) due to differences in sex, ethnicity, age, or in those taking gender-affirming hormone therapy the functionality of muscle stores is also ignored. |
| | Accurate measurement of height/weight is required – use of surrogate/self-reported can over- or underestimate BMI. Significant changes in hydration, presence of ascites, oedema, or amputations will affect accuracy |
| | BMI should be used in combination with more specific markers of fat, muscle, and function |
| Involuntary (unplanned/ unintentional) weight loss (IWL) | Reflects acute changes in nutritional status |
| | Significant predictor of length of stay, morbidity, and mortality |
| | Weight loss 5–10% over the last 3–6 mo is an early indicator of increased risk independent of BMI status. Weight loss >10% is clinically significant and warrants nutritional intervention |
| | Significant changes in hydration, presence of ascites, or oedema should be considered when calculating and interpreting |
| Mid-upper arm circumference (MUAC) | MUAC is a marker of fat mass and lean tissue mass that can be used to identify malnutrition. It has been shown to be a predictor of mortality in hospitalised patients |
| | Although it can be used to estimate BMI in the absence of weight and height, results should be interpreted with caution and not used as a sole measurement to determine risk [17] |
| | If MUAC <23.5 cm, BMI is likely to be <20 kg/m$^2$ |
| | If MUAC >32.0 cm, BMI is likely to be >30 kg/m$^2$ |
| Mid-arm muscle circumference (MAMC) | Marker of upper-body muscle stores. Determined from the measurements of MUAC and triceps skinfold thickness (TSF) as follows: |
| | MAMC (cm) = MUAC (cm) − (TSF [mm] × 0.3142) |
| | The measurement of skinfolds requires the use of a reliable skinfold caliper, training, and skill to ensure accuracy of the derived MAMC |
| | Appropriate centiles can be used to interpret results |

(Continued)

**TABLE 2.4**    (Continued)

| | |
|---|---|
| Calf circumference (CC) | Indirect marker of muscle stores highly correlated with direct measurements of skeletal muscle mass [33]. Maximal circumference is measured in a seated position Recent diagnostic cut-offs derived from US data [33] are as follows: <br>• Males: moderately low CC 34 cm, severely low 32 cm <br>• Females: moderately low CC 33 cm, severely low 31 cm <br>Presence of oedema should be considered when measuring/interpreting BMI adjustment factors (based on ethnicity and sex) outside the range of BMI 18.5–24.9 kg/m² are available, potentially increasing the utility of CC in practice [33] |
| Handgrip strength (HGS) | Measures upper-extremity grip strength using a calibrated handheld dynamometer. Portable and inexpensive method shown to predict outcome independent of muscle stores <br>Considered to be a crucial assessment of strength for patients with suspected sarcopenia [15] <br>Consideration of how measurements are taken (e.g. lying, sitting, standing); the type of dynamometer used; presence of comorbidities, e.g. impaired cognition, arthritis, depression, inflammation, myopathy, and neuropathy, is needed when interpreting findings UK population centiles are available [34], with a weak handgrip defined as follows: <br>• Males <27.0 kg <br>• Females <16.0 kg |
| Sit to stand (chair rise) | Functional performance test of lower limbs demonstrating a stronger relationship with muscle strength than muscle mass <br>Several versions of the test exist, e.g. time taken to undertake five transitions or number of transitions completed within 30 or 60 s. The timed five sit to stands may be more practical for older adults. Results can be interpreted using relevant population data or diagnostic cut-offs, e.g. >15 s for five chair rises [8] |
| Gait speed | Measure of functional performance (mobility) <br>Commonly measured as an individual's usual walking pace over a level 4 m distance A usual gait speed of <0.8 m/s has been proposed as a diagnostic cut-off in older adults [8] |

Source: Adapted from [5, 35].

# REFERENCES

1. Gillis, C. and Wischmeyer, P.E. (2019). Pre-operative nutrition and the elective surgical patient: why, how and what? *Anaesthesia* 74 (Suppl 1): 27–35.

2. Cederholm, T., Barazzoni, R., Austin, P. et al. (2017). ESPEN guidelines on definitions and terminology of clinical nutrition. *Clin. Nutr.* 36 (1): 49–64.

3. Sheenan, P., Gonzalez, C., Prado, C.M. et al. (2019). American Society for parenteral and enteral nutrition clinical guidelines: the validity of body composition assessment in clinical populations. *J. Parenter. Enteral. Nutr.* 44 (1): 12–43.

4. Addison, O., Marcus, R.L., Lastayo, P.C., and Ryan, A.S. (2014). Intermuscular fat: a review of the consequences and causes. *Int. J. Endocrinol.* 2014: 309570.

5. Smith, S. and Madden, A.M. (2016). Body composition and functional assessment of nutritional status in adults: a narrative review of imaging, impedance, strength and functional techniques. *J. Hum. Nutr.* 29 (6): 714–732.

6. Desborough, J.P. (2000). The stress response to trauma and surgery. *Br. J. Anaesth.* 85 (1): 109–117.

7. Cederholm, T. and Jensen, G.L. (2019). GLIM criteria for the diagnosis of malnutrition: a consensus report from the global clinical nutrition community. *Clin. Nutr.* 38: 1–9.

8. Cruz-Jentoft, A.J., Bahat, G., Bauer, J. et al. (2019). Sarcopenia: revised European consensus on definition and diagnosis. *Age and Ageing* 48: 16–31.

9. Donini, L.M., Busetto, L., Bauer, J.M. et al. (2022). Definition and diagnostic criteria for sarcopenic obesity: ESPEN and EASO consensus statement. *Clin. Nutr.* 41 (4): 990–1000.

10. Evans, W.J., Morley, J.E., Argiles, J. et al. (2008). Cachexia: a new definition. *Clin. Nutr.* 27: 793–799.

11. Fried, L.P., Tangen, C.M., Walston, J. et al. (2001). Frailty in older adults: evidence for a phenotype. *J. Parenter. Enteral. Nut.* 56 (3): M146–M156.

12. Mori, H. and Tokuda, Y. (2019). Differences and overlap between sarcopenia and physical frailty in older community-dwelling Japanese. *Asia Pac. J. Clin. Nutr.* 28 (1): 157–165.

13. Faxén-Irving, G., Luiking, Y., Grönstedt, H. et al. (2021). Do malnutrition, sarcopenia and frailty overlap in nursing-home residents? *J. Frailty & Aging* 10 (1): 17–21.

14. Gingrich, A., Volkert, D., Kiesswetter et al. (2019). Prevalence and overlap of sarcopenia, frailty, cachexia and malnutrition in older medical inpatients. *BMC Geriatr.* 19: 120.

15. Jensen, G.L. and Cederholm, T. (2018). The malnutrition overlap syndromes of cachexia and sarcopenia: a malnutrition conundrum. *Am. J. Clin. Nutr.* 108: 1157–1158.

16. Miller, J., Wells, L., Nwulu, U. et al. (2018). Validated screening tools for the assessment of cachexia, sarcopenia, and malnutrition: a systematic review. *Am. J. Clin. Nutr.* 108 (6): 1196–1208.

17. Todorovic, V., Russell, C.A., and Elia, M. (2011). *The 'MUST' Explanatory Booklet. A Guide to the Malnutrition Universal Screening Tool (MUST) for Adults.* Redditch: BAPEN.

18. Detsky, A.S., McLaughlin, J.R., Baker, J.P. et al. (1987). What is subjective global assessment of nutritional status? *J. Parenter. Enteral. Nutr.* 11 (1): 8–13.

19. Reber, E., Schönenberger, K.A., Vasiloglou, M.F., and Stanga, Z. (2021). Nutritional risk screening in cancer patients: the first step toward better clinical outcome. *Front. Nutr.* 8: 603936.

20. Ottery, F.D. (1996). Definition of standardized nutritional assessment and interventional pathways in oncology. *Nutrition* 12 (1): S15–S19.

21. Kondrup, J., Allison, S.P., Elia, M. et al. (2003). Educational and clinical practice committee, European Society of Parenteral and Enteral Nutrition (ESPEN). ESPEN guidelines for nutrition screening 2002. *Clin. Nutr.* 22 (4): 415–421.

22. Kaiser, M.J., Bauer, J.M., Ramsch, C. et al. (2009). Validation of the mini nutritional assessment short-form (MNA-SF): a practical tool for identification of nutritional status. *J. Nutr. Health Aging* 13 (9): 782–788.

23. Huhmann, M.B., Perez, V., Alexander, D.D., and Thomas, D.R. (2013). A self-completed nutrition screening tool for community-dwelling older adults with high reliability: a comparison study. *J. Nutr. Health Aging* 17 (4): 339–344.

24. Malmstrom, T.K. and Morley, J.E. (2013). SARC-F: a simple questionnaire to rapidly diagnose sarcopenia. *J. Am. Med. Direct. Assoc.* 14 (8): 531–532.

25. Bahat, G., Ozkok, S., Kilic, C., and Karan, M.A. (2021). SARC-F questionnaire detects frailty in older adults. *J. Nutr. Health Aging* 25 (4): 448–453.

26. Lu, J.L., Ding, L.Y., Xu, Q. et al. (2021). Screening accuracy of SARC-F for sarcopenia in the elderly: a diagnostic meta-analysis. *J. Nutr. Health Aging* 25: 172–182.

27. Barbosa-Silva, T.G., Menezes, A.M.B., Bielemann, R.M. et al. (2016). Enhancing SARC-F: improving sarcopenia screening in the clinical practice. *J. Am. Med. Direct. Assoc.* 17: 1136–1141.

28. Rockwood, K., Song, X., MacKnight, C. et al. (2005). A global clinical measure of fitness and frailty in elderly people. *Can. Med. Assoc. J.* 173 (5): 489–495.

29. Darvall, J.N., Loth, J., Bose, T. et al. (2020). Accuracy of the clinical frailty scale for perioperative frailty screening: a prospective observational study. *Can. J. Anaesth.* 67 (6): 694–705.

30. Davidson, H.I.M. and Smith, S. (2004). Nutritional screening: pitfalls of nutritional screening in the injured obese patient. *Proc. Nutr. Soc.* 63: 421–425.

31. Balstad, T.R., Bye, A., Jenssen, C.R. et al. (2019). Patient interpretation of the patient-generated subjective global assessment (PG-SGA) short form. *Pat. Prefer. Adher.* 13: 1391–1400.

32. Gillis, C., Hasil, L., Kasvis, P. et al. (2021). Nutrition care process model approach to surgical Prehabilitation in oncology. *Front. Nutr.* 8: 644706.

33. Gonzalez, M.C., Mehrnezhad, A., Razaviarab, N. et al. (2021). Calf circumference: cutoff values from the NHANES 1999-2006. *Am. J. Clin. Nutr.* 113 (6): 1679–1687.

34. Dodds, R.M., Syddall, H.E., Cooper, R. et al. (2014). Grip strength across the life course: normative data from twelve British studies. *PLoS One* 9 (12): e113637.

35. Madden, A.M. and Smith, S. (2016). Body composition and morphological assessment of nutritional status in adults: a review of anthropometric variables. *J. Hum. Nutr. Diet.* 29: 7–25.

# CHAPTER 3

# Nutritional Considerations Prior to Surgery

Oonagh Griffin

*Department of Nutrition and Dietetics, St Vincent's University Hospital, Dublin, Ireland*
*School of Physiotherapy, Public Health and Sports Science, University College Dublin, Dublin, Ireland*

---

**KEY POINTS**

- Malnutrition is prevalent in surgical populations, especially in patients with underlying malignant disease.
- Both malnutrition and sarcopenia increase the risk of post-operative morbidity and reduce overall survival.
- Pre-operative nutrition screening should be universally applied to allow timely identification and treatment of malnutrition.
- The goal of nutritional support should focus on appropriate nutritional therapy to optimise surgical readiness, minimise starvation, prevent post-operative malnutrition, and support anabolism for recovery.

---

Malnutrition is prevalent in pre-operative patients, with studies demonstrating that nearly half of all patients are malnourished on admission to hospital [1, 2]. International collaborative projects such as 'NutritionDay' have allowed annual surveys of the nutritional status of hospitalised inpatients, demonstrating significant determinants of malnutrition as predictors of prolonged length of stay, morbidity, and mortality [3, 4]. Recently the Global Leadership Initiative on Malnutrition (GLIM) consensus criteria for the diagnosis of malnutrition have been developed and proposed by the European Society for Clinical Nutrition and Metabolism (ESPEN), moving the diagnostic criteria beyond phenotypical criteria such as weight loss or low body mass index (BMI), and considering the impact of aetiological criteria such as malabsorption and inflammation [5] (see Chapter 2). Indeed, surgical illness is often an instance where both the phenotypical and aetiological causes of malnutrition occur

*Nutritional Management of the Surgical Patient*, First Edition. Edited by Mary E. Phillips.
© 2023 John Wiley & Sons Ltd. Published 2023 by John Wiley & Sons Ltd.

**TABLE 3.1**  Aetiology of malnutrition in surgical patients.

| Inadequate nutritional intake | Malabsorption | Impaired nutrient assimilation |
|---|---|---|
| Pain | Gastrointestinal resection | Sepsis |
| Dysphagia | Autoimmune disease e.g. inflammatory bowel disease, coeliac disease | Insulin resistance |
| Hypermetabolism | Ischaemia | Cancer cachexia |
| Nausea and vomiting (disease or treatment induced) | Pancreatic insufficiency | Refeeding syndrome |
| Anorexia | Radiation enteropathy | |
| Food aversion/dietary restrictions, including unpleasant eating environment | Biliary obstruction | |
| Psychosocial factors e.g. underlying disability, poverty, inadequate food supply | Significant small bowel oedema | |
| Emotional distress and anxiety | | |

simultaneously, especially where there is underlying cancer or autoimmune disease. The aetiology of malnutrition in surgical patients is outlined in Table 3.1.

Malnutrition in surgical patients typically manifests as decreased nutritional intake, unintentional weight loss, and/or loss of muscle mass and function (or sarcopenia). Regardless of baseline BMI, sarcopenia has been shown to be a negative prognostic factor for patients undergoing major abdominal surgery [6], while cancer patients with both obesity and sarcopenia [7] endured the most severe outcomes [8–10]. Sarcopenic obesity has recently been defined as the coexistence of excess adiposity and low muscle mass/function [11, 12]. In addition to sarcopenic obesity, increased adipose deposition in both muscle and lean tissue structures such as muscle – manifesting as myosteatosis – is recognised as an adverse prognostic feature, with studies suggesting that computed tomography (CT)-based muscle radiodensity or attenuation may be superior to CT-based muscle mass assessment as a surrogate for muscle function and strength [13]. Muscle attenuation or radiodensity is reduced by adipose tissue infiltration of muscle, a known consequence of ageing. Increased accumulation of lipid within muscle has also been

demonstrated in patients with increased inflammation associated with cachexia [14], and is associated with reduced muscle contractility and power [13]. Transcriptomic analysis of rectus abdominal muscle biopsies taken from patients at the time of cancer resection highlighted that sarcopenia and myosteatosis are distinct biological profiles; increased inflammation and decreased muscle synthesis were observed in patients with sarcopenia, while disruption of oxidative phosphorylation and lipid accumulation were seen in patients with low muscle radiodensity [15]. Nevertheless, the revised European Working Group on Sarcopenia in Older People diagnostic criteria for sarcopenia prioritise measurement of strength and function over mass when assessing for sarcopenia [16].

## MALNUTRITION AND SARCOPENIA

### Incidence

The incidence of malnutrition in hospitalised patients ranges from 15% to 60%, with higher estimates seen in patients with cancer (in excess of 70%) [17]. Up to 54% of patients undergoing surgery for head and neck cancer have been found to be malnourished prior to surgery, while 53% were sarcopenic [18]. One-third of patients with resectable lung cancer were sarcopenic prior to surgery [19], while the prevalence of pre-operative sarcopenia in patients undergoing transcatheter aortic valve implantation ranged between 21% and 70% [20]. Applying the GLIM criteria, one-third of patients undergoing major abdominal surgery for cancer were found to be malnourished [21]. Two different nutritional assessment tools (Patient-Generated Subjective Global Assessment [PG-SGA] and Nutritional Risk Screening [NRS 2002]) were used to prospectively evaluate the nutritional status of nearly 1500 patients with oesophageal cancer and it was found that the incidence of malnutrition was 76% and 50%, respectively [22]. A systematic review evaluating the prevalence of sarcopenia in patients with gastrointestinal (GI) and hepato-pancreato-biliary (HPB) cancers found wide variation in the reported prevalence of sarcopenia (17–79%) [23]. More than half (52%) of patients with oesophageal cancer undergoing oesophagectomy were found to be sarcopenic [24]. The prevalence of sarcopenia among patients prior to surgery for gynaecological malignancy ranged between 38% and 55% [25].

## Impact of Malnutrition and Sarcopenia on Surgical Outcomes

### Malnutrition

A study that prospectively assessed the nutritional status of patients with GI cancer undergoing major abdominal surgery found that pre-operative malnutrition, assessed using the GLIM criteria, was an independent predictor of post-operative pulmonary complications. Moreover, patients diagnosed with severe malnutrition had an increased risk of 90-day all-cause mortality [21]. Another study evaluated the prevalence of pre-operative malnutrition, assessed using the NRS 2002, in patients undergoing GI cancer surgery who were in treated in the intensive care unit (ICU) post surgery. The authors found that 85% of patients were malnourished,

with multivariable regression analysis showing that malnutrition was an independent risk factor for higher complications, infections, mortality, prolonged ventilator dependence, and ICU stay [26]. Malnutrition, assessed using GLIM criteria combined with serum albumin, was independently associated with higher post-operative morbidity and mortality in patients who underwent emergent GI surgery [27]. Malnutrition has been shown to increase the risk of surgical site infection following spinal surgery [28].

### Sarcopenia and Sarcopenic Obesity

A retrospective cohort study evaluating the impact of pre-operative sarcopenic obesity, assessed by CT, was associated with an increased risk of gastric leak after sleeve gastrectomy [29]. One study evaluating both pre-operative body composition and longitudinal changes post oesophagectomy for adenocarcinoma found that pre-operative sarcopenia was associated with an increased risk of major post-operative morbidity, while those with pre-operative sarcopenic obesity endured prolonged hospitalisation post surgery [30]. Sarcopenia was found to be an independent unfavourable prognostic factor for patients with non-small cell lung cancer treated surgically [19]. A meta-analysis evaluated the impact of sarcopenia on survival in head and neck cancers, and found that sarcopenia was an adverse prognostic factor for patients treated surgically [31]. Patients with rectal cancer who proceeded to surgery following neo-adjuvant chemoradiotherapy were evaluated by researchers who sought to investigate the impact of pre-operative muscle measures on post-operative outcome. Patients with sarcopenic obesity and low muscle attenuation endured a higher rate of post-operative complications [32]. A systematic review evaluating the impact of pre-operative nutritional status on post-operative complications in bladder cancer found that increased BMI and sarcopenia increased the rate of complications after radical cystectomy for bladder cancer; sarcopenia was also identified as an adverse prognostic indicator for five-year survival [33]. Sarcopenic obesity was an independent risk factor for 30-day mortality in critically ill patients with intra-abdominal sepsis who required surgical intervention [34], and reduced survival in patients undergoing liver transplantation [35]. Sarcopenia was associated with poorer clinical functional outcome following surgery for distal radial fractures [36], and an increased risk of inpatient, 30-day, and one-year mortality in trauma patients [37].

## PRE-OPERATIVE NUTRITIONAL TREATMENT STRATEGIES

Surgical trauma induces a state of metabolic activation that parallels the extent of surgery, and is characterised by hormonal, haematological, metabolic, and immunological changes [38, 39]. Adequate pre-operative physiological reserve is required to meet the functional demands of the surgical stress response, including increased cardiac output and delivery of oxygen [39–41]. Nutritionally relevant clinical consequences of the surgical stress response include hyperglycaemia and whole-body protein catabolism [39]. In the peri-operative period, nutritional goals should focus on evaluating the patient for pre-existing malnutrition, and nutritional therapy to optimise surgical readiness, minimise starvation, prevent post-operative malnutrition, and support anabolism for recovery [40].

While there has been significant interest in the physiological and pharmacological management of the surgical patient, the importance of peri-operative nutrition optimisation is poorly recognised [42]. A key recommendation of multiple surgical nutrition guidelines is the integration of routine nutrition screening (using a validated nutrition screening tool) in pre-operative assessment [43–45]. Where patients are identified as being nutritionally at risk, patients should be referred to a registered dietitian for comprehensive nutritional assessment and an individualised nutrition care plan [38, 45]. Where possible the enteral route should be used for the provision of any necessary nutrition support, including oral nutritional supplements and enteral tube feeding [44]. ESPEN recommends that all patients undergoing surgery for cancer, whether curative or palliative, should be managed within an enhanced recovery after surgery (ERAS) programme [46, 47], and for upper GI patients suggests that pre-operative oral/ enteral immuno-nutrition should be considered (arginine, omega-3 fatty acids, and nucleotides). A Cochrane review that evaluated pre-operative nutrition support in patients undergoing GI surgery raised concerns about the impact of bias on studies that evaluated the impact of pre-operative immuno-nutrition, alongside the potential for detrimental effects in patients who required critical care support post-operatively [48]. Pre-operative parenteral nutrition should only be used in patients with malnutrition where energy requirements cannot be adequately or safely met with enteral nutrition, and a period of 7–14 days is recommended [45]. Contraindications to enteral nutrition for surgical patients include intestinal obstruction or ileus, severe shock, intestinal ischaemia, high-output fistula, and severe intestinal haemorrhage [44].

### Carbohydrate Loading

Pre-operative carbohydrate loading the evening prior to and the morning of surgery is designed to ameliorate post-operative insulin resistance in non-diabetic patients and any subsequent need for aggressive insulin therapy. While no influence has been shown in post-operative complication rates, pre-operative carbohydrate loading has been shown to reduce post-operative length of stay [44], and to improve insulin resistance and indices of patient comfort following surgery [49], and has thus been incorporated into many ERAS protocols (see Chapter 5).

### Liver Shrinkage Diets

For some (non-time sensitive) major elective surgery, a delay may be appropriate to allow patients with class II or III obesity (BMI > 35 kg/m$^2$) to achieve weight loss [43]. Very low-calorie diets (VLCD), or so-called liver shrinkage diets, are commonly employed prior to bariatric surgery. The rationale is that the resultant loss of hepatic steatosis will allow reduction in the left lobe of the liver, improving the mobility of the liver to allow safer laparoscopic access to the stomach [50], with a randomised control trial demonstrating that a pre-operative VLCD reduced the difficulty of surgery and improvement in long-term outcomes [51]. The optimal composition of VLCD is not established, with typical daily caloric prescription varying from 450 to 800 kcal and duration lasting between 10 and 63 days [52, 53]. The main risk of VLCDs in this setting is the rapid loss of lean tissue [54], with increasing awareness of the negative impact of sarcopenic obesity. A recent systematic review concluded that calorie provision between 800 and 1200 kcal (defined by the authors as a low-calorie diet rather than VLCD) for two to four weeks prior to bariatric surgery should be recommended [55]. With the emergence of hepatic steatosis as the most common parenchymal disorder of the liver in western countries, and the increased risk of morbidity and mortality seen in patients with hepatic steatosis who undergo liver resection, VLCD prior to hepatectomy has been shown to reduce body weight and BMI, with some preliminary studies reporting reductions in steatosis and intra-operative blood loss [50]. Furthermore, some institutions use VLCD prior to cholecystectomy, with clinical reports suggesting that this improves the visibility of the biliary structures and thus potentially reduces the risk of bile duct injuries [56].

## PRIORITIES FOR FUTURE RESEARCH

While the advent of CT-based body composition has sparked increasing interest in the impact of malnutrition in clinical populations, the use of non-validated methods by non-nutrition professionals and arbitrary population-specific cut-offs have limited the systematic evaluation of the impact of body composition on post-operative outcomes [57, 58]. Future studies evaluating the impact of sarcopenia should focus on strength and functional measurements rather than rely on muscle mass alone [16]. Nutrition screening tools used in the peri-operative setting should consider the need to identify both sarcopenia and sarcopenic obesity. While the GLIM criteria offer much-needed diagnostic criteria for the assessment of malnutrition, there is a need to validate these in surgical populations. Prehabilitation (Chapter 4) has emerged as an important priority across the cancer continuum, with increasing recognition that multimodal, rather than unimodal (i.e. diet or exercise alone), interventions are necessary [59].

## REFERENCES

1. Torosian, M.H. (1999). Perioperative nutrition support for patients undergoing gastrointestinal surgery: critical analysis and recommendations. *World J. Surg.* 23 (6): 565–569.

2. Beattie, A.H., Prach, A.T., Baxter, J.P., and Pennington, C.R. (2000). A randomised controlled trial evaluating the use of enteral nutritional supplements postoperatively in malnourished surgical patients. *Gut* 46 (6): 813–818.

3. Cardenas, D., Bermúdez, C., Pérez, A. et al. (2020). Nutritional risk is associated with an increase of in-hospital mortality and a reduction of being discharged home: results of the 2009-2015 NutritionDay survey. *Clin. Nutr. ESPEN* 38: 138–145.

4. Zheng, H., Huang, Y., Shi, Y. et al. (2016). Nutrition status, nutrition support therapy, and food intake are related to prolonged hospital stays in China: results from the NutritionDay 2015 survey. *Ann. Nutr. Metab.* 69 (3–4): 215–225.

5. Cederholm, T., Jensen, G.L., Correia, M.I.T.D. et al. (2019). GLIM criteria for the diagnosis of malnutrition – a consensus report from the global clinical nutrition community. *Clin. Nutr.* 38 (1): 1–9.

6. Jones, K., Gordon-Weeks, A., Coleman, C., and Silva, M. (2017). Radiologically determined sarcopenia predicts morbidity and mortality following abdominal surgery: a systematic review and meta-analysis. *World J. Surg.* 41 (9): 2266–2279.

7. Bibby, N. and Griffin, O. (2021). Nutritional considerations for the management of the older person with hepato-pancreatico-biliary malignancy. *Eur. J. Surg. Oncol.* 47 (3 Pt A): 533–538.

8. Tan, B.H., Birdsell, L.A., Martin, L. et al. (2009). Sarcopenia in an overweight or obese patient is an adverse prognostic factor in pancreatic cancer. *Clin. Cancer Res.* 15 (22): 6973–6979.

9. Pecorelli, N., Capretti, G., Sandini, M. et al. (2018). Impact of sarcopenic obesity on failure to rescue from major complications following pancreaticoduodenectomy for cancer: results from a multicenter study. *Ann. of Surg. Oncol.* 25 (1): 308–317.

10. Prado, C.M., Lieffers, J.R., McCargar, L.J. et al. (2008). Prevalence and clinical implications of sarcopenic obesity in patients with solid tumours of the respiratory and gastrointestinal tracts: a population-based study. *Lancet Oncol.* 9 (7): 629–635.

11. Donini, L.M., Busetto, L., Bischoff, S.C. et al. (2022). Definition and diagnostic criteria for sarcopenic obesity: ESPEN and EASO consensus statement. *Clin. Nutr.* 41 (4): 990–1000.

12. Donini, L.M., Busetto, L., Bischoff, S.C. et al. (2022). Definition and diagnostic criteria for sarcopenic obesity: ESPEN and EASO consensus statement. *Obes. Facts.* 15 (3): 321–335.

13. Goodpaster, B.H., Carlson, C.L., Visser, M. et al. (2001). Attenuation of skeletal muscle and strength in the elderly: the health ABC study. *J. Appl. Phys. (1985).* 90 (6): 2157–2165.

14. Stephens, N.A., Skipworth, R.J., Macdonald, A.J. et al. (2011). Intramyocellular lipid droplets increase with progression of cachexia in cancer patients. *J. Cachexia. Sarcopenia. Muscle.* 2 (2): 111–117.

15. Stretch, C., Aubin, J.M., Mickiewicz, B. et al. (2018). Sarcopenia and myosteatosis are accompanied by distinct biological profiles in patients with pancreatic and periampullary adenocarcinomas. *PLoS One* 13 (5): e0196235.

16. Cruz-Jentoft, A.J., Bahat, G., Bauer, J. et al. (2019). Sarcopenia: revised European consensus on definition and diagnosis. *Age Ageing.* 48 (1): 16–31.

17. Tobert, C.M., Hamilton-Reeves, J.M., Norian, L.A. et al. (2017). Emerging impact of malnutrition on surgical patients: literature review and potential implications for cystectomy in bladder cancer. *J. Urol.* 198 (3): 511–519.

18. Caburet, C., Farigon, N., Mulliez, A. et al. (2020). Impact of nutritional status at the outset of assessment on postoperative complications in head and neck cancer. *Eur. Ann. Otorhinolaryngol. Head Neck Dis.* 137 (5): 393–398.

19. Deng, H.Y., Hou, L., Zha, P. et al. (2019). Sarcopenia is an independent unfavorable prognostic factor of non-small cell lung cancer after surgical resection: a comprehensive systematic review and meta-analysis. *Eur. J. Surg. Oncol.* 45 (5): 728–735.

20. Bertschi, D., Kiss, C.M., Schoenenberger, A.W. et al. (2021). Sarcopenia in patients undergoing transcatheter aortic valve implantation (TAVI): a systematic review of the literature. *J. Nutr. Health Aging.* 25 (1): 64–70.

21. Kakavas, S., Karayiannis, D., Bouloubasi, Z. et al. (2020). Global leadership initiative on malnutrition criteria predict pulmonary complications and 90-day mortality after major abdominal surgery in cancer patients. *Nutrients* 12 (12): 3726.

22. Cao, J., Xu, H., Li, W. et al. (2021). Nutritional assessment and risk factors associated to malnutrition in patients with esophageal cancer. *Curr. Probl. Cancer.* 45 (1): 100638.

23. Levolger, S., van Vugt, J.L., de Bruin, R.W., and JN IJ. (2015). Systematic review of sarcopenia in patients operated on for gastrointestinal and hepatopancreatobiliary malignancies. *Br. J. Surg.* 102 (12): 1448–1458.

24. Deng, H.Y., Zha, P., Peng, L. et al. (2019). Preoperative sarcopenia is a predictor of poor prognosis of esophageal cancer after esophagectomy: a comprehensive systematic review and meta-analysis. *Dis. Esophagus.* 32 (3): doy115.

25. Li, Y.X., Xia, W.W., and Liu, W.Y. (2021). The influence process of sarcopenia on female cancer: a systematic review and meta-analysis. *J. Obstet. Gynaecol. Res.* 47 (12): 4403–4413.

26. Shpata, V., Prendushi, X., Kreka, M. et al. (2014). Malnutrition at the time of surgery affects negatively the clinical outcome of critically ill patients with gastrointestinal cancer. *Med. Arch.* 68 (4): 263–267.

27. Haines, K.L., Lao, W., Nguyen, B.P. et al. (2021). Evaluation of malnutrition via modified GLIM criteria for in patients undergoing emergent gastrointestinal surgery. *Clin. Nutr.* 40 (3): 1367–1375.

28. Tsantes, A.G., Papadopoulos, D.V., Lytras, T. et al. (2020). Association of malnutrition with surgical site infection following spinal surgery: systematic review and meta-analysis. *J. Hosp. Infect.* 104 (1): 111–119.

29. Gaillard, M., Tranchart, H., Maitre, S. et al. (2018). Preoperative detection of sarcopenic obesity helps to predict the occurrence of gastric leak after sleeve gastrectomy. *Obes. Surg.* 28 (8): 2379–2385.

30. Fehrenbach, U., Wuensch, T., Gabriel, P. et al. (2021). CT body composition of sarcopenia and sarcopenic obesity: predictors of postoperative complications and survival in patients with locally advanced Esophageal adenocarcinoma. *Cancers (Basel)* 13 (12): 2921.

31. Takenaka, Y., Takemoto, N., Oya, R., and Inohara, H. (2021). Prognostic impact of sarcopenia in patients with head and neck cancer treated with surgery or radiation: a meta-analysis. *PLoS One* 16 (10): e0259288.

32. Berkel, A.E.M., Klaase, J.M., de Graaff, F. et al. (2019). Patient's skeletal muscle radiation attenuation and sarcopenic obesity are associated with postoperative morbidity after neoadjuvant chemoradiation and resection for rectal cancer. *Dig. Surg.* 36 (5): 376–383.

33. Ornaghi, P.I., Afferi, L., Antonelli, A. et al. (2021). The impact of preoperative nutritional status on post-surgical complication and mortality rates in patients undergoing radical cystectomy for bladder cancer: a systematic review of the literature. *World J. Urol.* 39 (4): 1045–1081.

34. Ji, Y., Cheng, B., Xu, Z. et al. (2018). Impact of sarcopenic obesity on 30-day mortality in critically ill patients with intra-abdominal sepsis. *J. Crit. Care* 46: 50–54.

35. Kamo, N., Kaido, T., Hamaguchi, Y. et al. (2019). Impact of sarcopenic obesity on outcomes in patients undergoing living donor liver transplantation. *Clin. Nutr.* 38 (5): 2202–2209.

36. Artiaco, S., Fusini, F., Pennacchio, G. et al. (2020). Sarcopenia in distal radius fractures: systematic review of the literature and current findings. *Eur. J. Orthop. Surg. Traumatol.* 30 (7): 1251–1255.

37. Xia, W., Barazanchi, A.W.H., MacFater, W.S., and Hill, A.G. (2019). The impact of computed tomography-assessed sarcopenia on outcomes for trauma patients - a systematic review and meta-analysis. *Injury* 50 (9): 1565–1576.

38. Weimann, A., Braga, M., Carli, F. et al. (2017). ESPEN guideline: clinical nutrition in surgery. *Clin. Nutr.* 36 (3): 623–650.

39. Gillis, C. and Carli, F. (2015). Promoting perioperative metabolic and nutritional care. *Anesthesiology* 123 (6): 1455–1472.

40. Gillis, C. and Wischmeyer, P.E. (2019). Pre-operative nutrition and the elective surgical patient: why, how and what? *Anaesthesia* 74 (Suppl 1): 27–35.

41. Fearon, K.C., Jenkins, J.T., Carli, F., and Lassen, K. (2013). Patient optimization for gastrointestinal cancer surgery. *Bri. J. Sur.* 100 (1): 15–27.

42. Williams, J.D. and Wischmeyer, P.E. (2017). Assessment of perioperative nutrition practices and attitudes-a national survey of colorectal and GI surgical oncology programs. *Am. J. Surg.* 213 (6): 1010–1018.

43. McClave, S.A., Kozar, R., Martindale, R.G. et al. (2013). Summary points and consensus recommendations from the North American surgical nutrition summit. *JPEN J. Parenter. Enteral. Nutr.* 37 (5 Suppl): 99S–105S.

44. Weimann, A., Braga, M., Carli, F. et al. (2021). ESPEN practical guideline: clinical nutrition in surgery. *Clin. Nutr.* 40 (7): 4745–4761.

45. Wischmeyer, P.E., Carli, F., Evans, D.C. et al. (2018). American Society for Enhanced Recovery and Perioperative Quality Initiative Joint Consensus Statement on nutrition screening and therapy within a surgical enhanced recovery pathway. *Anesth. Analg.* 126 (6): 1883–1895.

46. Muscaritoli, M., Arends, J., Bachmann, P. et al. (2021). ESPEN practical guideline: clinical nutrition in cancer. *Clin. Nutr.* 40 (5): 2898–2913.

47. Munn, Z., Moola, S., Lisy, K. et al. (2017). Systematic reviews of prevalence and incidence. In: *Joanna Briggs Institute Reviewer's Manual*, 4e (ed. E. Alenzi). Adelaide: Joanna Briggs Institute, ch. 5.

48. Burden, S., Todd, C., Hill, J., and Lal, S. (2012). Pre-operative nutrition support in patients undergoing gastrointestinal surgery. *Cochrane Database Syst. Rev.* 11: CD008879.

49. Bilku, D.K., Dennison, A.R., Hall, T.C. et al. (2014). Role of preoperative carbohydrate loading: a systematic review. *Ann. R Coll. Surg. Engl.* 96 (1): 15–22.

50. Hitchins, C.R., Jones, R.M., Kanwar, A., and Aroori, S. (2022). Is there a role for preoperative liver reducing diet in hepatectomy? A systematic review. *Langenbecks. Arch. Surg.* 407 (4): 1357–1367.

51. Van Nieuwenhove, Y., Dambrauskas, Z., Campillo-Soto, A. et al. (2011). Preoperative very low-calorie diet and operative outcome after laparoscopic gastric bypass: a randomized multicenter study. *Arch. Surg.* 146 (11): 1300–1305.

52. Delbridge, E. and Proietto, J. (2006). State of the science: VLED (very low energy diet) for obesity. *Asia Pac. J. Clin. Nutr.* 15 (Suppl): 49–54.

53. Holderbaum, M., Casagrande, D.S., Sussenbach, S., and Buss, C. (2018). Effects of very low calorie diets on liver size and weight loss in the preoperative period of bariatric surgery: a systematic review. *Surg. Obes. Relat. Dis.* 14 (2): 237–244.

54. Sivakumar, J., Chong, L., Ward, S. et al. (2020). Body composition changes following a very-low-calorie preoperative diet in patients undergoing bariatric surgery. *Obes. Surg.* 30 (1): 119–126.

55. Romeijn, M.M., Kolen, A.M., Holthuijsen, D.D.B. et al. (2021). Effectiveness of a low-calorie diet for liver volume reduction prior to bariatric surgery: a systematic review. *Obes. Surg.* 31 (1): 350–356.

56. Burnand, K.M., Lahiri, R.P., Burr, N. et al. (2016). A randomised, single blinded trial, assessing the effect of a two week preoperative very low calorie diet on laparoscopic cholecystectomy in obese patients. *HPB.* 18 (5): 456–461.

57. Griffin, O.M., Bashir, Y., O'Connor, D. et al. (2022). Measurement of body composition in pancreatic cancer: a systematic review, meta-analysis and recommendations for future study design. *Dig. Surg.* 39 (4): 141–152.

58. Ozola Zalite, I., Zykus, R., Francisco Gonzalez, M. et al. (2015). Influence of cachexia and sarcopenia on survival in pancreatic ductal adenocarcinoma: a systematic review. *Pancreatol.* 15 (1): 19–24.

59. Santa Mina, D., van Rooijen, S.J., Minnella, E.M. et al. (2020). Multiphasic prehabilitation across the cancer continuum: a narrative review and conceptual framework. *Front. Oncol.* 10: 598425.

# CHAPTER 4

# Prehabilitation Programmes and Their Impact on Surgical Outcomes

Helen McNamara

*Department of Occupational Therapy, Royal Surrey NHS Foundation Trust, Guildford, UK*

> **KEY POINTS**
> - Prehabilitation should be multimodal.
> - Prehabilitation targets should be individualised to the patient.
> - More research is required to analyse the outcomes and most effective treatment strategies.

## A BRIEF HISTORY OF PREHABILITATION

The concept of prehabilitation has been available for some time to those undergoing elective surgery for orthopaedic and cardiac procedures as well as those diagnosed with cancer. There are proven benefits for pre-operative preparation, but it is widely acknowledged that more research is required to investigate the impact of prehabilitation on clinical outcomes.

In 2013 Demeules et al. demonstrated significant improvements in lower-limb function, following a prehabilitation intervention programme for patients with severe hip and knee arthritis awaiting surgery. This included improved walking pace and timed ascent and descent of stairs [1]. Other studies reported the effect of prehabilitation on quality of life (QOL), noting that those having total knee arthroplasty demonstrated considerable improvement in QOL three months post surgery compared to those who had not participated in prehabilitation. It was also suggested that the functional ability of those receiving prehabilitation appeared to be better than those who did not, but this did not reach significance [1].

Pre-operative physical therapy in those having elective cardiac surgery has been demonstrated to result in a significant reduction in post-operative lung complications and a reduction in length of stay (LOS) [2].

In 2013, a narrative review of cancer prehabilitation suggested that physical preparation is beneficial for newly diagnosed cancer patients to optimise

*Nutritional Management of the Surgical Patient*, First Edition. Edited by Mary E. Phillips.
© 2023 John Wiley & Sons Ltd. Published 2023 by John Wiley & Sons Ltd.

their health prior to and during treatment. This study identified the need for multimodal approaches including psychological input, which was found to be more effective than simply addressing physical fitness alone. This study indicated that adherence to treatment might also be improved, and provided suggestions for clinical outcomes measures for further research. There was some evidence for a reduction in admissions and other associated costs, with research recommendations made in these areas [3].

## DEFINING PREHABILITATION

Prehabilitation has since been established in several different clinical fields, using a range of approaches both in hospitals and in community settings. However, there has not been a clear and accepted definition or model to define prehabilitation programmes. This was acknowledged by Macmillan cancer support, who published a review of evidence and insights in 2018. The review has helped to clarify the definition of prehabilitation, the most appropriate time to intervene, and the multiprofessional provision of service [4]. Macmillan made the following statements:

- *Definitions of prehabilitation:*
  - For non-cancer patients: 'The process of enhancing the functional capacity of the individual to enable him or her to withstand a stressful event' [5].
  - For cancer patients: 'A process on the cancer continuum of care that occurs between the time of cancer diagnosis and the beginning of acute treatment and includes physical and psychological assessments that establish a baseline functional level, identify impairments, and provide interventions that promote physical and psychological health to reduce the incidence and/or severity of future impairments' [6].
- *Prehabilitation is made up of three stages*:
  - Baseline assessment including identification of risk factors for poor clinical outcome.

- Interventions including physical activity, dietary support, and psychological well-being.
- Post-treatment assessment to measure progress and refer for long-term follow-up if required.
- *Prehabilitation is part of a continuum.* It is the first stage of optimisation of fitness and well-being in readiness for surgery or other treatments.
- *Prehabilitation should be personalised* to the needs of the patient, allowing for varying timescales, as well as ensuring it is accessible for everyone.
- *Interventions most commonly include physical activity, dietary support, and psychological support*; occasionally other services have been included such as smoking cessation, respiratory exercise, managing lymphoedema and other comorbidities.
- *Physiotherapists, dietitians and psychologists* were most commonly present in the services reviewed, though it is suggested that all healthcare professionals may be able to provide basic advice to patients for areas such as activity or stress management. Occupational therapists, though not often mentioned in services to date, were acknowledged by the report to be well placed to offer support for fatigue and pain management as well as supporting those with moderate psychological difficulties. Many other health workers and specialists were identified as potential members of a prehabilitation service, thus ensuring a holistic approach to patient care [4].

## STRATIFIED CARE AND PREHABILITATION

A stratified approach to care was developed by NHS Improvement in conjunction with the National Cancer Survivorship Initiative to ensure that cancer patients receive care that is appropriate to their diagnosis and level of function. Although initially developed for specific tumour sites, it provides a generic pathway that can be used to guide the implementation of pathways for other specialties and is useful when considering the development of prehabilitation services. The stratified approach allows patients to be supported and monitored at a level that is in line with their diagnosis, health status, and functional ability. It recognises that some patients can independently manage their condition and its effects, while others need targeted support from healthcare professionals. This document also recognised that there were patients whose needs are complex and require specialist management [7].

General information can be provided to all patients about stress management; however, patients who are experiencing deterioration in their mental health such as increased anxiety or low mood may benefit from personalised support from an occupational therapist. Others who may have a history of severe and enduring mental health difficulties will require the care of a psychologist or psychiatrist. The model recommends regular review of patients using a needs assessment, to ensure that their needs have not changed and that they are continuing to receive the appropriate level of care. The model includes all aspects of living with cancer, such as clinical needs, physical fitness, education, and other areas such as financial advice or complementary therapies [7].

By establishing services in this way, resources are targeted to where they are most needed. This may not only be financially more efficient, but also allows patients to increase their sense of control and autonomy, and where possible empowering them to take responsibility for their own health. A prehabilitation programme based on these principles ensures that patients have access to a multidisciplinary team who can address the broad range of concerns that arise, and at the same time empowers patients to take some responsibility for their health and well-being.

## ENHANCED RECOVERY AFTER SURGERY AND PREHABILITATION

Using enhanced recovery after surgery (ERAS) as part of a surgical pathway has been shown to reduce the risks of post-operative complications, lower LOS, and improve cost-effectiveness for major surgeries such as those considered for prehabilitation [8–10] (see Chapter 5). Recommendations from the National Institute of Health and Care Excellence (NICE) are for peri-operative, intra-operative, and post-operative protocols to be in place, which may include medicine adherence, nutritional assessment, and fluid, glucose, and pain management [11]. ERAS protocols have demonstrated significant improvements in LOS and post-operative complications for patients receiving both open and laparoscopic procedures [12, 13]. Thus, LOS should not be the main aim of the prehabilitation programme, but instead prehabilitation should complement the protocols already in place, by focusing on physical fitness, nutritional optimisation, psychological preparedness, and practical preparation, as indicated in the Macmillan report [4].

## HOLISTIC AND PERSON-CENTRED APPROACHES TO PREHABILITATION

Prehabilitation embraces the principles of person-centred care by using the skills and expertise of a range of professionals to consider all aspects of patients' lives that may have impacts on their adherence to the programme and their recovery. Examples of this might be their daily functioning, work, education, social support, relationships, emotional well-being, environment, or hobbies.

Research has begun to consider the effects of a more holistic and multimodal approach to prehabilitation rather than earlier work that focused on exercise targets only.

A meta-analysis assessing outcomes of bladder, breast, and lung cancer surgery reported beneficial outcomes in mood, QOL, post-operative complications, and LOS. This paper recommended further research to provide robust evidence in other tumour sites, and to explore the cost-effectiveness of prehabilitation programmes [14].

Studies in prostate cancer recommended that prehabilitation programmes should include exercise, pelvic floor muscle training, nutritional advice, and support with anxiety, depression, and sexual well-being [15].

Although specific to the tumour sites, these studies demonstrate the need to address all aspects of a patient's life in preparation for surgery.

## PSYCHOLOGICAL PREPARATION

The multimodal approaches already described acknowledge the need for psychological preparation as well as physical and nutritional support; however, there is less data for psychological support. Narrative reviews indicate decreases in post-operative anxiety and depression and improvements in wound healing, pain management, and physical recovery in the first four weeks post surgery [16]. Further research, particularly in relation to anxiety, depression, QOL, and self-efficacy, will support the design and provision of prehabilitation in the future.

## PREHABILITATION TO SUPPORT BEHAVIOUR CHANGE

A fundamental aspect of the prehabilitation programme at the Royal Surrey (PRIME programme) is the assistance provided to patients to support behaviour change and make lifestyle choices that will improve their outcomes and recovery. The health belief model is a useful tool to inform practice that enables clinicians to see patients as at the centre of the service. This acknowledges the internal assessments that patients make about the costs and benefits of participation, as well as their perceptions of the severity of disease and treatments. Together, these inform the choices that patients make about their health behaviours. The model also reminds clinicians of the importance of self-efficacy and how this may affect participation [17]. It is therefore important for those working closely with patients to understand what each patient's priorities are, what motivates them to participate, and what their barriers are to making changes. Clinicians and health professionals may benefit from gaining a better understanding of enabling behaviour change to increase engagement and improve outcomes.

## FRAMEWORKS FOR PREHABILITATION

Santa Mina et al. recognised the need for a conceptual framework to support service development [18]. Their review suggested that prehabilitation should not be limited to surgical patients, but should be offered to those undergoing other treatments that have impacts on functional capacity, starting from diagnosis and continuing through neo-adjuvant chemotherapy, surgical intervention, and in preparation for adjuvant treatment. These approaches aim to prepare and enable patients to cope with late or long-term effects of treatment. Prehabilitation should therefore aim to embrace these principles as part of its development, and ensure that it is available to patients along the continuum of their diagnosis and treatment [18].

There is much to be gained by using the time prior to treatment and surgery to fully prepare patients by not only ensuring that they are physically fit and nutritionally prepared, but also have realistic expectations of post-operative care, recovery, and survivorship.

## PRIME PREHABILITATION FOR SURGERY AT THE ROYAL SURREY HOSPITAL FOUNDATION TRUST

The development of the prehabilitation programme at the Royal Surrey Hospital Foundation Trust (RSFT) sought to embrace the available evidence and suggested approaches already mentioned, to provide a robust service for surgical patients with a cancer diagnosis. Following a promising pre-pilot, using exercise as the only intervention for surgical oncology patients, and a two-year Macmillan-funded pilot that included dietetics and occupational therapy, a permanent service was instigated. The programme was offered to patients referred for major surgeries primarily due to a cancer diagnosis, under the care of urology, gynae-oncology, oesophageal, or hepato-pancreato-biliary surgeons.

This holistic service offers a range of interventions, which aim to reach as many patients as possible, for whom access may be challenging due to geography, physical or mental health, finances, work and family commitments, or education. This has meant remaining flexible and open to different ways of working to ensure that all patients receive equitable levels of education and support about what to expect and what they can do to improve their outcomes.

## INTERVENTIONS OF PRIME PREHABILITATION

Interventions offered by the PRIME team of therapists include face-to-face, telephone, and virtual contacts.

### Group Programmes

There is a five-week face-to-face rolling programme consisting of an exercise class and education sessions covering fatigue, sleep, mental health, nutrition, and preparing for admission. During these sessions, opportunities are given to practise stress management techniques such as relaxation and mindfulness.

A consolidated version of the five-week educational programme was offered once per month at another site for those who lived outside of the local area.

Due to the Covid-19 pandemic a virtual version of the five-week programme was made available that consisted of pre-recorded talks, an exercise session, and relaxation videos. Patient experience videos have also been recorded by past service users who wish to offer hope and encouragement to those going through prehabilitation and anticipating surgery.

### One-to-One Consultations

One-to-one consultations are primarily carried out by telephone call, but also take place on hospital wards, in patients' homes, and using video technology. Telephone support is used as a way of monitoring patients and providing advice and emotional support on a regular basis without the necessity of patients coming to the hospital. On occasion, it is necessary to offer greater support using face-to-face options for those who are struggling to cope, or where communication is impaired.

### Home Exercise Programmes

Patients are encouraged to develop a routine of regular exercise and are supported by a tailored programme provided by the physiotherapist. This ensures that each patient understands how to exercise at an appropriate level of intensity, based on their health and fitness.

For those patients who do not use technology, in addition to the video recordings and face-to-face sessions they also have the option to receive written resources.

### Friends and Family

It was clear from interactions with patients and their families that the diagnosis and treatment plans given to patients had impacts not only on the patients but also on their wider social support. PRIME therefore encourages the inclusion of partners, family members, and supporters to participate in the programme. Friends and family can often assist patients to implement recommendations and support them to stay motivated, as well as benefit personally by attending the programme.

### Nutritional Support

Generalised nutritional advice can be provided for patients requiring weight maintenance in the pre-operative setting, focusing on healthy eating advice. However, many patients may require screening and treatment for malnutrition, with others needing optimisation of glycaemic control, and in some cases pre-operative weight loss is indicated. In some tumour sites other considerations include pre-operative enteral feeding, management of pancreatic exocrine insufficiency, modified consistency or fibre modification, and identification of patients who require admission for nutritional intervention (see Chapter 3).

## Peer Support

One of the strengths of group activities is the opportunity for patients to meet others in similar circumstances and share experiences. The benefits of this are frequently observed by therapists and reported by patients and their families. A number of patients have enjoyed staying in contact with the new friends that they made during the programme. This has been enhanced by a buddy system that allows for current patients to be put in contact with past patients for advice and support.

## PRIME OUTCOME DATA

During the pilot of PRIME, outcomes were audited by the physiotherapist and occupational therapist at first and last contact, to measure the effectiveness of the interventions and the service. The variance in how many weeks patients participated in prehabilitation means that statistical analysis is not reliable. However, the overall trend was positive, with improvements in functional tests.

A bespoke questionnaire developed by the occupational therapy team demonstrated a 16% increase in preparedness, reduction of 13% in anxiety, improvement in sleep quality of 5%, and patients' understanding of nutritional advice increased by

13%. A mean of 3.4 of a possible 5 sessions were attended, and patients made an average of 2.6 of 5 possible changes within eight weeks (n = 44; unpublished data).

## CONCLUSION

Prehabilitation plays a key role in preparing patients for surgery and neo-adjuvant treatment. However, clear guidance is required on the optimal mode of delivery, and support needed for the development of a fully multidisciplinary team.

The provision of a broad range of interventions along with the flexible approach of therapists builds on the evidence for prehabilitation, supports the idea of patient-centred care, and helps to facilitate positive behaviour change. It is of paramount importance that therapists engage with patients at their level, acknowledging what their anxieties or past experiences are. This is what often shapes their behaviour, motivation, and interactions with the team. Evidence of this is best demonstrated by feedback and case studies of patients who have completed the programme, as well as the data gathered during the pilot.

Further evidence is required to improve the evidence base for psychological interventions. Prehabilitation is an exciting area in which to work and has been embraced and valued by those who have received it. Further research will help to ensure that it continues to develop and enable clinicians to facilitate thorough and holistic preparation for their patients.

---

### Case Studies

**Mr A – a 69-year-old man prior to pancreatico-duodenectomy**

Mr A was a widower who lived alone on a low income, with a supportive family nearby. He led a sedentary lifestyle and was not highly educated. His daughter attended all prehabilitation sessions and appointments with him to assist with retaining and disseminating information.

*Intervention*

He attended 10 gym classes and 5 education groups.

His outcomes were as follows:

|  | Pre intervention | Post intervention |
|---|---|---|
| 6 min walk test (m) | 307.5 | 445 |
| 60 s sit to stand | 18 | 32 |
| Handgrip strength (kg) | 42.4 | 41.93 |
| Group questionnaire | 30 | 32 |

Mr A's daughter regularly sought advice and support from the prehabilitation team and in particular the occupational therapist. She was anxious that her father's home environment was unsuitable for him to return to on discharge: he did not have a proper bed and his home was unkempt and soiled since his wife passed away. The occupational therapist was able to apply for grants to provide a bed, carpet, and curtains as well as referring the daughter to carer's support to ensure she was able to continue supporting Mr A.

Mr A had surgical post-operative complications that extended his hospital stay to 22 days. However, he said, 'I don't think I would have recovered as well if I hadn't done that prehab, it was really good.'

His daughter said, 'The support and advice has been invaluable.'

Mr A was seen participating in a patient support day 18 months later with his daughter and was continuing to keep well.

## Mr B – a 72-year-old man prior to oesophagectomy

Mr B lived with his wife some distance from RSFT. He was an educated man who lived a full life but was not particularly active. When referred to prehabilitation, he was assessed as unfit for surgery and he completed neo-adjuvant chemotherapy.

### Intervention

Mr B attended the satellite education session, which on the feedback questionnaire he scored as 6/6 for helpfulness. This along with contacts with the team appeared to spur him on to attend the hospital gym despite the distance required to travel. He attended 10 gym classes.

His outcomes were as follows:

|  | Pre intervention | Post intervention |
| --- | --- | --- |
| 6-min walk test (m) | 513 | 567 |
| Handgrip strength (kg) | 35.73 | 36.37 |

Following reassessment, Mr B was assessed as fit for surgery. His surgery was successfully completed and, despite a post-operative chest infection, his hospital stay was 14 days. Mr B was very grateful for the holistic support he had received and agreed to be a buddy to others preparing for oesophagostomies. He has since supported several other patients.

## REFERENCES

1. Demeules, F., Hall, J., and Woodhouse, L.J. (2013). Prehabilitation improves physical function of individuals with severe disability from hip or knee osteoarthritis. *Physiother. Can.* 65 (2): 116–124.

2. Humphrey, R. and Malone, D. (2015). Effectiveness of preoperative physical therapy for elective cardiac surgery. *Phys. Ther.* 95 (2): 160–166.

3. Silver, J.K. and Baima, J. (2013). Cancer prehabilitation: an opportunity to decrease treatment-related morbidity, increase cancer treatment options, and improve physical and psychological health outcomes. *Am. J. Phys. Med. Rehabil.* 92 (8): 715–727.

4. Bloom, E. (2018). *Prehabilitation Evidence and Insight.* London: Macmillan Cancer Support.

5. Jensen, B.T., Petersen, A.K., Jensen, J.B. et al. (2015). Efficacy of a multiprofessional rehabilitation programme in radical cystectomy pathways: a prospective randomized controlled trial. *Scand. J. Urol.* 49 (2): 133–141.

6. Silver, J.K. (2015). Cancer prehabilitation and its role in improving health outcomes and reducing care costs. *Sem. Oncol. Nurs.* 31 (1): 13–30.

7. NHS Improvement (2016). *Innovation to Implementation: Stratified Pathways of Care for People Living with Cancer. A 'How to' Guide.* London: NHS.

8. Lee, Y., Yu, J., Doumouras, A.G. et al. (2020). Enhanced recovery after surgery (ERAS) versus standard recovery for elective gastric cancer surgery: a meta-analysis of randomized controlled trials. *Surg. Oncol.* 32: 75–87.

9. Pisarska, M., Małczak, P., Major, P. et al. (2017). Enhanced recovery after surgery protocol in oesophageal cancer surgery: systematic review and meta-analysis. *PLoS One* 12 (3): e0174382.

10. Roulin, D. and Demartines, N. (2020). Evidence for enhanced recovery in pancreatic cancer surgery. *Langenbeck's Arch. Surg.* 405 (5): 595–602.

11. NICE (2020). Perioperative care in adults. NICE guideline NG180. London: NICE. https://www.nice.org.uk/guidance/ng180/resources/perioperative-care-in-adults-pdf-66142014963397. (Accessed 20 Aug 2021)

12. Jones, C., Kelliher, L., Dickinson, M. et al. (2013). Randomized clinical trial on enhanced recovery versus standard care following open liver resection. *Br. J. Surg.* 100: 1015–1024.

13. Levy, B.F., Scott, M.J.P., Fawcett, W.J., and Rockall, T.A. (2009). 23-hour-stay laparoscopic colectomy. *Dis. Colon. Rectum.* 52 (7): 1239–1243.

14. Treanor, C., Kyaw, T., and Donnelly, M. (2018). An international review and meta-analysis of prehabilitation compared to usual care for cancer patients. *J. Cancer Surviv.* 12: 64–73.

15. Paterson, C., Roberts, C., and McKie, A. (2020). Prostate cancer prehabilitation and the importance of multimodal interventions for person-centred care and recovery. *Sem. Oncol. Nurs.* 36: 151048.

16. Levett, D.Z.H. and Grimmett, C. (2019). Psychological factors, prehabilitation and surgical outcomes: evidence and future directions. *Anaesthesia* 76 (1): 36–42.

17. Jain, R., Gibson, L., and Coburn, N. (2018). Prehabilitation for surgical oncology patients: empowering patient volition. *Support. Care Cancer* 26: 3665–3667.

18. Santa Mina, D., van Rooijen, S.J., Minnella, E.M. et al. (2021). Multiphasic prehabilitation across the cancer continuum: a narrative review and conceptual framework. *Front. Oncol.* 10: 598425.

# CHAPTER 5

# Enhanced Recovery after Surgery

Neil Bibby, Rebekah Lord, and Ashleigh Maske

*Department of Nutrition and Dietetics, Manchester University Hospitals NHS Foundation Trust, Manchester, UK*

---

### KEY POINTS

- Enhanced recovery after surgery (ERAS) programmes are multidisciplinary, multimodal care pathways aimed at reducing the surgical stress response and accelerating patient recovery.
- Studies have shown improved programme adherence to be associated with earlier recovery, decreased complications, and shorter length of hospital stay.
- A key aspect of the ERAS protocols is avoiding long periods of fasting and current guidelines recommend initiating oral intake on the first post-operative day in most cases.
- Peri-operative oral nutrition support, including oral nutritional supplements, is important for patients who are malnourished or at high nutritional risk.
- Following upper gastrointestinal and pancreatic surgery, patients struggle to meet nutritional requirements orally and longer-term enteral feeding may be beneficial.
- Immuno-nutrition is recommended by some ERAS guidelines, but the exact dose, timing, and product remain unclear.

---

Enhanced recovery after surgery (ERAS) programmes are multidisciplinary, multimodal care pathways aimed at reducing the surgical stress response and accelerating patient recovery. The ERAS pathways span the pre-operative, intra-operative, and post-operative periods [1]. ERAS pathways were initially established in colorectal surgery; however, guidelines have now been extended to liver, pancreatic, upper gastro-intestinal (UGI), thoracic, urological, gynaecological, head and neck, orthopaedic, cardiac, bariatric, and emergency surgery [2].

Most ERAS programmes consist of 15–20 recommended components (see Table 5.1), although the relative contribution of each component

*Nutritional Management of the Surgical Patient*, First Edition. Edited by Mary E. Phillips.
© 2023 John Wiley & Sons Ltd. Published 2023 by John Wiley & Sons Ltd.

**TABLE 5.1**    Core elements of enhanced recovery after surgery (ERAS) care, with the nutritional components highlighted in bold.

| Pre-operative | Intra-operative | Post-operative |
| --- | --- | --- |
| Pre-admission counselling | Minimally invasive surgical techniques | Early mobilisation |
| **Nutrition screening/ support** | Standardised anaesthesia, avoiding long-acting opioids | **Early intake of oral fluids and solids Oral nutritional supplements** |
| Prehabilitation/medical optimisation | Restrictive use of surgical site drains | Early removal of urinary catheters and intravenous fluids |
| No routine use of mechanical bowel preparation | Maintaining fluid balance to avoid over- or underhydration | Use of chewing gums and laxatives and peripheral opioid-blocking agents |
| **No prolonged fasting** | Administer vasopressors to support blood pressure control | Multimodal approach to opioid-sparing pain control |
| **Carbohydrate loading (see Chapter 2)** | Epidural anaesthesia for open surgery | Multimodal approach to control of nausea and vomiting |
| Antibiotic prophylaxis | Removal of nasogastric tubes | Prepare for early discharge |
| Thrombosis prophylaxis | Control of body temperature | Audit of outcomes and process in a multidisciplinary team |

Source: Adapted from [1].

remains unknown. Many components lack definitive evidence regarding improved outcomes, but it is believed that it is the combination of each of the different elements, rather than a single element, that produces the greatest effect [3]. Some components may be procedure specific and should not be applied across all surgical procedures.

Studies have reported that ERAS can reduce length of hospital stay (LOS) and cost of hospitalisation, reduce post-operative complications, and improve patient satisfaction [4]. Additional benefits have been demonstrated, including a reduction in insulin resistance and the inflammatory response syndrome caused by surgery and earlier return of gastrointestinal (GI) function [4]. However, most ERAS studies are cohort studies that demonstrate variation in protocols, making interpretation of results difficult. There have been three Cochrane reviews (in colorectal, gynaecological, and UGI/ liver/pancreas surgery) performed to evaluate ERAS protocols [5–7]

In colorectal surgery four randomised control trials (RCTs) demonstrated a decrease in LOS by 2.9 days, without increasing readmissions, and a reduction in overall complications, but no difference in major complications [5].

The review in UGI/liver/pancreas surgery included 10 studies and concluded that ERAS may reduce LOS and costs (primarily because of reduction in hospital stay) [6]. However, both reviews raised concerns regarding the poor quality of the studies, the risk of bias, and lack of sufficient outcome measures and concluded that more high-quality RCTs were required.

A Cochrane review found no high-quality studies to support or refute the use of ERAS programmes in gynaecological cancer surgery [7].

The lack of evaluation of compliance within ERAS protocols is a weakness of many studies, despite ERAS guidelines highlighting regular audit as a core component [1]. Studies have shown improved programme adherence to be associated with earlier recovery, decreased complications, and shorter LOS, therefore compliance is a vital consideration when interpreting ERAS research [8, 9].

It has been suggested that longer-term outcomes are needed in future RCTs, and that they should incorporate measures of quality of life (QOL) and functional recovery [5, 6]. Surgery is often part of a multimodal treatment regimen and a faster, improved recovery may increase the number of patients getting to their intended adjuvant oncological therapy, but this requires further investigation [10].

## EARLY ORAL FEEDING

A key aspect of the ERAS protocols is avoiding long periods of fasting and current guidelines recommend initiating oral intake on the first post-operative day in most cases. A 2018 Cochrane review, including 17 RCTs with 1437 participants undergoing lower GI surgery, concluded that early enteral feeding may lead to reduced post-operative LOS. However, findings for all other outcomes, such as post-operative complications and QOL, were inconclusive. Moreover, studies were of low quality, with significant heterogeneity and risk of bias [11]. A recent study by Pu et al. [12] suggested that the limited findings of this review were due to a pooled assessment of protein-containing diets with non-protein liquid diets. They evaluated studies with an intervention of oral or enteral intake initiated within 24 hours of surgery that contained calories and protein, compared to any form of nutrition commenced more than 24 hours after surgery [12].

Two RCTs established early oral intake by using a protein-enriched drink, two RCTs provided enteral nutrition (EN) via a feeding tube, and four RCTs commenced a solid diet containing protein. This study concluded that the early intervention groups had significantly reduced mortality (odds ratio [OR] 0.31, P = 0.02), surgical site infection rate (OR 0.39, P = 0.002), post-operative nausea and vomiting (PONV; OR 0.62, P = 0.04), and serious post-operative complications (OR 0.60, P = 0.01). Limitations of this study include the small sample size of the individual studies, a low mortality rate within studies, and a lack of quantification of oral intake. Another RCT in colorectal surgery reported that a low-residue diet, rather than a clear liquid diet, is associated with less nausea, faster return of bowel function, and a shorter hospital stay without increasing post-operative morbidity [13]. Future trials should investigate the effect of differing post-operative dietary regimens on outcomes.

A Cochrane review of early post-operative oral feeding after major abdominal gynaecological surgery found that it appeared to be safe without increased GI morbidities or other post-operative complications. The benefits of this approach included faster recovery of bowel function, lower rates of infectious complications, shorter hospital stay, and higher satisfaction [14]. Within UGI cancer surgery, early oral feeding has raised concerns due to the risk of anastomotic leaks. Some studies suggest that the incidence of leaks may be higher with early oral feeding, but this may be heavily modulated by the surgical approach [15]. A systematic review in this area found that an early oral diet reduced post-operative LOS and did not increase post-operative complications. However, the optimal timing for the introduction of an early oral diet could not be established, and the type of feeding varied considerably across studies [16].

The European Society for Clinical Nutrition and Metabolism (ESPEN) advises post-operative protein and energy requirements of 1.5 g/kg/day and 25–30 kcal/kg/day, respectively [17], but only a few studies have reported nutritional adequacy following major surgery [18]. Following pancreatic cancer surgery, one study showed a median daily energy intake of 588 kcal and 27 g protein during the period from resuming oral diet to the day of discharge. Symptoms affecting nutritional intake were prevalent, with 51.6% of patients having 2–4 symptoms and 12.9% having $\geq$5 symptoms [19]. A further study of 50 patients after major open abdominal cancer surgery found that the mean daily protein and energy intake was $0.61 \pm 0.44$ g/kg/day and $9.58 \pm 3.33$ kcal/kg/day within the first post-operative week, respectively. Protein and energy intakes were insufficient in 90% and 82% of the 50 patients [20]. Patients with Clavien-Dindo grade $\geq$III complications consumed less daily protein compared with the group of patients without complications and patients with grade I or II complications [20]. It is important to consider that poor compliance with other ERAS elements, including management of PONV and fluid management, is likely to hinder tolerance to an early oral diet. Suboptimal fluid administration can result in intestinal oedema and reduced GI motility, contributing to PONV and postoperative ileus [21]. An observational study involving 806 patients in a colorectal ERAS programme found PONV on day 2 to be associated with poor oral intake, delayed tolerance of solid food, and mean increased LOS of two days [22].

## NUTRITIONAL SUPPORT AND ORAL NUTRITION SUPPLEMENTS

Peri-operative nutritional support is important for patients who are malnourished or at high nutritional risk. Peri-operative oral nutrition supplements (ONS) should be considered for those who are not expected to eat for five days or for those who are expected to meet less than 50% recommended nutritional intake for seven days post surgery [17]. There is a higher risk of mortality when there has been inadequate oral intake for more than 14 days post surgery [23]. Those who develop post-operative complications are at higher nutritional risk, as there may be delay in the initiation/tolerance of oral nutrition [24].

An RCT involving 100 patients using post-operative ONS resulted in significantly improved nutritional intake, less weight loss (P <0.001), and maintenance of handgrip strength (P <0.01). Subjective levels of fatigue increased significantly above pre-operative levels in control patients, but not in the supplemented group (P <0.01). Twelve patients in the control group developed complications compared with four in the supplemented group (P <0.05) [25]. In another RCT of ONS versus standard care in 101 malnourished surgical patients, the intervention group experienced fewer reductions in weight, anthropometry (triceps skinfold thickness, mid-arm muscle circumference), grip strength, and QOL (P <0.001). Fewer patients in the treatment group (7/52) required antibiotic prescriptions compared with the control group (15/49; P <0.05) [26].

In a larger American study using a nationwide administrative-financial database in colorectal patients following surgery, a propensity-matched sample of early ONS provision (n = 267) versus no nutritional intervention (n = 534) experienced significantly lower infectious complications (P <0.03), reduced rates of pneumonia, intensive care unit admissions (P <0.04), and GI complications (P <0.05) in the nutritional intervention group [27].

## ENTERAL NUTRITION

Following UGI and pancreatic surgery, patients struggle to meet nutritional requirements orally. Early EN (within 24 hours) should be initiated in those who cannot start early oral nutrition or in those who are not expected to meet >50% nutritional requirements by day 7 post surgery [17]. A meta-analysis of 18 studies [28] found that patients who underwent oesophagectomies experienced 5–12% weight loss at six months post-operatively. More than half of patients experienced >10% weight loss at 12 months. In pancreatic surgery, weight loss in the region of 10% in the first few months after surgery has been linked to failure to complete adjuvant chemotherapy and worse prognosis [29, 30].

Despite that, use of enteral feeding tubes remains controversial after GI surgery. Within pancreatic ERAS guidelines, the routine use of enteral feeding tubes is not recommended, but these guidelines are based predominantly on extrapolated data from other specialties, and the level of evidence for this recommendation is very low [31]. Subsequently, the International Study Group on Pancreatic Surgery (ISGPS) position paper, published six years later, concluded that in malnourished patients, or patients at high risk of developing malnutrition and those who develop severe post-operative complications early after operation, supplementary artificial nutrition should be considered a key supportive intervention [32].

Many benefits have been shown with placing nasojejunal tubes (NJT) or needle catheter jejunostomy (NCJ) at the time of surgery in malnourished patients undergoing major UGI or pancreatic surgery [33–36], and they can remain in place following hospital discharge for longer-term nutrition support. A systematic review of nine RCTs involving 757 patients evaluated the short-term outcomes of EN at home in cancer patients following oesophagectomy [37]. When compared to an oral diet, EN was associated with significantly increased body weight, body mass index, and physical function. No significant differences were found in GI adverse reactions and nausea, vomiting, and fatigue were all reduced in patients receiving EN [37]. Although rare in this patient group, bowel ischaemia is a significant complication and is a barrier to tube insertion [32].

If less than 50% of caloric requirements are being met for more than seven days post surgery by the oral and enteral route, European guidelines recommend that a combination of enteral and parenteral nutrition (PN) is used [17]. The enteral route for nutrition should always be preferred unless contraindicated, such as with intestinal obstruction/ileus, high-output fistula, intestinal ischaemia, severe shock, and severe intestinal haemorrhage. In these cases, PN may be appropriate.

## IMMUNO-NUTRITION

Immuno-nutrition (IN) denotes the delivery of specific substrates such as arginine, ω-3 fatty acids, glutamine, and nucleotides in supra-physiological doses [38]. These substrates are added to standard nutrition preparations with the aim of modulating the host's inflammatory response and thus improve clinical outcomes. The role and implementation of IN within ERAS pathways remain unclear and conflicting. The 2016 ERAS protocol investigating peri-operative standard ONS versus IN in patients undergoing colorectal resection concluded that immuno-nutrient-enriched supplements reduce complications in patients undergoing colorectal resection [39]. However, strong conclusions could not be drawn as the study was underpowered. Although this was a multicentre study, participants were all from one country, thus limiting external validity in other healthcare systems. A later study in 2017 comprising 3375 elective colorectal surgery patients concluded that the use of IN pre surgery reduced LOS and improved the quality of surgical care [39]. Patients were issued with a pre-operative checklist recommending that they consume IN three times a day for five days prior to their surgical resection. Despite the results, the study design had several limitations. It was only conducted in centres in Washington State and was a non-controlled trial. Furthermore, compliance of IN was not recorded, regulated, or reported by the investigators [40].

A 2014 meta-analysis found no significant difference in preoperative IN versus standard ONS on clinical outcomes in patients undergoing GI surgery [41]. Moreover, recent ERAS guidelines for peri-operative care in patients undergoing oesophagectomies concluded that evidence for patients undergoing surgery for oesophageal cancer is conflicting and the routine use of IN cannot be supported at present [42].

The dosage and timing of IN supplementation in surgery are not clear. There are concerns with limited reporting of exact volumes of IN/control formula administered in each intervention group. It is possible that there may be potential to demonstrate greater clinical benefit in an intervention group receiving nutrition closer to adequate or goal requirements. Thus, data should be analysed by both intention to treat and actual intake.

When comparing IN to standard supplement/no intervention, research is limited in determining efficacy of application of IN in the ERAS pathway. In various studies, IN is compared to no nutritional intervention or to control products that contain 50–80% less protein than the product being investigated [43–47], thus possibly resulting in beneficial effects from improved protein provision in the intervention group, independent of the immune-modulating components.

In summary, drawing conclusions from published data is not possible, as IN is administered to heterogeneous patient groups, at different time periods in relation to surgery, in different combinations and dosages, and often compared with control preparations that are not always isonitrogenous [48].

Studies investigating the benefits of IN are often funded by commercial entities that produce the product being tested [49]. Given the increased cost associated with IN versus standard formula and the potential for any advantageous effects to be obscured by peri-operative factors (related to low morbidity and severe surgical complications), patients should be assessed and selected on an individual basis. Future trials should be conducted with single immune-enhancing substances. Mortality, LOS, and post-operative complications should not be the only outcomes measured. With increasing financial constraints and inadequate resources available, the economic costs for healthcare systems should also be considered.

## Case Studies

### Routine Case

| Patient | Mrs A, age 75 yr |
|---|---|
| Presenting complaint | Abdominal pain and altered bowel habit for 3 mo |
| Past medical history | Hypertension |
| Social history | Lives with husband. Retired nurse. Nil alcohol and never smoked |
| Investigation | Colonoscopy and computed tomography (CT) |
| Oral intake | Before surgery eating well with no reduction in appetite or food intake |
| Anthropometrics | Nutrition screening pre-operatively and on admission for surgery<br>Weight 75 kg, height 1.6 m, body mass index (BMI) 29.3 kg/m$^2$<br>No weight loss in past 6 mo<br>Malnutrition Universal Screening Tool (MUST) 0 |
| Bowel function | Opening daily or every few days. Alternating between constipation and diarrhoea |
| Diagnosis | Stage 2 colon cancer |
| Surgical plan | Cardiopulmonary exercise testing to determine fitness for surgery<br>Referral to community prehabilitation service and hospital surgery school |
| Nutritional plan | Allowed to eat up to 6 h before surgery and clear fluids up to 2 h before surgery, including carbohydrate loading drinks (800 ml evening before and 400 ml up to 2 h before anaesthesia) |
| Admission | Underwent right hemi-colectomy<br>No nasogastric tube (NGT) post-operatively and normal diet started from day of surgery |
| Nutrition support | Reduced appetite and some nausea post surgery causing suboptimal oral intake (estimated 1000 kcal and 40 g protein)<br>Started on 1.5 kcal/ml high-protein oral nutritional supplement twice a day as per ERAS protocol and continued until discharge |
| Outcome | Uneventful recovery and patient discharged home on day 5 |
| Long-term prescriptions | No oral nutritional supplements provided beyond discharge as patient MUST 0<br>Not seen by a dietitian and expected to improve oral intake at home |
| Follow-up | Appetite and food intake improved over 1–2 wk at home with a 4% weight loss reported before stabilising |

## Complex case

| Patient | Mr B, age 63 yr |
|---|---|
| Presenting complaint | Dysphagia and vomiting |
| Past medical history | Gastritis, reflux, oesophagitis, depression |
| Social history | Lives alone. Ex-waiter. Drinks occasionally (~2 units/wk)<br>Ex-smoker – quit 5 yr ago |
| Investigations | CT scan showed D2/D3 stricture causing gastric outlet obstruction. Endoscopy demonstrated a duodenal stricture. NJT inserted |
| Oral intake | No food intake for 2 wk pre-operatively due to vomiting<br>NJ feeding tube dislodged during vomiting episode 4 d later<br>Admitted for pre-operative PN for 12 d |
| Anthropometrics | Pre-operative weight 45.3 kg, height 1.7 m, BMI 15.7 kg/m$^2$, 22.7% weight loss over past 6 mo<br>Mean grip strength in dominant hand 19.7 kg (44% of normal for age and sex) |
| Bowel function | Bowel not open past 4 d |
| Diagnosis | Duodenal cancer with gastric outlet obstruction |
| Surgical plan | Laparotomy with pancreatico-duodenectomy or palliative bypass depending on operative findings |
| Nutritional plan | Given severe malnutrition (as evidenced by significant weight loss and BMI), NJT insertion at surgery for post-operative nutrition support |
| Admission | Underwent pylorus preserving pancreatico-duodenectomy for a large D2 mass infiltrating the pancreas<br>Followed Whipple ERAS pathway post-operatively, with additional NJ feeding |
| Nutritional support | Day 1: NJ feeding started, 1.0 kcal peptide feed, increasing gradually over 3 d to target 1000 ml (1000 kcal and 40 g protein)<br>Days 1–2: Free fluids orally<br>Day 3: Ryles NGT removed and commenced on soft diet and oral nutritional supplements with ongoing NJ feeding<br>Started on Creon® (Viatris Pharmaceuticals, Canonsburg, PA, USA) 75 000 units with meals and 50 000 units with snacks and milky drinks/nutritional supplements |
| Outcome | Made an uneventful recovery, discharged home on day 14 post-operatively<br>Tolerating small amounts of soft diet (800 kcal, 30 g protein), 1 nutritional supplement daily (300 kcal, 12 g protein)<br>Decision to continue overnight NJ feed (700 ml 1.5 kcal/ml, peptide feed providing 1050 kcal, 52.5 g protein) to promote weight gain before potential adjuvant chemotherapy |
| Long-term prescriptions | Creon 25 000 units: 3 capsules with meals, 2 capsules with snacks and nutritional supplements<br>Multivitamin and mineral once a day (for prevention of micronutrient deficiencies)<br>Proton pump inhibitor<br>Paracetamol and codeine for pain control |
| Follow-up | Patient reviewed in clinic at 1 and 2 mo post-operatively. At 2 mo good progress and decision to remove NJT as tolerating sufficient diet. Weight 53 kg, BMI 18.3 kg/m$^2$ (increase of 8.3 kg from admission weight) |

# REFERENCES

1. Ljungqvist, O., Scott, M., and Fearon, K.C. (2017). Enhanced recovery after surgery: a review. *JAMA Surg.* 152 (3): 292–298.

2. Enhanced Recovery After Surgery (ERAS) Society. Guidelines. https://erassociety.org/guidelines. Accessed August 2021.

3. Fearon, K.C., Jenkins, J.T., Carli, F., and Lassen, K. (2013). Patient optimization for gastrointestinal cancer surgery. *Br. J. Surg.* 100 (1): 15–27.

4. Zhang, X., Yang, J., Chen, X. et al. (2020). Enhanced recovery after surgery on multiple clinical outcomes: umbrella review of systematic reviews and meta-analyses. *Medicine (Baltimore).* 99 (29): e20983.

5. Spanjersberg, W.R., Reurings, J., Keus, F., and van Laarhoven, C.J. (2011). Fast track surgery versus conventional recovery strategies for colorectal surgery. *Cochrane Database Syst. Rev.* (2): CD007635.

6. Bond-Smith, G., Belgaumkar, A.P., Davidson, B.R., and Gurusamy, K.S. (2016). Enhanced recovery protocols for major upper gastrointestinal, liver and pancreatic surgery. *Cochrane Database Syst. Rev.* (2): CD011382.

7. Lu, D., Wang, X., and Shi, G. (2015). Perioperative enhanced recovery programmes for gynaecological cancer patients. *Cochrane Database Syst. Rev.* (3): CD008239.

8. Berian, J.R., Ban, K.A., Liu, J.B. et al. (2019). Adherence to enhanced recovery protocols in NSQIP and association with colectomy outcomes. *Ann. Surg.* 269 (3): 486–493.

9. ERAS Compliance Group (2015). The impact of enhanced recovery protocol compliance on elective colorectal cancer resection: results from an international registry. *Ann. Surg.* 261 (6): 1153–1159.

10. Biagi, J.J., Raphael, M.J., Mackillop, W.J. et al. (2011). Association between time to initiation of adjuvant chemotherapy and survival in colorectal cancer: a systematic review and meta-analysis. *JAMA* 305 (22): 2335–2342.

11. Herbert, G., Perry, R., Andersen, H.K. et al. (2018). Early enteral nutrition within 24 hours of lower gastrointestinal surgery versus later commencement for length of hospital stay and postoperative complications. *Cochrane Database Syst. Rev.* 10 (10): CD004080. Update in: Cochrane Database Syst Rev. 2019 7:CD004080. .

12. Pu, H., Heighes, P.T., Simpson, F. et al. (2021). Early oral protein-containing diets following elective lower gastrointestinal tract surgery in adults: a meta-analysis of randomized clinical trials. *Perioper. Med. (Lond).* 10 (1): 10.

13. Lau, C., Phillips, E., Bresee, C., and Fleshner, P. (2014). Early use of low residue diet is superior to clear liquid diet after elective colorectal surgery: a randomized controlled trial. *Ann. Surg.* 260 (4): 641–647; discussion 647-9.

14. Charoenkwan, K. and Matovinovic, E. (2014). Early versus delayed oral fluids and food for reducing complications after major abdominal gynaecologic surgery. *Cochrane Database Syst. Rev.* 2014 (12): CD004508.

15. Zheng, R., Devin, C.L., Pucci, M.J. et al. (2019). Optimal timing and route of nutritional support after esophagectomy: a review of the literature. *World J. Gastroenterol.* 25 (31): 4427–4436.

16. Carmichael, L., Rocca, R., Laing, E. et al. (2022). Early postoperative feeding following surgery for upper gastrointestinal cancer: a systematic review. *J. Hum. Nutr. Diet.* 35 (1): 33–48.

17. Weimann, A., Braga, M., Carli, F. et al. (2017). ESPEN guideline: clinical nutrition in surgery. *Clin. Nutr.* 36 (3): 623–650.

18. Gillis, C., Nguyen, T.H., Liberman, A.S., and Carli, F. (2015). Nutrition adequacy in enhanced recovery after surgery: a single academic center experience. *Nutr. Clin. Pract.* 30 (3): 414–419.

19. Kang, J., Park, J.S., Yoon, D.S. et al. (2016 Oct). A study on the dietary intake and the nutritional status among the pancreatic cancer surgical patients. *Clin. Nutr. Res.* 5 (4): 279–289.

20. Constansia, R.D.N., Hentzen, J.E.K.R., Hogenbirk, R.N.M. et al. (2022). Actual postoperative protein and calorie intake in patients undergoing major open abdominal cancer surgery: a prospective, observational cohort study. *Nutr. Clin. Pract.* 37 (1): 183–191.

21. Thacker, J.K., Mountford, W.K., Ernst, F.R. et al. (2016). Perioperative fluid utilization variability and association with outcomes: considerations for enhanced recovery efforts in sample US surgical populations. *Ann. Surg.* 263 (3): 502–510.

22. Mc Loughlin, S., Terrasa, S.A., Ljungqvist, O. et al. (2019). Nausea and vomiting in a colorectal ERAS program: impact on nutritional recovery and the length of hospital stay. *Clin. Nutr. ESPEN* 34: 73–80.

23. Gustafsson, U.O., Scott, M.J., Hubner, M. et al. (2018). Guidelines for perioperative care in elective colorectal surgery enhanced recovery after surgery (ERAS) society recommendations: 2018. *World J. Surg.* 43 (3): 659–695.

24. Berkelmans, G.H.K., Fransen, L.F.C., Dolmans-Zwartjes, A.C.P. et al. (2020). Direct oral feeding following minimally invasiveesophagectomy (NUTRIENT II trial): an international, multicenter, open-label randomized controlled trial. *Ann. Surg.* 271: 41e7.

25. Keele, A.M., Bray, M.J., Emery, P.W. et al. (1997). Two phase randomised controlled clinical trial of

postoperative oral dietary supplements in surgical patients. *Gut.* 40 (3): 393–399.

26. Beattie, A.H., Prach, A.T., Baxter, J.P., and Pennington, C.R. (2000). A randomised controlled trial evaluating the use of enteral nutritional supplements postoperatively in malnourished surgical patients. *Gut.* 46 (6): 813–818.

27. Williams, D.G.A., Ohnuma, T., Krishnamoorthy, V. et al. (2020). Impact of early postoperative oral nutritional supplement utilization on clinical outcomes in colorectal surgery. *Perioper. Med. (Lond)* 9: 29.

28. Baker, M., Halliday, V., Williams, R.N., and Bowrey, D.J. (2016). A systematic review of the nutritional consequences of esophagectomy. *Clin. Nutr.* 35 (5): 987–994.

29. Hashimoto, D., Chikamoto, A., Ohmuraya, M. et al. (2015). Impact of postoperative weight loss on survival after resection for pancreatic Cancer. *JPEN.* 39 (5): 598–603.

30. Morita, Y., Sakaguchi, T., Kitajima, R. et al. (2019). Body weight loss after surgery affects the continuity of adjuvant chemotherapy for pancreatic cancer. *BMC Cancer* 19 (1): 416.

31. Lassen, K., Coolsen, M.M., Slim, K. et al.; ERAS® Society; European Society for Clinical Nutrition and Metabolism; International Association for Surgical Metabolism and Nutrition.(2012). Guidelines for perioperative care for pancreaticoduodenectomy: Enhanced Recovery After Surgery (ERAS®) Society recommendations. *Clin. Nutr.* 31 (6): 817–830.

32. Gianotti, L., Besselink, M.G., Sandini, M. et al. (2018). Nutritional support and therapy in pancreatic surgery: a position paper of the international study group on pancreatic surgery (ISGPS). *Surgery* 164 (5): 1035–1048.

33. Delany, H.M., Carnevale, N., Garvey, J.W., and Moss, G.M. (1977). Postoperative nutritional support using needle catheter feeding jejunostomy. *Ann. Surg.* 186 (2): 165–170.

34. Braga, M., Gianotti, L., Gentilini, O. et al. (2002). Feeding the gut early after digestive surgery: results of a nine-year experience. *Clin. Nutr.* 21 (1): 59–65.

35. Daly, J.M., Bonau, R., Stofberg, P. et al. (1987). Immediate postoperative jejunostomy feeding. Clinical and metabolic results in a prospective trial. *Am. J. Surg.* 153 (2): 198–206.

36. Sica, G.S., Sujendran, V., Wheeler, J. et al. (2005). Needle catheter jejunostomy at esophagectomy for cancer. *J. Surg. Oncol.* 91 (4): 276–279.

37. Dai, L., Fu, H., Kang, X.Z. et al. (2018). A retrospective comparative study of continuous pumping for home enteral nutrition after esophagectomy. *Zhonghua. Wai. Ke. Za. Zhi.* 56 (8): 607–610. Chinese.

38. Calder, P.C. (2007). Immunonutrition in surgical and critically ill patients. *Br. J. Nutr.* 98 (Suppl 1): S133–S139.

39. Moya, P., Soriano-Irigaray, L., Ramirez, J.M. et al. (2016). Perioperative standard oral nutrition supplements versus immunonutrition in patients undergoing colorectal resection in an enhanced recovery (ERAS) protocol: a multicenter randomized clinical trial (SONVI study). *Medicine (Baltimore).* 95 (21): e3704.

40. Thornblade, L.W., Varghese, T.K. Jr., Shi, X. et al. (2017 Jan). Preoperative immunonutrition and elective colorectal resection outcomes. *Dis. Colon. Rectum.* 60 (1): 68–75.

41. Hegazi, R.A., Hustead, D.S., and Evans, D.C. (2014). Preoperative standard oral nutrition supplements vs immunonutrition: results of a systematic review and meta-analysis. *J. Am. Coll. Surg.* 219 (5): 1078–1087.

42. Low, D.E., Allum, W., De Manzoni, G. et al. (2019). Guidelines for perioperative care in esophagectomy: enhanced recovery after surgery (ERAS®) society recommendations. *World J. Surg.* 43 (2): 299–330.

43. Heslin, M.J., Latkany, L., Leung, D. et al. (1997). A prospective, randomized trial of early enteral feeding after resection of upper gastrointestinal malignancy. *Ann. Surg.* 226 (4): 567–577; discussion 577–580.

44. Klek, S., Kulig, J., Sierzega, M. et al. (2008). The impact of immunostimulating nutrition on infectious complications after upper gastrointestinal surgery: a prospective, randomized, clinical trial. *Ann. Surg.* 248 (2): 212–220.

45. Chen, D.W., Wei Fei, Z., Zhang, Y.C. et al. (2005). Role of enteral immunonutrition in patients with gastric carcinoma undergoing major surgery. *Asian J. Surg.* 28 (2): 121–124.

46. Jiang, X.H., Li, N., Zhu, W.M. et al. (2004). Effects of postoperative immune-enhancing enteral nutrition on the immune system, inflammatory responses, and clinical outcome. *Chin. Med. J. (Engl).* 117 (6): 835–839.

47. Gunerhan, Y., Koksal, N., Sahin, U.Y. et al. (2009). Effect of preoperative immunonutrition and other nutrition models on cellular immune parameters. *World J. Gastroenterol.* 15 (4): 467–472.

48. Miyauchi, Y., Furukawa, K., Suzuki, D. et al. (2019). Additional effect of perioperative, compared with preoperative, immunonutrition after pancreaticoduodenectomy: a randomized, controlled trial. *Int. J. Surg.* 61: 69–75.

49. Lexchin, J., Bero, L.A., Djulbegovic, B., and Clark, O. (2003). Pharmaceutical industry sponsorship and research outcome and quality: systematic review. *BMJ* 326 (7400): 1167–1170.

# CHAPTER 6

# Surgical Terminology and Pre-operative Considerations: A Guide for Non-Surgeons

Rajiv Lahiri

*Department of HPB Surgery, Royal Surrey NHS Foundation Trust, Guildford, UK*

Surgical terminology can be complicated and confusing. Operations often derive their names from Latin or Greek terms and are composed of different units. While it can be daunting, a general understanding of surgical anatomy is essential to name procedures correctly. All surgeons work to the same nomenclature; therefore, a correct description of the operation will immediately inform another surgeon of exactly what procedure was performed. In some cases the operation is named after the surgeon who developed it, such as Whipple's and Hartmann's procedures that are discussed in other chapters.

## SURGICAL DESCRIPTORS

In surgery, the prefix usually refers to the organ being operated on. Since the advent of different surgical approaches (e.g. open, laparoscopic, robotic, endoscopy), the word describing the approach precedes the operation. To aid understanding in complex major operations, many surgeons will draw diagrams to accompany their written operation note. This is a common example of a surgical descriptor:

> Laparoscopic cholecystectomy
>
> = **Laparoscopic** ('keyhole') **cholecyst** ('gallbladder') **ectomy** ('removal of')
>
> = keyhole removal of gallbladder

## Key Suffixes in Surgical Terminology

The key suffixes in general surgery are defined as follows. These are used in the majority of surgical procedures.

- **Ectomy** – removal of
- **Otomy** – to open a structure, but not necessarily remove it
- **Plasty** – remodelling of a structure
- **Graphy** – imaging of part of the body
- **Scopy** – procedure performed with flexible or rigid scope
- **Stoma/ostomy** – artificial opening in hollow viscus

Here are examples of surgical procedures using these terms.

- Open right hemihepatectomy

  = **Open** ('open') **right hemi** ('right half') **hepat** ('liver') **ectomy** ('removal of')

  = open removal of the right liver

- Laparoscopic enterotomy

  = **Laparoscopic** ('keyhole') **enter** ('small bowel') **otomy** ('open structure')

  = keyhole opening of small bowel

- Percutaneous coronary angioplasty

  = **per** ('via') **cutaneous** ('skin') **coronary** ('cardiac arteries') **angio** ('blood vessel') **plasty** ('remodelling')

  = remodelling of cardiac arteries via the skin

- CT colonography

  = **CT** ('computer tomography') **colon** ('colon') **ography** ('imaging')

  = CT imaging of the colon

- Endoscopic oesophagogastroduodenoscopy

  = **Endoscopic** ('scope within') **oesophago** ('oesophagus') **gastro** ('stomach') **duoden** ('duodenum') **oscopy** ('performed with scope')

  = scope within the oesophagus, stomach, and duodenum

- Open feeding jejunostomy

  = **Open** ('open') **feeding** ('to feed') **jejun** ('jejunum') **ostomy** ('artificial opening')

  = artificial opening in the jejunum for feeding performed by open surgery

International standardisation of surgical nomenclature is not just confined to operations. All medical professionals use these terms and numerous abbreviations. Many of them are outside the scope of this text. However, some important definitions related to surgical nutrition will be discussed, although this is not an exhaustive list. An understanding of these terms is vital to ensure full understanding of complex patients who require nutritional support.

## Anatomical terminology

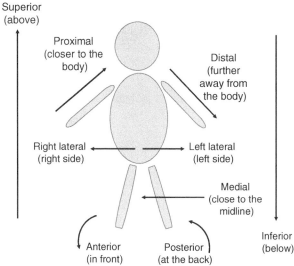

**FIGURE 6.1**   Anatomical terminology.

## Terms to Explain Positioning

There are key terms used to describe which portion of the body is being described, as shown in Figure 6.1. Proximal means closer to the trunk of the patient, whereas distal means further from the trunk. An example would be that the shoulder is proximal to the elbow. Superior can be used interchangeably with 'cranial' (closer to the skull) and inferior used interchangeably with 'caudal' (closer to the hind part of the body).

## PRE-OPERATIVE CONSIDERATIONS

*A good surgeon knows when to operate, a better surgeon knows when not to operate and the best surgeon knows the limit of his operability in inoperable cases. —Ahmedur Rahman*

Planning the right operation, at the right time, in the right patient is arguably the hardest skill for a surgeon to master. In the elective setting, the surgeon starts their assessment watching the patient walk into the clinic room. (Does the patient require a walking aid? Are they on oxygen? What is their exercise tolerance like?) These informal assessments can be all that is required, especially for minor surgery. However, for major surgery, objective assessments are available and should be used. A multidisciplinary team (MDT) approach should also be used in high-risk patients, not only to determine fitness for surgery but also to help optimise recovery [1].

## Frailty

As the population ages and treatments improve, high-risk surgery is now offered to patients who would have previously been considered too high risk. Assessing frailty has become essential in this age group. More frank discussions are now had with regard to resuscitation status both in hospital and in the community. Some patients present to surgical clinic with a community 'do not resuscitate' (DNR) order and this helps to frame the discussion regarding surgical suitability, certainly in the elective setting. There are formal frailty scores available for use, including the commonly used Rockwood frailty score (Figure 6.2) [2]. This score allows a patient to be assigned from 1 (very fit) to 9 (terminal frailty) that can help decide on whether surgery should be performed. The Charlston Age Comorbidity Index (CACI) is a validated tool used to predict patient outcomes based on their comorbidities [3]. It can be used to help predict outcomes following major

### Clinical Frailty Scale

 1  Very Fit – **People who are robust, active, energetic, and motivated.** These people commonly exercise regularly. They are among the fittest for their age.

 2  Well – **People who have no active disease** symptoms but are less fit than category 1. Often, they exercise or are very active occasionally, e.g. seasonally.

 3  Managing Well – **People whose medical problems are well controlled, but are not regularly active** beyond routine walking.

 4  Vulnerable – **While not dependent on others for** daily help, often **symptoms limit activities.** A common complaint is being, slowed up, and/or being tired during the day.

 5  Mildly Frail – **These people often have more evident slowing,** and need help in **high-order IADLs** (finances, transportation, heavy housework, medications). Typically, mild frailty progressively impairs shopping and walking outside alone, meal preparation, and housework.

 6  Moderately Frail – People need help with **all outside activities** and with **keeping house.** Inside, they often have problems with stairs and need **help with bathing** and might need minimal assistance (cuing, standby) with dressing.

 7  Severely Frail – **Completely dependent for personal care,** from whatever cause (physical or cognitive). Even so, they seem stable and not at high risk of dying (within ~6 months).

 8  Very Severely Frail – Completely dependent, approaching the end of life. Typically, they could not recover even from a minor illness.

 9  Terminally Il - Approaching the end of life. This category applies to people with **a life expectancy <6 months,** who are **not otherwise evidently frail.**

Scoring frailty in people with dementia

The degree of frailty corresponds to the degree of dementia. Common **symptoms in mild dementia** include forgetting the details of a recent event, though still remembering the event itself, repeating the same question/story, and social withdrawal.

In **moderate dementia,** recent memory is very impaired, even though they seemingly can remember their past life events well. They can do personal care with prompting.

In **severe dementia,** they cannot do personal care without help.

**FIGURE 6.2**   Rockwood score. IADL, instrumental activities of daily living. *Source*: Adapted from Rockwood, K., Wolfson, C., and McDowell, I. (2001). The Canadian Study of Health and Aging: organizational lessons from a national, multicenter, epidemiologic study. *Int. Psychogeriatr.* 13(Supp 1): 233–237; and Waite, I., Deshpande, R., Baghai, M. et al. (2017). Home-based preoperative rehabilitation (prehab) to improve physical function and reduce hospital length of stay for frail patients undergoing coronary artery bypass graft and valve surgery. *J. Card. Surg.* 12(1): 91. Licensed under CC BY-4.0.

surgery and inform pre-operative counselling. The Edmonton Frail Scale [4] is another validated tool that gives patients a score out of 17 and is safe and feasible for use by doctors who do not specialise in elderly care medicine. In addition to accurate scoring, formal review by a care of the elderly physician and high-risk anaesthetist should also be considered in high-risk cases.

## Anaemia

Anaemia is prevalent in surgical patients. Identifying anaemia pre-operatively has been improved by pre-assessment clinic and, if found, it should be addressed. The underlying cause of anaemia should be treated if possible. A common cause of anaemia is iron deficiency. If found on a haematinics screen, it is generally treated either with oral iron replacement or intravenous iron infusion. However, the recent PREVENTT randomised control trial showed no reduction in death or blood transfusion in patients undergoing major abdominal surgery [5].

## Previous Surgical History

A detailed history is the bedrock of all medical practice and surgery is no exception. In addition to understanding the implications of medical comorbidities (particularly cardiovascular and respiratory disease, diabetes mellitus, and a smoking history) for planned surgery, a comprehensive past surgical history is essential to avoid unexpected findings in surgery. The date, surgical approach, and previous complications must be elucidated. In addition, any other treatment related to the surgery (e.g. chemotherapy, radiotherapy) should be known given the implications it can have for planned surgery. Multiple previous open abdominal operations can preclude a minimally invasive approach and make it generally more technically demanding due to intra-abdominal *adhesions* (bands of scar tissue formed after surgery, infection, trauma, or radiation) and distorted anatomy. Multiple previous laparotomies can lead to a so-called *frozen abdomen* with dense intra-abdominal adhesions that significantly increase the risk of post-operative complications.

Incisional hernias can occur following major surgery and can have a significant impact on quality of life and planning further surgery. Many incisional hernias require mesh repair for definitive repair, and concurrent repair while performing major abdominal surgery needs to be individualised to each patient.

Complication rates are known to be increased in patients undergoing *revisional surgery* (a second operation at the same site, typically undertaken to rectify a post-operative complication) and the incidence of ileus is higher [6], which can have implications for nutrition post-operatively. Patients identified as at high risk of ileus following major abdominal surgery based on their history and examination should have a plan in place for their post-operative nutrition, which can take the form of enteral feeding (e.g. naso-jejunal tube) or total parenteral nutrition (TPN) (see Chapter 19).

## Completion of Multimodal Therapy

Another important consideration before embarking on major surgery is the patient's ability to complete multimodal therapy. This generally refers to treatment before or shortly after major cancer surgery. Patients undergoing oesophagogastrectomy for adenocarcinoma of the oesophagus are generally offered *neo-adjuvant* (before surgery) and *adjuvant* (after surgery) chemotherapy along with surgery [7]. Multiple studies have shown that patients who complete multimodal treatment have significantly longer disease-free and overall survival compared to surgery alone. It is therefore essential that the surgeon and MDT assess whether the patient will be able to complete multimodal treatment. While major post-operative complications may prevent a patient from completing adjuvant treatment, this is unforeseen. However, selecting patients for major surgery who are too frail to complete multimodal treatment even without surgical complications is poor patient selection.

This is also an important consideration in pancreatic surgery. There is evidence that only 50% of patients complete adjuvant chemotherapy after major pancreatic resection [8]. This is due to the magnitude of surgery, the incidence of post-operative complications, and the toxicity of the chemotherapy regime used in pancreatic cancer. It is essential that patients who have undergone major pancreatic resection have regular input from their hepato-pancreatico-biliary (HPB) surgeon, oncologist, HPB clinical nurse specialist (CNS), specialist dietitian, and endocrinologist (if necessary) to maximise the chances of the patient completing adjuvant chemotherapy.

## PREHABILITATION

Prehabilitation refers to the practice of improving a patient's functional capacity prior to surgery, which can lead to improved post-operative outcomes. It is important to identify which patients are most likely to benefit from prehabilitation as it is currently not widely available. It is a multifaceted process and aims to address the patient's physical (muscle mass, respiratory), nutritional (dietary advice and optimisation), and psychological (anxiety, concerns regarding recovery) needs to improve post-operative outcomes. Supporting patients who are enrolled in prehabilitation programmes is essential, therefore patients generally require regular contact with specialist nurses, physiotherapists, and dietitians [9].

A recent randomised control trial demonstrated that prehabilitation during neo-adjuvant therapy prior to oesophagogastrectomy led to patients retaining cardiopulmonary fitness and more patients completing full-dose neo-adjuvant therapy. This thereby indicates that more patients undergoing prehabilitation will complete multimodal treatment [10] (see Chapter 4).

As highlighted earlier, a thorough multidisciplinary, pre-operative assessment is essential to optimise outcomes for patients undergoing major surgery. These approaches have led to patients who would have previously been deemed unfit for major surgery receiving full multimodal treatment. In addition, if patients are objectively too frail for surgery or unable to complete prehabilitation, this can be used to help explain to patients why major surgery may not be in their best overall interests.

## ASSESSING SURGICAL RISK

### Emergency Patients

Many of the pre-operative considerations described are related to elective surgery, where patients can be optimised in the outpatient setting over time. This is not the case with emergency surgery, as the decision for surgery can be made within minutes in cases of life-threatening illness. It is essential that the patient and their family are fully informed of the risks involved with major emergency surgery and that their wishes are considered during all decision making. If possible, an MDT discussion should take place between the patient, their family, and the operating surgeon, consultant anaesthetist, and consultant intensivist. This will allow ceilings of care to be established (if appropriate) and can give both the patient and their family realistic expectations for recovery.

There are scoring systems for patients undergoing major emergency surgery. These systems are easy to access and use pre-operative data to calculate the estimated morbidity and mortality. These scores can be used to help guide discussions pre-operatively and allow patients to attribute a value to the 'surgical risk' they are undertaking. Two of the most commonly used scoring systems for emergency surgery are pPOSSUM (Portsmouth Physiological and Operative Severity Score for the enUmeration of Mortality and morbidity) [11] and the NELA (National Emergency Laparotomy Audit) risk calculator [12].

The pPOSSUM score estimates morbidity and mortality using:

- Physiological factors (age, clinical observations, blood tests, electrocardiogram [ECG], cardiorespiratory comorbidities).
- Operative severity (magnitude of surgery, peritoneal soiling [contamination of the peritoneal cavity, usually related to a bowel perforation], blood loss, presence of malignancy).

The NELA risk calculator uses similar parameters to calculate estimated morbidity and mortality:

- Physiological factors (clinical observations, ASA [performance status determined by physical parameters determined by the American Society of Anesthiolesiologists], cardiorespiratory comorbidities, ECG, blood tests).
- Operative severity (magnitude of surgery, peritoneal soiling, blood loss, presence of malignancy).

These scoring systems should be used allied to clinical judgement, not to dictate it. They also provide valuable data, as the NELA risk calculator has been developed from data gathered in the National Emergency Laparotomy Audit between 2014 and 2016.

## High-Risk Patients

Advances in peri-operative care allied to the development of minimally invasive complex operations have led to patients being offered operations for which they were previously deemed unfit. It is essential that the merits of a particular surgical procedure are weighed up for each individual patient. 'High-risk' patients are generally called so due to comorbidities or frailty and often require further evaluation to assess if major surgery is feasible and safe. Two of the most common assessments of high-risk patients are detailed in the following.

High-risk anaesthetic clinics (HRAC) are run by senior anaesthetists with an interest in peri-operative medicine [13]. Patients are reviewed clinically and with relevant investigations to assess their fitness for surgery. Further investigations such as echocardiography and lung function tests can be requested during this clinic and an individualised risk calculated for the patient based upon previously mentioned scores such as the Rockwood frailty score and pPOSSUM. The Duke Activity Status Index (DASI) [13] is also commonly used to give an estimate of the patient's functional capacity. The results of these investigations give the patient an estimate of their personal 'surgical risk' and facilitate shared decision making with the patient. The high-risk anaesthetic clinic can also work synergistically with other pre-operative interventions such as prehabilitation to highlight and then improve patient function prior to surgery. HRAC can also facilitate discussions with the intensivists with regard to post-operative level 2 (high dependency) or level 3 (intensive care) management.

In addition to HRAC, many centres offer targeted cardiopulmonary exercise (CPEX) testing for high-risk patients for whom major surgery is planned. This is a safe, non-invasive tool that provides comprehensive data regarding the cardiovascular status of the patient [14]. CPEX assesses a number of physiological parameters including anaerobic threshold, peak and max $VO_2$ (oxygen uptake), maximum voluntary ventilation, and ventilation–perfusion mismatch. Detailed knowledge of these parameters is beyond the scope of this chapter. However, with regard to major abdominal surgery, an anaerobic threshold less than 11 ml/kg/min is associated with a higher risk of morbidity and mortality after surgery. Once again, this single value should not supersede clinical judgement, but it should be considered with all other pre-operative data.

## Intra-operative Risk Assessment

For patients undergoing complex abdominal surgery, findings at the time of surgery can influence the risk of complications after surgery. Being cognisant of these intra-operative findings can help surgeons predict possible complications, and modify the post-operative plans in these patients to try to mitigate this risk. This is very important in the current era of enhanced recovery after surgery (ERAS), where standardised post-operative management may not be suitable for patients with specific intra-operative risk. The best-known intra-operative scoring system is the pancreatic fistula risk score. This is used in patients undergoing pancreaticoduodenectomy for head-of-pancreas masses. Pancreaticoduodenectomy is a complex major operation with significant morbidity attached (Chapter 14). The pancreatic fistula risk score [15] consists of simple intra-operative findings and calculates an estimated risk of leakage of pancreatic juice, which can lead to further complications. Patients with a documented high pancreatic fistula risk score can have their post-operative management tailored to this fact, with the aim of minimising the risk of developing a clinically relevant pancreatic fistula.

## POST-OPERATIVE COMPLICATIONS

Complications following surgery can have a detrimental effect on a patient's nutritional state. This in turn can lead to further complications and poor surgical outcomes. While an exhaustive list of these issues is beyond the scope of this chapter, a good understanding of surgical complications that have an impact on nutrition is important.

### Fistula

A fistula is defined as 'an abnormal connection that connects two (or more) structures that are not usually in continuity'. The commonest fistulas in the human body are ear piercings. These and some surgical fistulae are iatrogenic (caused by medical treatment or examination):. However, fistulas in the gastrointestinal tract often require management by the MDT due to the complex surgical and nutritional needs of these patients.

The site of the fistula typically dictates the management strategy, as does which two organs are abnormally connected. Fistulae can be formed by disease processes (e.g. diverticulitis) and iatrogenically (e.g. end colostomy following sigmoid colectomy). Some fistulae require immediate surgical or radiological intervention in order to save life, while others are managed over months prior to definitive intervention. The management of different gastrointestinal fistulae is beyond the scope of this chapter. However, to fully understand how different fistulae are named, these are examples:

Enterocutaneous fistula
= **entero** ('small bowel') **cutaneous** ('skin') **fistula** ('abdominal connection')

= abnormal connection between the small bowel and skin

### Collections

A collection in the context of surgery refers to a collection of fluid or material that occurs following surgery. A post-operative collection is generally 'organised'. This means that the collection of fluid is confined to a certain anatomical part of the body and is walled off. This differs from 'free fluid', which can move throughout a body compartment. An example of a post-operative collection is a pelvic collection following an appendicectomy for perforated appendicitis. In this case, the collection usually contains infected fluid and can develop into an abscess. An abscess is defined as a 'collection of pus' and is generally resistant to antibiotic therapy and normally requires drainage. An intra-abdominal abscess can have a significant impact on a patient's nutritional state as chronic sepsis can lead to a catabolic state.

Collections can lead to peritonitis, referring to inflammation of the peritoneum that lines the abdomen. This is most commonly caused by infection or perforation of an abdominal organ. The peritoneum has a rich nerve supply; therefore, peritonitis is extremely painful and leads to the patient exhibiting classic examination findings (e.g. lying still, involuntary guarding [involuntary response to touch causing rigidity of the abdomen], absent bowel sounds). The finding of peritonitis should trigger immediate senior surgical review and management.

### Anastomotic Leak

An anastomotic leak refers to the partial or full *dehiscence* (opening up of the surgical wound) of a surgical anastomosis, with spillage of the contents of the anastomosis into the peritoneal cavity.

An anastomotic leak can have devastating consequences for the patient. Once again, an understanding of operative terminology is essential to understand the implications for the patient and also why surgeons are more concerned about certain anastomoses compared to others. An example of a high-risk anastomosis is an end-to-side pancreatico-jejunostomy (an anastomosis between the end of the pancreas and the side of the jejunum). This anastomosis is at high risk of leakage (between 10% and 20%) [16] and can have severe implications for the patient's recovery and nutritional state, as a large leak may require TPN. A low-risk anastomosis would be a side-to-side jejuno-jejunostomy (side of jejunum to side of jejunum), as it is well vascularised and under minimal tension. Most surgeons would institute oral feeding early in this case.

Anastomotic leaks can have a significant impact on the patient's recovery. Many anastomotic leaks require either surgical (re-operative) or radiological (drainage) management. The spillage of gastrointestinal contents (e.g. gastric secretions, bile, pancreatic juice, or faeces) can be life threatening and predisposes the patient to peritonitis, ileus, and obstruction. These patients require senior surgical management and an MDT approach (including intensive care unit input) to try to optimise outcomes from these devastating complications.

## Chyle Leak

Chyle is a milky fluid that is rich in fat. It travels in lymphatics from the small intestine to the cisterna chyli and thoracic duct to enter the main circulation. Lymphatic drainage can be disrupted during major surgery as part of a lymphadenectomy to remove lymph nodes and lymphatic tissue. Lymphatics are generally *ligated* (tied) during surgery, or are so small that they do not require this. On occasion, patients can have persistent chyle leaks after surgery. This can have significant implications, as they can become immunocompromised due to leucopenia. Chyle leaks are perpetuated by fat in the diet and are commonly treated with a very low-fat diet or TPN.

## CONCLUSION

An understanding of surgical terminology is important for any health care professional. Being able to understand the details in an operation note will allow understanding of the post-operative plans of the operating surgeon and why these plans may change. The assessment of surgical risk is a complex, MDT issue. It begins at the time of first consultation and can even be ongoing during the operation itself. Identifying patients who are likely to benefit from an operation, and the timing of the operation, is a difficult skill to master.

## ACKNOWLEDGEMENTS

Thank you to Judith Tomlinson, Consultant Anaesthetist, Royal Surrey Hospital, for her help with this chapter.

## REFERENCES

1. Pearse, R.M., Harrison, D.A., James, P. et al. (2006). Identification and characterisation of the high-risk surgical population in the United Kingdom. *Crit. Care* 10: R81.
2. Rockwood, K., Song, X., MacKnight, C. et al. (2005). A global clinical measure of fitness and frailty in elderly people. *CMAJ* 173: 489–495.
3. Charlson, M., Szatrowski, T.P., Peterson, J., and Gold, J. (1994). Validation of a combined comorbidity index. *J. Clin. Epidemiol.* 47 (11): 1245–1251.
4. Rolfson, D.B., Majumdar, S.R., Tsuyuki, R.T. et al. (2006). Validity and reliability of the Edmonton frail scale. *Age Ageing* 35 (5): 526–529.
5. Richards, T., Baikady, R.R., Clevenger, B. et al. (2020). Preoperative intravenous iron to treat anaemia before major abdominal surgery (PREVENTT): a randomised, double-blind, controlled trial. *Lancet* 396 (10259): 1353–1361.
6. Strik, C., Stommel, M.W.J., Schipper, L.J. et al. (2016). Risk factors for future repeat abdominal surgery. *Langenbecks. Arch. Surg.* 401 (6): 829–837.
7. Cunningham, D., Allum, W.H., Stenning, S.P. et al. (2006). Perioperative chemotherapy versus surgery alone for resectable gastroesophageal cancer. *N. Engl. J. Med.* 355 (1): 11–20.
8. DePeralta, D.K., Ogami, T., Zhou, J.-M. et al. (2020). Completion of adjuvant therapy in resected pancreatic cancer. *HPB (Oxford)* 22 (2): 241–248.
9. Hughes, M.J., Hackney, R.J., Lamb, P.J. et al. (2019). Prehabilitation before major abdominal surgery: a systematic review and meta-analysis. *World J. Surg.* 43 (7): 1661–1668.

10. Allen, S.K., Brown, V., White, D. et al. (2021). Multimodal prehabilitation during neoadjuvant therapy prior to esophagogastric cancer resection: effect on cardiopulmonary exercise test performance, muscle mass and quality of life-a pilot randomized clinical trial. *Ann. Surg. Oncol.* 29 (3): 1839–1850.

11. Copeland, G.P., Jones, D., and Walters, M. (1991). POSSUM: a scoring system for surgical audit. *Br. J. Surg.* 78: 355–360.

12. Eugene, N., Oliver, C.M., Bassett, M.G. et al., on behalf of the NELA collaboration.(2018). Development and internal validation of a novel risk adjustment model for adult patients undergoing emergency laparotomy surgery: the National Emergency Laparotomy Audit risk model. *Br. J. Anaesth.* 121 (4): 739–748.

13. Tomlinson, J.H. and Moonesinghe, S.R. Risk assessment in anaesthesia. *Clin. Anaesth.* 17 (10): 486–491.

14. Chambers, D.J. and Wisely, N.A. (2019). Cardiopulmonary exercise testing: a beginner's guide to the nine-panel plot. *BJA Educ.* 19 (5): 158e164.

15. Callery, M.P., Pratt, W.B., Kent, T.S. et al. (2013 Jan). A prospectively validated clinical risk score accurately predicts pancreatic fistula after pancreatoduodenectomy. *J. Am. Coll. Surg.* 216 (1): 1–14.

16. Crippa, S., Salvia, R., Falconi, M. et al. (2007). Anastomotic leakage in pancreatic surgery. *HPB (Oxford)* 9 (1): 8–15.

# CHAPTER 7

# Operating on the Malnourished Patient

Katy O'Rourke and Chris Jones

*Department of Anaesthetics, Royal Surrey NHS Foundation Trust, Guildford, UK*

---

**KEY POINTS**

- Many surgical patients have biochemical abnormalities relating to malnutrition and underlying surgical pathology.
- Up to 30% of surgical patients are anaemic pre-operatively.
- Obesity and hyperglycaemia are becoming more prevalent in the general population and therefore the surgical population.
- Obesity and sarcopenic obesity pose a multitude of risks for the peri-operative period and are independently associated with worse surgical outcomes.

---

Many surgical patients have a degree of malnutrition on presentation that can have significant effects on peri-operative management. This chapter discusses typical biochemical and haematological abnormalities relating to common surgical pathologies that may be seen in the acute and elective surgical patient and the impact of these on peri-operative care, in particular anaesthesia.

## ANAEMIA

Anaemia is defined by the World Health Organization (WHO) as a haemoglobin concentration of less than 130 g/dl for men and less than 120 g/dl for non-pregnant women, and is a state in which the oxygen-carrying capacity of red blood cells is unable to meet physiological demands [1]. There is an

*Nutritional Management of the Surgical Patient*, First Edition. Edited by Mary E. Phillips.
© 2023 John Wiley & Sons Ltd. Published 2023 by John Wiley & Sons Ltd.

estimated prevalence of anaemia in the surgical population of up to 30% internationally [2].

Pre-operative anaemia is independently associated with an increased risk of 30-day morbidity and mortality in patients undergoing both cardiac and non-cardiac surgery [3]. The international consensus statement on management of peri-operative anaemia published in 2017 [4] recommends investigation of anaemia for all surgical procedures with an expected blood loss of 500 ml or more. Causes of anaemia are summarised in Table 7.1.

Iron-deficiency anaemia is the most common cause of anaemia and may be due to dietary insufficiency, chronic inflammatory conditions, or chronic bleeding, which are frequently present in surgical patients. It is often asymptomatic and therefore may not have been recognised pre-operatively. The most sensitive and specific test for investigation of iron-deficiency anaemia pre-operatively is the presence of a serum ferritin level <30 μg/l, which indicates low iron stores within the body. Ferritin is an acute-phase protein that can be falsely elevated in infection or inflammation. As the daily absorption of iron is limited to 1–2 mg/d, most of the iron required for metabolic processes is taken from macrophages recycling iron from these stores [5]. The majority of iron is stored in haemoglobin, but small amounts are also found in muscle tissue, liver, macrophages, and bone marrow. Transferrin saturation can also be used as an indicator of iron available for normal production of red blood cells; a transferrin saturation less than 20% is inadequate. A transferrin saturation of less than 20% with serum ferritin >100 μg/l indicates that iron sequestration (inappropriate mobilisation of iron from stores to bone marrow) or functional iron deficiency (seen with use of erythropoietic drugs) is occurring [4]. Interpretation of the serum ferritin level is summarised in Table 7.2.

A deficiency of iron within the body has impacts on several crucial processes at the cellular level, including delivery of oxygen to tissues, and a decrease in activity of iron-dependent enzymes such as electron transfer reactions and cellular immunity.

**TABLE 7.1** Causes of anaemia.

| Cause of anaemia | Clinical examples |
| --- | --- |
| Iron deficiency | Increased demand, e.g. pregnancy |
| | Limited supply, e.g. malnutrition, poor dietary intake, malabsorption, gastric resection |
| | Increased loss from bleeding (acute or chronic) |
| | Iron sequestration (decreased mobilisation of iron from stores in inflammation) |
| Nutritional deficiencies | Vitamin A, folate, or B12 deficiency due to malabsorption, gastric resection, or poor dietary intake |
| | Folate deficiency |
| | Vitamin B12 deficiency |
| Inflammation | Rheumatoid arthritis Connective tissue disorders |
| Infection | Malaria Mononucleosis |
| Inherited or acquired disorders | Sickle cell anaemia Thalassaemia Hereditary spherocytosis |

**TABLE 7.2** Interpretation of serum ferritin levels.

| Ferritin | Transferrin saturations | Cause |
| --- | --- | --- |
| <30 μg/l | <20% | Iron deficiency |
| <100 μg/l | 20–50% | Low iron stores (Consider supplementation before surgery with moderate to high blood loss expected) |
| 30–300 μg/l | 20–50% | Normal |
| 100–500 μg/l | <20% | Functional iron deficiency (Check folate and B12 levels) |
| >100 μg/l | <20% | Iron sequestration |

The symptoms of iron deficiency are non-specific and include fatigue, weakness, and concentration difficulties. Peri-operatively, low iron stores are associated with an increase in the systemic inflammatory response caused by surgery, higher rates of post-operative infections in abdominal and orthopaedic surgery, and a requirement of post-operative critical care for longer periods.

The management of iron-deficiency anaemia is in replacement of depleted iron stores and aims for a pre-operative haemoglobin of over 130 g/l in both males and females, which reduces the likelihood of complications arising from blood transfusion [6]. If possible all patients should be treated, but those undergoing major surgery should be particularly focused on. Daily or alternate daily oral iron replacement together with dietary advice may be appropriate if it is not contra-indicated, there is at least four to six weeks until the proposed surgery date, and there is no active bleeding present [6]. For patients with chronic bleeding, inflammation, or functional iron deficiency, intravenous (IV) iron infusion is likely to be more beneficial, with effects on haemoglobin seen from three days and maximal at three weeks after transfusion. An iron infusion in the fortnight prior to surgery has been shown to have decreased rates of post-operative complications such as acute kidney injury, infection, and decreased hospital stay [7]. Liver dysfunction and ongoing inflammation are relative contraindications to iron supplementation, and constipation is common with oral supplements.

## ELECTROLYTE ABNORMALITIES

Total body weight comprises 60% water, which is split between intracellular (approximately 60%) and extracellular (30%) fluid compartments [8, 9]. The extracellular compartment further consists of intravascular volume and interstitial fluid. These compartments are maintained in a state of equilibrium through the movement of water by osmosis from an area of low solute concentration to one of high solute concentration. These osmotic forces are controlled by the dominant cations in each compartment: sodium in the extracellular fluid compartment and

potassium in the intracellular fluid compartment. Sodium and potassium are unable to freely cross the lipid cell membrane and rely on voltage-gated protein channels for movement. Within the extracellular fluid compartment, the capillary endothelium is freely permeable to ions as well as water, so interstitial fluid and plasma have similar solute concentrations. Therefore, as proteins are too large to pass through the endothelium, plasma oncotic pressure is maintained by the presence of proteins such as albumin [8].

### Sodium

The regulation of sodium is through the actions of anti-diuretic hormone (ADH) and aldosterone in the kidneys, systemic catecholamine production, and myocardial release of natriuretic peptides [10]. In the healthy person, thirst mechanisms ensure adequate water intake and renal function controls water loss, maintaining serum sodium concentrations between 138 and 142 mmol/l.

Abnormal sodium occurs when there is a defect in the dilutional capacity of the kidneys with excess water intake, causing hyponatraemia, or defective urinary concentration with inadequate water intake, causing hypernatraemia [11]. Deviations in baseline sodium of more than 5 mmol/l are associated with an increased mortality rate in hospitals [10], despite few patients undergoing investigation for abnormal sodium levels in the peri-operative period.

### Hyponatraemia

Investigation and treatment of hyponatraemia (serum sodium <136 mmol/l) are important due to the possibility of underlying disorders causing hyponatraemia that may have negative implications for post-operative recovery such as diabetes, heart failure, malignancy, and adrenal insufficiency. Hyponatraemia may be worsened by fluid shifts occurring intra-operatively, and inappropriate large amounts of fluid can rapidly reverse serum hyponatraemia and lead to cerebral oedema and cortical demyelination.

When approaching a patient with hyponatraemia, several factors must be considered.

- *Osmolality*: Plasma osmolality is the presence of solutes such as sodium or glucose in the extracellular fluid compartment that are unable to freely shift to the intracellular fluid compartment, and therefore influence the movement of water. Unlike hypernatraemia, which is always associated with hyperosmolality, hyponatraemia can be associated with low, normal, or high osmolality [12]. A hypoosmolar hyponatraemia is a dilutional hyponatraemia and is the most common cause of hyponatraemia, occurring when water intake exceeds the capacity of the kidneys to excrete water. High plasma osmolality in hyponatraemia is less common and may be caused by the presence of other solutes like glucose, mannitol, and glycine.
- *Fluid status*: Hyponatraemia can be hypovolaemic, euvolaemic, or hypervolaemic. This usually relates to the release and activity of ADH by the body and may indicate the underlying cause of hyponatraemia.
- *Chronicity*: Hyponatraemia can be defined as acute (established within the past 48 hours) or chronic.
- *Symptoms*: Symptoms of hyponatraemia are usually in proportion to the deficit or acuity of the deficit and include drowsiness, confusion, nausea and vomiting, weakness, and seizures. However, many patients presenting with hyponatraemia will be asymptomatic, particularly if the onset has been insidious or chronic and the serum sodium remains above 125 mmol/l [12].

Acute, symptomatic hyponatraemia should be promptly treated due to the high risk of cerebral oedema, which occurs as a result of water shift from the extracellular fluid compartment to the intracellular fluid compartment. Serum sodium should be raised by 2 mmol/l every hour until symptoms resolve, usually by the administration of hypertonic saline [10]. A diuretic such as frusemide may be co-administered to counteract the subsequent expansion of the extracellular fluid compartment.

Chronic symptomatic hyponatraemia should be carefully managed due to the risk of cortical demyelination, which occurs when plasma osmolality increases suddenly in a brain that has adapted to low sodium levels with a loss of intracellular solutes such as potassium in order to maintain equilibrium. In these patients, sodium should be raised slowly, and should not exceed 10 mmol/l in 24 hours [13].

Patients presenting for surgery with asymptomatic hyponatraemia should be assessed as already discussed and the cause of the hyponatraemia should be determined and managed prior to surgery.

## Hypernatraemia

Hypernatraemia (serum sodium >145 mmol/l) results from a defect in urinary concentrating mechanisms or excessive loss of hypotonic fluids [10]. These patients will have high plasma osmolality, but their fluid status can be used to ascertain the cause of hypernatraemia.

Hypovolaemic patients lose both sodium and water, but water losses exceed sodium. The cause of this is usually renal, but can be gastrointestinal or other fluid losses (excessive sweating, burns). Euvolaemic hyponatraemia may be a result of a defect in the production or release of ADH, or a failure of the kidneys to respond to it, or either central or nephrogenic diabetes insipidus [10].

Neurological symptoms are more common in hypernatraemia than hyponatraemia, and hypernatraemia may present with altered mental status, lethargy, pyrexia, hyperreflexia, nausea and vomiting, and excessive thirst.

The management of hypernatraemia is by restoring normal plasma osmolality; this is usually by replacement of the lost body water with oral water, 5% dextrose, or 0.45% saline. Diabetes insipidus is managed with desmopressin, a synthetic analogue of ADH [10].

## Potassium

Potassium within the extracellular fluid compartment is tightly controlled by insulin and glucagon, which increase transport into the intracellular space, and aldosterone, which increases active transport of potassium into the distal convoluted tubule in the kidneys for excretion [8]. Like sodium, potassium is vitally important in maintaining the voltage across cell membranes, which means that disorders of potassium balance can have severe complications within excitatory tissues like nerves and cardiac muscle [14].

### Hypokalaemia

Hypokalaemia (serum potassium <3.5 mmol/l) can occur due to increased gastrointestinal or renal losses, or reduced dietary intake [15]. Symptoms include muscle weakness, arrhythmias, and electrocardiogram (ECG) abnormalities such as T-wave inversion, development of U-waves, and ST depression.

Management is by identification and correction of the underlying cause with replacement of potassium ions, either orally or IV. IV potassium can cause localised inflammation when given peripherally in concentrated solutions, although it can be given in more concentrated solution centrally, and the maximum rate of infusion should be 10–20 mmol/h.

### Hyperkalaemia

Hyperkalaemia (serum potassium >5.5 mmol/l) is associated with dangerous cardiac conduction abnormalities and can cause life-threatening arrhythmias, including ventricular fibrillation and asystole. ECG changes include peaked T-waves, decreased R-wave amplitude, and widened QRS complexes.

Management of hyperkalaemia is treated as a medical emergency in the presence of ECG changes. IV insulin (usually administered alongside glucose infusion) and beta receptor agonists like inhaled salbutamol help drive potassium intracellularly. Cation exchange resins like calcium resonium can be used to bind and accelerate potassium loss from the gut. Renal replacement therapy can also be used as haemodialysis, haemofiltration, or peritoneal dialysis. Serum potassium levels can be falsely elevated if the sample is haemolysed; and plasma potassium, rather than serum potassium, levels should be used if platelet levels are high.

## Calcium

Calcium in plasma may be in one of three forms: as a free ion, bound to plasma proteins (the majority of which is albumin), or bound to anions, which can diffuse across cell membranes. Calcium is an important factor in muscular contraction and various endocrine and exocrine processes. Regulation of calcium within the body is tightly regulated by hormonal control of the kidneys, bone, and intestines, particularly by parathyroid hormone and 1,25 di-hydroxyvitamin D3 [16].

### Hypocalcaemia

Hypocalcaemia can present with muscle spasm, tetany, tingling in feet and hands, and seizures. ECG changes include prolonged QT interval and even heart block.

Management of hypocalcaemia is by identification and management of the underlying cause. Oral calcium supplements can be given to chronic, asymptomatic patients, along with vitamin D to increase absorption. In the acute setting, IV calcium replacement can be instituted, with 10% calcium gluconate or 10% calcium chloride. Both are irritant and rapid infusion can cause hypotension, flushing, nausea, and vomiting [16].

### Hypercalcaemia

Hypercalcaemia is usually the result of increased calcium influx into the extracellular space exceeding the efflux to bone, intestine, and kidneys. Symptoms may be neurological (confusion, drowsiness, coma), intestinal (abdominal pain, renal calculi, constipation, gastric ulcers, pancreatitis), or cardiac (arrhythmias, shortened QT interval).

Milk alkali syndrome (hypercalcaemia with metabolic alkalosis) occurs when high levels of calcium are consumed alongside an alkali, and was defined in the 1930s when peptic ulcer disease was treated with milk and sodium bicarbonate.

Again, the management of hypercalcaemia depends on the underlying cause and severity. In an outpatient setting with mild hypercalcaemia, general measures such as cessation of drugs (e.g. thiazide diuretics), avoidance of immobilisation, and emphasis on the importance of hydration can be used. The mainstay of management of acute severe hypercalcaemia involves dilution of plasma calcium with IV sodium chloride infusion and loop diuretic drugs to increase excretion.

Primary hyperparathyroidism with severe hypercalcaemia needs assessment for surgical resection. Bisphosphonates and glucocorticoids can also be used, depending on the underlying cause [16].

## Magnesium

Magnesium is one of the most abundant cations and has an important role in physiological and pharmacological processes within the body [17]. Most absorption of dietary magnesium occurs in the small intestine, with some absorption occurring in the large intestine. Most magnesium in the body is stored in bones, skeletal muscle, and soft tissue, while 0.3% of total magnesium is found in serum, 66% ionised and 33% protein bound.

### Hypomagnesaemia

Hypomagnesaemia (serum magnesium <0.7 mmol/l) can be common in the peri-operative setting and symptoms range from asymptomatic to life-threatening cardiovascular compromise [18]. Defining symptoms may be neuromuscular or cardiovascular and include muscle weakness, tingling or paraesthesia, tremor, and seizure. ECG changes include prolonged PR interval, widened QRS, and torsades de pointes (an uncommon, life-threatening distinctive form of polymorphic ventricular tachycardia [VT] associated with sudden cardiac death). It is common to find hypokalaemia in patients with low magnesium.

Management of hypomagnesaemia is with supplementation, either orally or IV.

## Hypermagnesaemia

Hypermagnesaemia (serum magnesium >1.6 mmol/l) is relatively rare and usually occurs following supplementation of magnesium, for example in patients undergoing renal replacement therapy or obstetric patients having treatment for pre-eclampsia. Symptoms include hypotension, respiratory depression, loss of deep tendon reflexes, and cardiac arrest. Management is with respiratory and circulatory support and IV calcium administration [18].

## Phosphate

Phosphate has important roles in physiological processes, especially in combination with calcium, to which its ionised form will bind readily. Most dietary phosphate is absorbed in the gut, with up to 70% absorbed in the duodenum and jejunum [19].

### Hypophosphataemia

Hypophosphataemia (serum phosphate <0.8 mmol/l) is common in the post-operative phase, especially in critically ill patients [19], and is often seen in patients on the intensive care unit (ICU). (Refeeding syndrome is covered in the next section.)

Hypophosphataemia may be asymptomatic, but symptoms are varied and can include hypoxia due to reduced oxygen delivery to tissues, respiratory failure or difficulty weaning mechanical ventilation, arrythmias including supraventricular tachycardia or VT, acute heart failure, muscle weakness, altered mental state, confusion, or seizures [20]. Treatment is by oral or IV replacement of phosphate; however, rapid correction of hypophosphataemia can lead to displacement of calcium and subsequent hypocalcaemia and hypomagnesaemia. In oral replacement, vitamin D should be considered to aid intestinal absorption [21].

## Hyperphosphataemia

Symptoms of hyperphosphataemia (serum phosphate >1.46 mmol/l) include tetany and other symptoms of hypocalcaemia (see earlier) due to deposition of calcium into soft tissues. Treatment is by identification and management of the underlying cause. In rapid severe cases such as rhabdomyolysis, renal replacement therapy may be required.

Electrolyte abnormalities are summarised in Table 7.3.

## REFEEDING SYNDROME

Refeeding syndrome was first documented at the end of the Second World War, when hypophosphataemia and oedema were observed in prisoners of war undergoing refeeding after their rescue from concentration camps. It is a state of severe electrolyte abnormalities following an abrupt carbohydrate load in patients who have had greatly reduced nutritional intake for five days or more [20]. As such,

**TABLE 7.3**  Causes of electrolyte abnormalities.

| Electrolyte | Cause |
| --- | --- |
| Hyponatraemia | Medication: thiazide diuretics, angiotensin-converting enzymes (ACE) inhibitors, non-steroidal anti-inflammatories (NSAIDs), selective serotonin reuptake inhibitors (SSRIs), proton pump inhibitors (PPIs) |
| | Polydipsia (excessive thirst) |
| | Adrenal dysfunction |
| | Syndrome of inappropriate antidiuretic hormone secretion (SIADH) |
| | Heart failure |
| | Liver cirrhosis |
| Hypernatraemia [10] | Defect in urinary concentrating mechanisms |
| | Excessive loss of hypotonic fluids |
| Hypokalaemia [14] | Medication: diuretics (thiazide, loop, osmotic), steroids, beta-adrenergic receptor agonists, laxatives, penicillin |
| | Gastrointestinal losses: diarrhoea/high-output stoma, excessive vomiting, bowel obstruction |
| | Poor intake |
| | Metabolic abnormalities: diabetes mellitus, Cushing syndrome |
| | Hypomagnesiumia |
| Hyperkalaemia | Medication: succinylcholine, digoxin, ACE inhibitors, angiotensin receptor antagonists, diuretics, antibiotics |
| | Insulin deficiency |
| | Addison's disease |
| | Metabolic acidosis |
| | Rhabdomyolysis |
| | Renal failure |

(Continued)

**TABLE 7.3**   (Continued)

| Electrolyte | Cause |
| --- | --- |
| Hypocalcaemia | Hypoparathyroidectomy – following parathyroidectomy or hereditary hypoparathyroidectomy |
| | Hypomagnesaemia |
| | Vitamin D deficiency |
| | Hypoalbuminaemia |
| | Hyperphosphataemia |
| Hypercalcaemia | Primary hyperparathyroidism |
| | Malignancy from direct bone destruction, paraneoplastic syndrome, or secondary hyperparathyroidism |
| | Medication: vitamin D, lithium, thiazide diuretics, calcium supplements |
| | Granulomatous disease: sarcoidosis, tuberculosis, leprosy |
| Hypomagnesaemia | Medication: thiazide diuretics, aminoglycosides, cisplatin, tacrolimus, laxatives, ACE inhibitors |
| | Decreased oral intake |
| | Alcohol dependency |
| | Redistribution into intracellular compartment: refeeding syndrome, diabetic ketoacidosis, pancreatitis |
| | Increased losses: diarrhoea, high-output stoma, vomiting, short bowel syndrome, pancreatic exocrine insufficiency |
| Hypophosphataemia [22] | Redistribution: respiratory alkalosis, refeeding syndrome |
| | Decreased absorption: vitamin D deficiency, diarrhoea, vomiting, low-phosphate diet |
| | Increased renal excretion: metabolic acidosis, use of diuretics, glucocorticosteroids, aminoglycosides |
| Hyperphosphataemia [21] | Increased phosphate load: phosphate-containing medication, phenytoin, laxatives, tumour lysis syndrome, rhabdomyolysis |
| | Reduced renal clearance: acute kidney disease, chronic kidney disease, hypoparathyroidism |
| | Cellular redistribution: hyperglycaemia, diabetic ketoacidosis, lactic acidosis |
| | Pseudohyperphosphataemia: inaccurate laboratory results due to the presence of heparin, haemolysis, hyperlipidaemia, or hyperbilirubinaemia |

patients who are malnourished pre-operatively due to existing pathology such as cancer (for example head and neck cancers, oesophageal cancers) are at increased risk (see Table 7.4).

During periods of starvation, there is a shift to fat metabolism from the usual carbohydrate metabolism. Reintroduction of carbohydrates leads to a rapid increase in insulin, which subsequently causes movement of phosphate, magnesium, and potassium into cells, resulting in hypophosphataemia, hypomagnesaemia, and hypokalaemia [24]. These electrolyte abnormalities can be severe and

**TABLE 7.4**  Risk factors for refeeding syndrome.

| Risk factor | Clinical examples |
| --- | --- |
| Malnutrition | One or more of the following:<br>• BMI <16 kg/m²<br>• Weight loss >15% in past 3–6 mo<br>• Little or no nutritional intake for 10 d<br>• Low potassium; phosphate or magnesium prior to feeding<br><br>Two or more of the following:<br>• BMI <18.5 kg/m²<br>• Weight loss >10% in past 3–6 mo<br>• History of risk factors listed below |
| Additional risk factors | |
| Drugs | Chemotherapy |
| | Insulin |
| | Diuretics |
| | Antacids |
| Alcohol abuse | |
| Cancer | Head and neck cancers |
| | Oesophageal or gastrointestinal cancers |
| | Nausea and vomiting (as a result of cancer or side effect of chemotherapy) |
| | Radiotherapy side effect |
| | Mucositis |
| Psychiatric disorders | Anorexia nervosa |
| | Dementia |
| | Depression |
| Elderly or vulnerable patients | |
| Obstetrics | Hyperemesis gravidarum |
| Obesity | Previous bariatric surgery |

Source: Adapted from [23].

cause multiorgan failure and death. The electrolyte shifts also cause movement of sodium out of cells in exchange for potassium, which can lead to retention of water, and pulmonary and peripheral oedema [25]. Hypophosphataemia can be especially pronounced in refeeding syndrome due to the requirement of phosphate for glycolysis. Thiamine is also required in this process and is not stored in significant amounts within the body, so should be supplemented when refeeding syndrome is suspected.

The management of refeeding syndrome is summarised into three categories [23, 25]:

- *Prevention*: detection of at-risk patients; minimising IV dextrose; slow instigation of nutritional support (5–10 kcal/kg initially) with B vitamin supplementation.

- *Monitoring*: daily electrolyte monitoring (including magnesium and phosphate); strict fluid balance; and cardiac monitoring in very high-risk patients.
- *Treatment*: prompt and effective management of electrolyte abnormalities and hyperglycaemia.

## Hyperglycaemia

There is a well-established link between peri-operative morbidity and worse outcomes in patients with hyperglycaemia, particularly those who require insulin therapy [26].

The stress response stimulated by surgery involves activation of the sympathetic nervous system with associated immunological and endocrinological changes. This leads to an increase in circulating catecholamines and inflammatory cytokines, and a decrease in anabolic hormones like insulin in order to aid in glucose mobilisation and production [26]. There is a subsequent rise in free fatty acids that contribute to a state of relative insulin resistance in the peri-operative period, which is pronounced in the first 24 hours after surgery but can persist for several days post-operatively. The magnitude of the stress response is related to the surgical approach, length, and anaesthetic techniques. Major, open-cavity surgical procedures are associated with a more pronounced stress response, and regional anaesthetic techniques have been shown to reduce it [27]. Many enhanced recovery programmes recommend the use of carbohydrate loading pre-operatively (see Chapter 5). This has the benefit of reduced starvation time and subsequently reduction in catecholamines released in the catabolic state, and has also been shown to decrease insulin resistance peri-operatively [28].

The International Diabetic Federation currently estimates the worldwide prevalence of diabetes mellitus (DM) to be 1 in 11 people, and this rises to 1 in 5 people over the age of 65 years. Some 90% of people with diabetes have type 2 DM, typically associated with insulin resistance. Surgical patients with DM have been found to have higher rates of post-operative complications (infections, myocardial infarction, acute kidney injury), longer lengths of stay, and higher mortality rates when compared to patients without DM in both the elective and emergency surgical populations [29]. These outcomes are worse in those patients who have not been formally diagnosed with diabetes, possibly due to less vigilance in monitoring of blood glucose and recognition of complications [30]. Glycated haemoglobin (HbA1$_c$) is recommended for monitoring of diabetes and investigation of suspected diabetes, and should be checked in all patients undergoing major surgery who are at risk of diabetes. HbA1$_c$ should be between 48 and 58 mmol/mol to ensure optimal glycaemic control pre-operatively [31].

In the UK, a national patient safety audit identified that DM was poorly managed in the pre-operative setting, and recommendations were made to support early identification of patients with DM; assessment of additional risk factors; timely referral for optimisation of glycaemic control prior to patients undergoing elective surgery; and close monitoring of blood glucose levels during and after surgery [32].

Patients who take insulin are also at risk of developing diabetic ketoacidosis during the perioperative period. For this reason, the 2015 guidelines from the Association of Anaesthetists of Great Britain and Ireland [33] on perioperative management of the surgical patient with diabetes recommend continuing basal insulin at a reduced dose. Any patients who are found to have a blood glucose level of 12 mmol/l or more intra-operatively should also have their capillary blood ketones measured and, if these are over 3 mmol/l, be treated as diabetic ketoacidosis.

Hyperglycaemia management intra-operatively should be with subcutaneous insulin or variable-rate insulin infusion [33]. When giving IV fluids with a variable-rate insulin infusion, care should be taken to avoid hyponatraemia by excessive administration of hypotonic solutions such as 5% glucose. Insulin also aids in transport of potassium into cells and potassium may need replacement IV. In order to minimise disruption to diabetic control, usual medications should be reinstated as soon as possible, and starvation times should be minimised.

## IMPACT OF BODY HABITUS ON ANAESTHESIA

### Obesity

With 68% of men and 60% of women in the UK now considered overweight or obese [34], the challenges of obesity in the peri-operative period are increasingly relevant.

The WHO classifies obesity according to body mass index (BMI), dividing BMI into class 1, 2, and 3 with BMI of 30–34.9, 35–39.9, and $>40\,kg/m^2$, respectively [35].

In addition to BMI, the distribution of body fat is an important indicator of risk of complications such as metabolic syndrome and cardiovascular compromise. Centrally located fat or an 'apple'-shaped distribution is higher risk, while peripheral obesity or a 'pear'-shaped distribution is lower risk.

The presence of sarcopenia in the obese patient is increasingly recognised and identified as a surgical risk factor in several fields (see Chapter 3).

### Consequences of Obesity during Anaesthesia

- Reduced functional residual capacity (FRC) and alveolar atelectasis.
- Increased oxygen demand due to high metabolic rate and work of breathing.
- High risk of hypoxia on induction of anaesthesia or when critically ill.
- Increased risk of requirement for ventilatory support post-operatively [35].
- Increased risk of difficult intubation and ventilation under general anaesthesia.
- Obstructive sleep apnoea is associated with opiate-induced respiratory depression and the need for post-operative ventilation.
- Patients with obesity hypoventilation syndrome are particularly vulnerable to opiates and anaesthetic agents, and the associated respiratory depression. In addition, they may develop heart failure as a result of chronic hypoxaemia.

- Hypertension [36].
- Heart failure [35]; left ventricular failure in turn leads to pulmonary vasoconstriction and right heart failure; cor pulmonale.
- Ischaemic heart disease.
- Arrythmias secondary to underlying heart disease and increased catecholamines and infiltration of the conducting system in the heart by fatty tissue [36].
- Obesity is a pro-thrombotic state and there is a high risk of thrombotic events like myocardial infarction, stroke, and venous thromboembolism during the peri-operative period. Patients should all undergo risk assessment and initiation of appropriate prophylactic management such as compression stockings, intermittent pneumatic compression, and low molecular weight heparin.
- Under anaesthesia gastro-oesophageal reflux leads to an increased risk of aspiration of gastric contents.

### The Underweight Patient

Although perhaps not as prevalent as obesity, patients with a BMI of <18 are also at higher risk during the peri-operative period. Much of the research into BMI has focused on those with a higher BMI, but there is evidence that in fact patients who are underweight have higher rates of post-operative complications compared to normal BMI than those who are overweight [37]. Patients presenting for surgery who fall into the underweight category should have nutritional assessment and optimisation with parenteral or enteral nutritional supplementation if possible (see Chapter 3).

### Consequences of Malnutrition during Anaesthesia

- Sarcopenia and loss of muscle mass can lead to poor respiratory muscle function and increased risk of post-operative respiratory complications (in both the under- and overweight patient).

- Electrolyte disturbances may also result in life-threatening cardiac arrhythmias.
- Heart failure.
- Hypoglycaemia.
- Hypoalbuminaemia.

- Underweight patients may be more prone to pressure sores and neuromuscular injury from pressure areas during surgery, and theatre staff should be aware that careful positioning and padding of at-risk areas are required.
- Hypothermia.

## Case Study 7.1

| Patient | Mrs A, age 72 yr |
|---|---|
| Presenting complaint | Presented to GP with a history of tiredness and shortness of breath on exertion |
| Past medical history | Mild asthma; taking salbutamol as required<br>Hysterectomy (aged 49 yr)<br>No allergies |
| Social history | Non-smoker, rarely drinks alcohol<br>Retired librarian<br>Sedentary lifestyle, but independent at home and manages stairs |
| Investigations | Blood tests:<br>• Anaemia with haemoglobin (Hb) 101 g/l<br>• Iron studies showed ferritin 28 µg/l<br>• HbA1$_c$ 58 mmol/mol (7%)<br>• Fasting glucose 8.3 mmol/l<br>• Nil else of note on biochemistry<br>Colonoscopy showed a suspicious lesion in sigmoid colon, which was biopsied and confirmed malignant. Computed tomography (CT) chest, abdomen, and pelvis showed no evidence of lymph node involvement or metastatic disease |
| Oral intake | Three meals a day with frequent snacking in between on sugary snacks |
| Anthropometrics | Height 165 cm, weight 89 kg<br>BMI 32.6 kg/m$^2$<br>No weight loss |
| Bowel function | Bowels open 2–3 times per day on average |
| Diagnosis | Adenocarcinoma of sigmoid colon with associated iron-deficiency anaemia<br>Raised HbA1$_c$ and fasting glucose suggestive of undiagnosed type 2 DM |
| Surgical plan | Primary surgical resection via sigmoid colectomy |
| Nutritional plan | Referred to diabetic team and suggested commencing metformin 500 mg once daily<br>Counselling regarding low glycaemic index diet and increasing exercise<br>Commenced oral iron supplementation<br>Carbohydrate loading prior to surgery |
| Admission | Blood glucose 15.6 mmol/l on bedside monitoring. Given the malignancy and urgency of surgery, it was not felt appropriate to postpone and a variable-rate insulin infusion (VRII) was commenced. Once blood glucose was less than 12 mmol/l, surgery went ahead and laparoscopic resection occurred, with good surgical margins and primary anastomosis |

| Outcome | Patient remained on VRII overnight and once oral feeds were re-instigated on day 1, post-operative metformin was restarted and VRII stopped. Blood sugars remained between 10 and 12 mmol/l and inpatient referral to diabetic team was made. Metformin dose was increased to 500 mg twice a day with good effect. Mrs A was discharged home 3 days post-operatively |
|---|---|
| Follow-up | For 8 wk follow-up in surgical clinic<br>Diabetes team to follow-up in 12 wk with HBA1$_c$ and fasting glucose |

## Case Study 7.2

| Patient | Mr B, aged 54 yr |
|---|---|
| Presenting complaint | Acute presentation to A&E with bilious vomiting and feeling unwell. Bowels not opened for the past 10 d. Poor appetite for the past 2 wk with significantly reduced intake |
| Past medical history | Open appendicectomy (aged 15 yr)<br>Open umbilical hernia repair (aged 40 yr)<br>Hypertension on amlodipine 10 mg once daily |
| Social history | Ex-smoker, gave up 10 yr ago (previously 10/d for 20 yr)<br>Drinks approximately 15 units/week (wine)<br>Works as a solicitor<br>Cycles 5–10 miles every weekend |
| Investigations | CT abdomen and pelvis showed acute intestinal obstruction likely secondary to adhesions<br>Biochemistry:<br>• Potassium 2.5 mmol/l (reference range [RR] 3.5–5.5 mmol/l)<br>• Chloride 95 mmol/l (RR 95–108 mmol/l)<br>• pH 7.51 (RR 7.35–7.45)<br>• Magnesium 0.64 mmol/l (RR 0.7–1.0 mmol/l)<br>• Phosphate 0.5 mmol/l (RR 0.74–1.4 mmol/l)<br>• Lactate 2.5 mmol/l (RR 0.5–1 mmol/l)<br>• Creatinine 120 μmol/l (RR 50–120 μmol/l)<br>• All other electrolytes within normal range<br>Clinically dehydrated with dry mucous membranes and urine output <20 ml/h<br>Blood pressure 95/43 mmHg and heart rate 110 beats/min |
| Oral intake | Previously good diet with 3 meals a day<br>In past fortnight managing fluids only, mostly water and black tea |
| Anthropometrics | Height 177 cm, weight 73 kg<br>Unknown recent weight loss in last 2 wk, but some assumed.<br>BMI 23.3 kg/m$^2$ |
| Bowel function | Usually normal, not opened for 10 d |

| | |
|---|---|
| Diagnosis | Acute bowel obstruction likely secondary to adhesions or umbilical hernia recurrence |
| Surgical plan | Urgent laparotomy and adhesiolysis |
| Nutritional plan | Nasogastric tube inserted and 2 l bilious fluid drained<br>Central venous access established and IV infusions of potassium and magnesium commenced prior to induction of anaesthesia<br>Initial fluid resuscitation with 1 l of IV balanced crystalloid solution |
| Outcome | Significant adhesions found intra-operatively with twisting, requiring resection of approximately 10 cm of small bowel and primary anastomosis<br>Post-operatively transferred to ICU. Nasogastric tube left on free drainage and commenced parenteral nutrition via central line.<br>Made good progress and discharged to surgical ward day 2 post-operatively having commenced sips of oral fluid<br>On day 3 high nasogastric output noted and bowels not yet opened with no bowel sounds present. Diagnosed as post-operative ileus and commenced regular metoclopramide and erythromycin<br>Discharged on day 8 having re-established usual oral intake and weaned off parenteral nutrition with support from dietitian |
| Follow-up | 4 wk follow-up in surgical clinic – making good progress |

# REFERENCES

1. World Health Organization. (2011). Haemoglobin concentrations for the diagnosis of anaemia and assessment of severity. WHO/NMH/NHD/MNM/11.1. VMNIS Vitamin and Mineral Nutrition Information System. Geneva: World Health Organization. https://apps.who.int/iris/bitstream/handle/10665/85839/WHO_NMH_NHD_MNM_11.1_eng.pdf. Accessed August 2021.

2. Fowler, A.J., Ahmad, T., Abbott, T.E.F. et al. (2018). Association of preoperative anaemia with postoperative morbidity and mortality: an observational cohort study in low-, middle-, and high-income countries. *Br. J. Anaesth.* 121 (6): 1227–1235.

3. Musallam, K.M., Tamim, H.M., Richards, T. et al. (2011). Preoperative anaemia and postoperative outcomes in noncardiac surgery: a retrospective cohort study. *Lancet* 378 (9800): 1396–1407.

4. Muñoz, M., Acheson, A.G., Auerbach, M. et al. (2017). International consensus statement on the peri-operative management of anaemia and iron deficiency. *Anaesthesia* 72 (2): 233–247.

5. Camaschella, C. (2015). Iron-deficiency anemia. *N. Engl. J. Med.* 372 (19): 1832–1843.

6. Muñoz, M., Gómez-Ramírez, S., Kozek-Langeneker, S. et al. (2015). 'Fit to fly': overcoming barriers to preoperative haemoglobin optimization in surgical patients. *Br. J. Anaesth.* 115 (1): 15–24.

7. Muñoz, M., Gómez-Ramírez, S., Cuenca, J. et al. (2014). Very-short-term perioperative intravenous iron administration and postoperative outcome in major orthopedic surgery: a pooled analysis of observational data from 2547 patients: IV iron and postoperative outcome in Orthopedic surgery. *Transfusion* 54 (2): 289–299.

8. Rassam, S.S. and Counsell, D.J. (2005). Perioperative electrolyte and fluid balance. *Contin. Educ. Anaesth. Crit. Care Pain* 5 (5): 157–160.

9. Mahmood, U. (2019). *Fluid and Electrolyte Disorders.* London: IntechOpen.

10. Klinck, J., McNeill, L., Di Angelantonio, E., and Menon, D.K. (2015). Predictors and outcome impact of perioperative serum sodium changes in a high-risk population. *Br. J. Anaesth.* 114 (4): 615–22.

11. Kumar, S. and Berl, T. (1998). Sodium. *Lancet.* 352 (9123): 220–228.

12. Adrogué, H.J. and Madias, N.E. (2000). Hyponatremia. *N. Engl. J. Med.* 342 (21): 1581–1589.

13. Sterns, R.H. and Silver, S.M. (2016). Complications and management of hyponatremia. *Curr. Opin. Nephrol. Hypertens.* 25 (2): 114–119.

14. Parikh, M. and Webb, S.T. (2012). Cations: potassium, calcium, and magnesium. *Contin. Educ. Anaesth. Crit. Care Pain* 12 (4): 195–198.

15. Kardalas, E., Paschou, S.A., Anagnostis, P. et al. (2018). Hypokalemia: a clinical update. *Endocr. Connect.* 7 (4): R135–R146.

16. Bushinsky, D.A. and Monk, R.D. (1998). *Calc. Lancet.* 352 (9124): 306–311.

17. Ahmed, F. and Mohammed, A. (2019). Magnesium: the forgotten electrolyte—a review on hypomagnesemia. *Med. Sci. (Basel)* 7 (4): 56.

18. Herroeder, S., Schönherr, M.E., De Hert, S.G., and Hollmann, M.W. (2011). Magnesium—essentials for anesthesiologists. *Anesthesiology* 114 (4): 971–993.

19. Wadsworth, R.L. and Siddiqui, S. (2016). Phosphate homeostasis in critical care. *BJA Educ.* 16 (9): 305–309.

20. Macdonald, K., Page, K., Brown, L., and Bryden, D. (2013). Parenteral nutrition in critical care. *Contin. Educ. Anaesth. Crit. Care Pain* 13 (1): 1–5.

21. Rudolph, E.H. and Gonin, J.M. (2012). Disorders of phosphorus metabolism. In: *Nephrology Secrets* (ed. E.V. Lerma and A.R. Nissenson), 551–559. London: Elsevier.

22. Geerse, D.A., Bindels, A.J., Kuiper, M.A. et al. (2010). Treatment of hypophosphatemia in the intensive care unit: a review. *Crit. Care* 14 (4): R147.

23. National Institute for Health and Care Excellence (2017). Nutrition support for adults: oral nutrition support, enteral tube feeding and parenteral nutrition. Clinical guideline [CG32]. www.nice.org.uk/guidance/cg32/chapter/1-guidance#screening-for-malnutrition-and-the-risk-of-malnutrition-in-hospital-and-the-community. Accessed August 2021.

24. McCracken, J. (2012). Refeeding syndrome and the cancer patient. *Compl. Nutr.* 12 (2): 44–46.

25. Reber, E., Friedli, N., Vasiloglou, M.F. et al. (2019). Management of refeeding syndrome in medial inpatients. *J. Clin. Forensic Med.* 8 (12): 2022.

26. Duggan, E.W., Carlson, K., and Umpierrez, G.E. (2017). Perioperative hyperglycemia management: an update. *Anesthesiology* 126 (3): 547–560.

27. Desborough, J.P. (2000). The stress response to trauma and surgery. *Br. J. Anaesth.* 85 (1): 109–117.

28. Bilku, D.K., Dennison, A.R., Hall, T.C. et al. (2014). Role of preoperative carbohydrate loading: a systematic review. *Ann. R Coll. Surg. Engl.* 96 (1): 15–22.

29. Holman, N., Hillson, R., and Young, R.J. (2013). Excess mortality during hospital stays among patients with recorded diabetes compared with those without diabetes. *Diabet. Med.* 30 (12): 1393–1402.

30. Levy, N. and Dhatariya, K. (2019). Pre-operative optimisation of the surgical patient with diagnosed and undiagnosed diabetes: a practical review. *Anaesthesia* 74 (Suppl 1): 58–66.

31. Joint Diabetes Societies for Inpatient Care. (2016). Management of adults with diabetes undergoing surgery and elective procedures: Improving standards. Summary. www.diabetes.org.uk/resources-s3/2017-09/Surgical%20guideline%202015%20-%20summary%20FINAL%20amended%20Mar%202016.pdf. Accessed August 2021.

32. Alleway, R. (2018). Perioperative diabetes: High and lows. National Confidential Enquiry into Patient Outcome and Death. www.ncepod.org.uk/2018pd.html.

33. Barker, P., Creasey, P.E., Dhatariya, K. et al. (2015). Perioperative management of the surgical patient with diabetes 2015: Association of Anaesthetists of Great Britain and Ireland. *Anaesthesia* 70 (12): 1427–1440.

34. NHS Digital (2019). Health Survey for England 2019. https://digital.nhs.uk/data-and-information/publications/statistical/health-survey-for-england/2019. Accessed August 2021.

35. World Health Organization (2021). Obesity and overweight. www.who.int/news-room/fact-sheets/detail/obesity-and-overweight. Accessed August 2021.

36. Association of Anaesthetists of Great Britain and Ireland (2015). Peri-operative management of the obese surgical patient 2015. *Anaesthesia* 70 (7): 859–876.

37. Han, T.S. and Lean, M.E. (2016). A clinical perspective of obesity, metabolic syndrome and cardiovascular disease. *JRSM Cardiovasc. Dis.* 5: 2048004016633371.

# IMPACT OF SURGERY

# Nutritional Management of the Surgical Patient in Critical Care

Nárbhla Donnelly and Anne Langan

*Department of Nutrition and Dietetics, Guy's and St Thomas' NHS Foundation Trust, London, UK*
*Department of Nutrition and Dietetics, The Royal London Hospital, Barts Health NHS Trust, London, UK*

---

**KEY POINTS**

- Low-dose enteral feeding is required in the very early stages of critical illness.
- Careful consideration of both protein and energy requirements is required to optimise nutritional status.
- Consideration of gut perfusion is crucial in the safe management of enteral nutrition in critical illness.

---

There were approximately 69 000 surgical (either planned or unplanned, elective or emergency) admissions to critical care units in the UK in 2019/20. This represents around 40% of all admissions [1]. Unsurprisingly, there is a higher mortality rate following emergency surgery when compared with elective procedures, and a fivefold increase in mortality for patients undergoing urgent intra-abdominal surgery [2]. All major surgery carries risk of infection, sepsis, or triggering of the systemic inflammatory response syndrome (SIRS), with those undergoing complex abdominal surgery deemed at the greatest risk of developing complications [3]. Surgical admissions requiring critical care can have negative impacts on the nutrition status of patients and on post-operative outcomes. The accumulation of calorie and protein deficits in a prolonged critical care

stay has also been shown to negatively influence outcomes. Therefore, understanding and ensuring appropriate nutrition is an essential element of care of the post-operative, critically ill patient. This chapter will cover the metabolic response to stress, feeding the post-operative surgical patient in critical care, and determining estimated nutritional targets.

## METABOLIC RESPONSE TO STRESS

Major surgery elicits a series of reactions referred to as the stress response, which is characterised by hypermetabolism, hyperglycaemia, catabolism, increased lipolysis, and sodium and water retention [4]. The metabolic stress response to surgical injury results in increased circulation of catabolic

*Nutritional Management of the Surgical Patient*, First Edition. Edited by Mary E. Phillips.
© 2023 John Wiley & Sons Ltd. Published 2023 by John Wiley & Sons Ltd.

hormones, including cortisol, glucagon, and catecholamines, alongside a decrease in anabolic hormones, testosterone and insulin [5]. This stress response is thought to aid in survival by increasing cardiac output and oxygen consumption, maintaining fluid volume (sodium and water retention), causing catabolism of glycogen, skeletal muscle, and adipose tissue, resulting in substrate mobilisation (glucose, amino acids, and fatty acids), diverting them to supply energy to support vital organs, enhance immune response, and optimise wound healing [6, 7]. Overall, the magnitude of the response is determined by the extent of surgical trauma [8] and if this response is prolonged, significant muscle wasting ensues.

A study that investigated the metabolic response in critically ill patients with either major trauma or severe sepsis using indirect calorimetry found that resting energy expenditure (REE) increased to a maximum of 40% above normal in both groups over the first week. During the second week of intensive care admission, the total energy expenditure (TEE) of mainly mechanically ventilated patients was 70–80% higher than the REE, particularly in the trauma group. Prolonged hypermetabolism was evident in both groups three weeks later despite the rapid decrease of pro-inflammatory cytokines after week one [9].

Hyperglycaemia ensues due to increased production of endogenous glucose (gluconeogenesis) alongside insulin resistance [10]. The severity of post-operative insulin resistance correlates with the extent of the procedure and associated complications like sepsis [8]. Importantly, post-operative hyperglycaemia is associated with poor outcomes, including mortality and increased infection risk [6, 11]. While monitoring of glycaemic control is recommended, a conventional approach to management rather than tight glucose control is considered best practice [12, 13].

Elevated cortisol and cytokine concentrations post-operatively stimulate protein catabolism [10]. Increased protein turnover occurs in the surgical stressed state, where protein breakdown accelerates and exceeds protein synthesis, leading to significant muscle wasting [14]. Critically ill patients may lose up to 2% muscle mass per day [15]. Skeletal muscle wasting is significantly greater in those

experiencing multiorgan failure compared with single-organ failure [16] and this extensive muscle wasting likely has impacts on recovery from critical illness [17–21].

## FEEDING THE POST-OPERATIVE SURGICAL PATIENT IN CRITICAL CARE

The aims of feeding the post-operative surgical patient in critical care are:

- To minimise energy, protein, and micronutrient deficits in order to prevent malnutrition and loss of lean mass.
- To maintain gut integrity and reduce intestinal permeability.
- To help attenuate the inflammatory response and favourably modulate the immune system.
- To help regulate the metabolic response, thereby reducing insulin resistance [22].

The provision of early post-operative nutrition is associated with fewer complications and has positive impacts on outcomes such as return of bowel function, anastomotic leak, hospital length of stay (LOS), and mortality, compared to traditional delayed post-operative feeding practices in elective surgical patients [8]. While oral intake within 24 hours of surgery is the preferred route of nutrition in the immediate post-operative period [23, 24], this is often not possible or appropriate when critically ill and therefore enteral (EN) or parenteral nutrition (PN) is the alternative route for nutrition that can be considered.

### Enteral Nutrition

The type, timing, and amount of nutrition to provide to a critically ill patient are frequently debated and there are few data pertaining specifically to the surgical patient. However, consensus exists that EN is preferred over PN and this should start within 24–48 hours of admission to the intensive care unit (ICU), once no contraindications to doing so exist. Feeding early via the enteral route has been shown to reduce infectious complications significantly and has shown a trend towards reduction of mortality (but not LOS) in a variety of critically ill patient groups [23, 25]. Specifically in patients who have undergone gastrointestinal (GI) surgery, early EN may reduce post-operative LOS [26] and reduce anastomotic leaks as well as wound and chest infections [27].

The European Society of Intensive Care Medicine formulated clinical practice guidelines specifically on the use of early EN and concluded that it is safe for use in the majority of critically ill patients when initiated at a low rate [28]. There are a number of cases where it is not appropriate to start EN early (Table 8.1), some of which may require consideration in the post-operative patient, although these recommendations are based on expert opinion only due to a low evidence base. Importantly, there is no evidence to suggest that EN should be delayed in the absence of bowel sounds. It is imperative to continue to monitor the most appropriate time to commence enteral feeding to avoid the detrimental effects of underfeeding.

Prokinetics should be started in the case of enteral feeding intolerance, which is evidenced by persistent vomiting or high gastric residual volumes (GRVs) [23]. It is important to note that metoclopramide, a commonly used prokinetic, is contraindicated in the initial three to four days post GI surgery [29]. Post-pyloric feeding should be considered when prokinetic agents have failed [23]. In the case of other complications such as severe abdominal distension or anastomotic leak, EN should be ceased and PN considered.

## Parenteral Nutrition

Similar to the timing of EN, the ideal time to start PN post-operatively is much debated. Guideline recommendations vary from starting PN immediately or anywhere between days 3 and 10, depending on nutritional risk [23, 30]. Reasons for the variation between guidelines is the perceived risk associated with PN, which can include line- and metabolic-related complications [31], and also the conflicting evidence available from randomised control trials (RCTs).

**TABLE 8.1**  Summary of European Society of Intensive Care Medicine (ESICM) guidelines on when to delay enteral feeding.

| Reasons to delay enteral feeding | Comments |
| --- | --- |
| Uncontrolled shock with haemodynamic instability where tissue perfusion goals are not reached | Once shock is controlled with fluids and vasopressors/inotropes, low-dose enteral nutrition (EN) should be started |
| Severe hypoxaemia, hypercapnia, or acidosis | EN should be started in patients with stable hypoxaemia and compensated or permissive acidosis and hypercapnia |
| Presence of bowel ischaemia | Requires surgical evaluation |
| High-output intestinal fistula when feeding distal to the fistula is not possible | Feeding proximally may lead to electrolyte disturbance secondary to excessive losses in fistula output and could cause skin breakdown |
| Presence of abdominal compartment syndrome or in the case of rising intra-abdominal pressures secondary to feeding | Gut perfusion may be impaired |
| Active upper gastrointestinal bleeding | Feed can be restarted once bleeding stopped |
| Gastric residual volumes of >500 ml/6 h | Prokinetics should be started and feed should not be held for a prolonged period<br>Consider post-pyloric feeding |

Two large studies (CALORIES trial and NUTRIREA-2 [32, 33]) compared early EN to early PN and showed that infectious complications did not differ between routes, in the context of appropriate energy delivery. NUTRIREA-2 excluded patients with GI surgery in the month preceding randomisation, whereas the CALORIES trial did not exclude patients who had surgery once they could be fed using either the enteral or parenteral route. In another RCT, providing early PN when there is a short-term contraindication to enteral feeding (e.g. multiple scheduled surgeries, or surgical advice to avoid oral intake post-operatively) was not shown to affect 60-day mortality or infection rates [34].

Many of the trials supporting the ESPEN recommendation [23] do not include a surgical population and therefore recommendations specific to this group are difficult to make. A meta-analysis including over 3000 patients from 16 studies (including some surgical cohorts) by Tian et al. did not find a difference in outcome between early EN over PN, when PN was started within two to three days of ICU admission. Outcome measures included mortality, incidence of pneumonia, duration of mechanical ventilation, and length of ICU and hospital stay [35].

Despite the limited evidence available for practical recommendations, delaying PN unnecessarily in the context of contraindications to EN could lead to accumulation of nutritional deficits, which has been shown to negatively affect outcomes in ICU [36, 37]. In practice, the decision to provide PN should be made on a case-by-case basis after the risks and benefits have been considered. Additionally, patients who were on PN pre-operatively should continue post-operatively once there is no clinical suspicion of bacteraemia [30], until oral or enteral feeding can be established.

An updated systematic review carried out by Elke et al. [38] found no difference in mortality between EN- and PN-fed critically ill patients. In patients fed similar amounts of energy, there was also no difference between groups in infectious complications and ICU LOS.

The evidence base supporting the recommendation to start PN within three to seven days in the ESPEN guideline is based on low- to very low-grade evidence, with the authors noting that meta-analyses carried out only looked at studies comparing EN and PN within 48 hours of admission, as no studies were available comparing both during a later timeframe (i.e. day 3 onwards) [23].

## Feeding While Receiving Inotrope and Vasopressor Support

Controversy surrounds feeding the post-operative patient requiring vasoactive support, since the mechanism of action of these medicines leads to decreased intestinal blood flow [39]. An inotrope is a drug used to increase cardiac contractility, while a vasopressor creates vasoconstriction, with some vasoactive agents exerting both effects. These agents can be indicated in patients with haemodynamic instability in order to improve organ perfusion. Commonly used agents include noradrenaline, adrenaline, vasopressin, and dobutamine among others, and patients may be on one or more of these [40]. Providing feed in this context could increase the gut oxygen demand beyond availability, which may lead to bowel ischaemia [41]. Bowel ischaemia, also referred to as acute mesenteric ischaemia, is a complication of critical illness [42]. It has an estimated incidence of 0.09–0.2% in all acute surgical admissions, but mortality can be approximately 50% if untreated [43].

Multiple observational studies exist exploring the association between early EN and adverse outcomes, with varying results [44, 45]. For example, early EN provided to shocked, ventilated patients requiring low- (<0.1μg/kg/min) or medium-dose (0.1–0.3μg/kg/min) noradrenaline was associated with reduction in mortality; however, these findings did not apply to the high-dose (≥0.3μg/kg/min) group [46]. A recent nested cohort analysis compared EEN versus delayed enteral nutrition (DEN) in mechanically ventilated patients with circulatory shock. This study also found an association between EEN and improved outcomes in patients on an average of 0.3±0.6 μg/kg/min of noradrenaline when energy delivery was up to 13.5 kcal/kg/day. However, after controlling for severity of illness this association disappeared, with the authors suggesting that EEN is potentially most beneficial in patients with lower nutrition risk (mNUTRIC score <5), lower APACHE and SOFA scores [47].

A large RCT found that early EN compared with PN in mechanically ventilated patients receiving vasopressors for shock did not reduce mortality or the risk of secondary infections [33]. Early EN was, however, associated with an increased risk of adverse GI events (e.g. vomiting, diarrhoea, and bowel ischaemia) in those receiving high-dose noradrenaline [33]. These patients were on median doses of noradrenaline of 0.5 and 0.56 μg/kg/min in the parenteral and enteral groups, respectively. It is important to note that the GI outcomes were secondary and patients with recent surgery were excluded from this trial, therefore strong recommendations for practice cannot be made. Other large RCTs comparing different doses of EN or EN vs PN have either excluded patients on high doses of vasopressors [48, 49] or did not report vasopressor dose [32].

Based on the available data, experts suggest that enteral feeding is safe in the context of low vasopressor doses, but a cautious approach should be used in cases where vasopressor doses are high, for example starting feeding at trophic doses and awaiting clinical improvement prior to advancing the rate [41, 50]. In these recommendations, low dose is considered <0.1 μg/kg/h, medium dose 0.1–0.3 μg/kg/h, and high dose >0.3 μg/kg/min [46]. For patients on high or escalating doses of vasopressors, it is suggested that EN should be postponed and this is advocated in many of the ICU guidelines on nutrition, whereas trophic EN may be instigated and increased very slowly in those with a medium dose of vasopressors [28, 30]. It has also been suggested that patients on high doses of vasopressors may benefit from receiving full PN as opposed to full EN [50] until haemodynamic stability is achieved. It should be noted that much of the evidence pertaining to incidence of bowel ischaemia in enterally fed patients is in those who were fed jejunally [44, 51, 52]. An interventional trial is required to improve the evidence base for practice in this area, especially considering that ESPEN was unable to make an evidence-based recommendation due to the lack of interventional studies [23].

## NUTRITIONAL TARGETS

While early feeding is advocated, the optimal energy and protein targets for critically ill patients remain unknown, due to the heterogeneous nature of this population and lack of consensus on defining the different phases of critical illness. It is however recognised that nutritional targets should be specific to the individual patient, closely monitored, and amended accordingly to reflect any changes in clinical condition, including the extent of any surgery.

## Determining Energy Targets

There is universal consensus that indirect calorimetry (IC) is the 'gold standard' method to determine energy expenditure and prevent under- and overfeeding of the critically ill patient [23, 30, 53]. Recent IC advancements have attempted to overcome the previous limitations of inaccuracy, affordability, and time constraints [54]. While it's use is becoming more common in clinical practice, it is not widespread and so predictive equations are more commonly used (Table 8.2), with acknowledgement of the varying accuracy when compared with IC. While several predictive equations exist to estimate energy expenditure, the one from the Advanced College of Chest Physicians (ACCP; 25 kcal/kg) is the most common and the modified Penn State the most accurate [55].

Critical illness may elevate REE due to the hypermetabolic state following the activation of catabolic hormones [56]; however, sedatives, analgesics, mechanical ventilation, and prolonged bed rest may result in hypometabolism in the critically ill patient [54] and clinical judgement is often required when determining energy targets in the critically ill patient in the absence of IC (Table 8.3).

TABLE 8.2    Common predictive equations used in critical care.

| Equation | Formula |
|---|---|
| ACCP | $25 \text{ kcal} \times W$ |
| Penn State (m) | $(\text{Mifflin-St Jeor} \times 0.96) + (\text{Tmax} \times 167) + (\text{Ve} \times 31) - 6212$ |
| Mifflin-St Jeor | Males: $(10 \times W) + (6.25 \times H) - (5 \times A) + 5$ Females: $(10 \times W) + (6.25 \times H) - (5 \times A) - 161$ |

A, age in yr; ACCP, American College of Chest Physicians; H, height in cm; Tmax, maximum body temperature last 24 h; VE, minute ventilation in l/min at time of measurement; W, weight in kg.

**TABLE 8.3** Factors influencing resting energy expenditure (REE).

| Factors ↑ REE | Factors ↓ REE |
| --- | --- |
| Surgery | Sedation/anaesthesia |
| Pyrexia | Paralysing agents |
| Infection | Hypothermia |
| Disease state | Starvation |

## Dose of Energy

Hypocaloric feeding (defined as 70% of measured energy expenditure or 80% using a predictive equation) is recommended in the first week of ICU admission in the ESPEN guidelines [23]. This recommendation was recently strengthened by the NUTRIREA-3 trial [57–58] comparing low energy and protein delivery (6 kcal/kg and 0.2–0.4 g/kg) to target energy and protein delivery (25kcal/kg and 1.0–1.3g/kg) in ventilated patients with shock over the first 7 days of ICU admission with results showing a 1-day difference in time to readiness to ICU discharge in the patients receiving low energy and protein. However, it is important to consider the specific patient population included in this trial and that prolonged underfeeding is not recommended in the critically ill so regular monitoring and decision making regarding the increase to energy target is essential [37]. This may be particularly relevant to surgical patients as they have been shown to be more significantly underfed than their non-surgical counterparts [59], due to repeat trips to theatre, imaging studies, (re)intubation/extubation, and major bedside procedures (tracheostomy/percutaneous endoscopic gastrostomy [PEG] placement) [60]. In a retrospective, cohort study exploring target energy intake achievements for 279 patients treated in the surgical ICU, only 36.9% met their energy target and 48.4% achieved their protein target during their admission [61].

Moreover, a systematic review and meta-analysis of RCTs investigating the frequency and clinical consequences of enteral energy delivery above requirements (overfeeding) in critically ill adult patients found that overfeeding via the enteral route was a rare occurrence, and showed no difference in mortality, ventilatory support, or infectious complications [62]. Underprescribing energy targets beyond one week is not advised, due to the regular interruption of feed delivery, and this approach may not be suitable in those who are malnourished pre-operatively, as hypocaloric feeding post-operatively may exacerbate nutritional deficits, emphasising the need for an individualised nutrition assessment and plan.

## Protein Targets

Protein catabolism occurs following severe tissue injury and sepsis, resulting in an overall negative nitrogen balance [63]. Prolonged periods of sepsis or critical illness therefore lead to significant muscle wasting. In the initial post-operative phase, nutritional therapy may only minimally impede muscle protein catabolism, or not at all [8]. There is a paucity of RCTs investigating the link between different protein levels and muscle wasting and none specifically includes surgical patients. In one RCT investigating the effect of providing 0.8g/kg/d versus 1.2g/kg/d parenteral amino acids to mostly surgical participants, no difference was found in the primary outcome of handgrip strength at day 7 following ICU admission. However, patients receiving the higher dose of amino acids demonstrated reduced thigh and forearm muscle wasting [64].

The recent EFFORT Protein trial [65] revealed no benefit to delivering higher protein dose (≥ 2.2 g/kg/day) compared with usual dose (≤1.2 g/kg/day) to critically ill patients considered to be at high nutrition risk. Indeed, potential harm was shown in patients with greater severity of illness and baseline acute kidney injury. Noteworthy, this study did not explore the effect of protein dose on muscle mass or physical function, yet nonetheless highlights that higher protein doses, especially in particular subgroups of patients, may be harmful and should be avoided. Similar to energy dosing, individualised assessment and prescription should be considered and guideline [23] recommendations for protein followed (1.3g/kg/day), with higher targets for various clinical conditions who were not represented in the EFFORT Protein trial (Table 8.4).

**TABLE 8.4**  Protein recommendations for various clinical conditions in critical illness.

| Patient group | Protein target |
|---|---|
| General intensive care unit | 1.3 g/kg |
| Continuous renal replacement therapy | 1.5–1.7 g/kg |
| Burns | 1.5–2.0 g/kg |
| Trauma | 1.3–1.5 g/kg |

*Source: Adapted from [23].*

## AREAS FOR FUTURE RESEARCH/ QUESTIONS UNANSWERED

- The optimal blood glucose range in critically ill surgical patients remains unclear.
- Further studies investigating the use of EN at various vasopressor doses.
- Well-designed RCTs are required to determine optimal protein targets for the surgical critically ill population.

| Routine Case Study | |
|---|---|
| **Patient** | Mrs A, age 68 |
| **Presenting complaint** | Presented to dialysis session with abdominal distension and pain<br>Bowels not active 5 d<br>Vomiting × 2 per day for previous 4 d<br>Background of recent admission with obstruction secondary to hernia that was managed conservatively and resolved |
| **Past medical history** | Hypertension<br>Rheumatoid arthritis<br>Atrial fibrillation<br>Atrial valve replacement and mitral valve replacement<br>End-stage renal failure – on dialysis (Monday, Wednesday, Friday)<br>Congestive cardiac failure<br>Not on regular anticoagulation – warfarin stopped, receives heparin at dialysis<br>Femoral hernia managed conservatively |
| **Social history** | Lives with husband<br>Nil alcohol or smoking history<br>Rockwood frailty score: 3 (Managing well)<br>Can walk 50 m, climb stairs, sleeps upright at night |
| **Investigations** | Abdominal x-ray: prominent loops of small bowel. Clinical concern for obstruction and computed tomography (CT) recommended<br>CT abdomen: right-sided femoral hernia that contains small bowel loop where there is stricturing and upstream small bowel dilatation/obstruction |
| **Oral Intake** | Minimal intake for 7 d pre-admission<br>Nil by mouth on admission for surgery |

| | |
|---|---|
| **Anthropometrics** | Weight 54.2 kg on admission<br>Height 1.62 m<br>Body mass index (BMI) 20.7 kg/m²<br>Weight history 66 kg 6 mo ago |
| **Bowel function** | Bowels not active, not passing wind |
| **Diagnosis** | Small bowel obstruction secondary to hernia |
| **Surgical plan** | High-risk surgical candidate; however, patient decided to go ahead with surgery<br>Surgery: open right inguinal hernia repair and resection of 5 cm of dusky small bowel<br>Side-to-side anastomosis |
| **Nutritional plan** | Start EN postoperatively<br>Manage risk of refeeding syndrome |
| **Clinical assessment** | Intubated and ventilated post-operatively<br>Sedation: propofol 10 ml/h and fentanyl 200 µg/h<br>Cardiovascular system: 0.20 µg/kg/min noradrenaline<br>Renal function: anuric on renal replacement therapy<br>Blood glucose: 6.5 mmol/l<br>Bowels: not active, scant bowel sounds<br>Skin: intact<br>Relevant medications: lansoprazole, movicol, colecalciferol, sodium docusate, piperacillin/tazobactam |
| **Initial dietetic assessment** | Mrs A was reviewed 2 days post-operatively<br>Nasogastric tube (NGT) had been placed and 10 ml/h of a 1 kcal/ml enteral feed was started post-operatively<br>On review, GRVs were 500 ml (exceeding local threshold of 350 ml) and Mrs A had one episode of vomiting. NGT feed stopped and tube placed on free drainage with total of 1.6 l out in 24 h. Intravenous fluids commenced<br>Repeat CT scan showed appearances in keeping with ileus but no obstruction |
| **Dietetic impression** | At risk of refeeding syndrome due to evidence of weight loss and prolonged period of low intake pre-admission<br>Not tolerating EN, as evidenced by high GRVs and vomiting along with imaging showing ileus. Total parenteral nutrition (TPN) indicated to meet nutritional needs |
| **Nutritional requirements** | Energy: 1275 kcal (25 kcal/kg)<br>Penn State (modified, 2003): 1320 kcal (Mifflin 1061, Mv 8, Tmax 37.5)<br>Protein: 76.5–87 g/d (1.5–1.7 g/kg) ≡ 12.2–13.9 g $N_2$/d<br>Propofol providing approx. 250 kcal/24 h |
| **Nutritional support** | TPN commenced via central venous catheter<br>Day 1: 800 kcal and 6 g nitrogen<br>Day 2: 1200 kcal and 8 g nitrogen<br>Day 3: 1300 kcal and 9 g nitrogen<br>Pabrinex commenced on Day 1 |

| | |
|---|---|
| Outcome | Day 3 post-op: refeeding electrolytes dropped on commencing nutrition – $PO_4^{3-}$ 0.68 mmol/l (reference range [RR] 0.7–1.4 mmol/l), $K^+$ 3.1 mmol/l (RR 3.5–5.1 mmol/l), $Mg^{2+}$ 0.7 mmol/l (RR 0.8–1.3 mmol/l). However, this may have also been related to continuous renal replacement therapy. Electrolytes replaced and monitored closely |
| | Day 5 post-op: Mrs A was treated with antibiotics, noradrenaline was ceased as blood pressure improved and she was extubated |
| | Day 8: GRVs reduced and Mrs A tried sips of fluid orally. This was well tolerated and was progressed to free fluids as per surgical advice. Passing wind but bowels not yet active |
| | Day 9: Ryles tube removed. Started on 2 bottles/day of oral nutritional supplements (ONS) – 200 ml of 2 kcal/ml supplement providing 400 kcal and 20 g protein. PN weaned to meet 50% of nutritional requirements |
| | Day 10: Tolerating ONS, started on light diet, bowels now active |
| | Day 12: PN stopped. Meeting 90% of nutritional requirements with oral diet and ONS |
| | Received ongoing nutrition support on step down from ICU to surgical ward in view of weight loss. ONS discontinued as appetite improved and weight increased |
| Follow-up | Follow-up by renal dietitian as outpatient on dialysis unit |

| Complex Case Study | |
|---|---|
| Patient | **Ms B, age 35** |
| Presenting complaint | Hypoxic respiratory failure – infective exacerbation of underlying interstitial lung disease (ILD)<br>Septic shock with myocardial dysfunction – acute kidney injury (AKI) and mesenteric ischaemia |
| Past medical history | Suspected ILD<br>Mononeuritis multiplex<br>?Monoclonal gammopathy of undetermined significance (MGUS)<br>Anxiety and depression<br>Obesity |
| Social history | Has been working from home<br>Lives alone –> minimal contact outside and with friends/family due to Covid-19 concerns<br>No travel history<br>Smokes ~10/d<br>No alcohol or illicit drug use |

| Anthropometrics | Weight ~155 kg, Height ~1.68 m, BMI ~55 kg/m² (obese class III) |
| --- | --- |
| | Ideal body weight (IBW, based on BMI 23 kg/m²) = 65 kg |
| | IBW based on BMI 25 kg/m² = 71 kg |
| | Adjusted body weight (actual weight − IBW based on BMI 23 kg/m²) × 0.25 + IBW = 87.5 kg |
| Estimated nutritional targets | Energy ~1562–1775 kcal (BMI >50 kg/m² = ~22–25 kcal/kg IBW 25 kg/m²) |
| | Protein ~98–130 g protein/~15.6–20.8 g nitrogen (BMI >50 kg/m² + renal replacement therapy ~1.5–2.0 g/kg IBW 23 kg/m²) |
| Investigations | CT scan of abdomen/pelvis initially showed terminal ileitis of uncertain aetiology. Further CT scans and discussion at inflammatory bowel disease (IBD) multidisciplinary meeting suggested terminal ileal/caecum ischaemia with small bowel dilatation likely representing an ileus/secondary to the ischaemia |
| Bowel function | Pre-op: ileus |
| | Post-op: high-output ileostomy |
| Diagnosis | Multiple pan-colic abscesses and perforations including terminal ileum, >3 m of small bowel viable, stomach/duodenum viable |
| Surgical plan | Initial surgical decision for conservative management due to surgical risk with morbid obesity |
| | At further surgical review, decision for surgery was made due to episodes of melaena and ongoing drops in haemoglobin (Hb) requiring daily blood transfusions. Patient underwent emergency laparotomy, total colectomy, and abdomen was left open |
| | Two days later patient returned to theatre for further laparotomy, washout, and ileostomy formation. Surgeon reports estimated bowel remaining ~1–2 m (not accurately measured) |
| Nutritional plan | Due to high gastric aspirates (>300 ml/4 h), vomiting, ileus (despite prokinetics and aperients), and CT showing terminal ileal ischaemia, enteral feed was ceased and TPN commenced. Pre and post surgery, patient required bespoke TPN to meet high protein targets while not overfeeding calories. Ryles tube remained on free drainage |
| | After 18 days on TPN, commenced rotating lipid/lipid-free bags on alternate days for liver protection and trialled some trophic enteral feed via NGT |
| | Prior to stepping down to the ward, NGT removed as patient managing small amounts of modified diet as per speech and language therapist (SLT; level 5 diet and level 2 fluids) and reported discomfort from NGT. High-output stoma required her to remain on PN to meet estimated nutritional targets within a fluid restriction |
| Nutritional support in ICU/ high-dependency unit (HDU) | TPN: Patient-specific lipid-free bags 5 d/wk; lipid-containing bags 2 d/wk: |
| | • Lipid-free: providing ~2 l, 1650 kcal, 18 g nitrogen, 300 g glucose, zero lipid, 60 mmol Na⁺, 40 mmol K⁺, 2 mmol Ca²⁺, 12 mmol Mg²⁺, 6 mmol $PO_4^{3-}$ plus vitamins, minerals, and trace elements |
| | • Lipid-containing: providing ~1.75 L, 1950 kcal, 18 g nitrogen, 250 g glucose, 50 g SMOFlipid, 60 mmol Na⁺, 40 mmol K⁺, 2 mmol Ca²⁺, 12 mmol Mg²⁺, 6 mmol $PO_4^{3-}$ plus vitamins, minerals, and trace elements |
| | Low-fibre diet (modified consistency as per SLT) and fluid restriction for high-output ileostomy |

| Outcome | After prolonged ICU/HDU stay and 3 wk post stepdown to the ward, PN was successfully weaned and patient was upgraded to normal diet/fluids, hence discharged from SLT. Lower gastrointestinal (LGI) dietitians recommended continuing low-fibre diet and fluid restriction to manage high-output ileostomy, with variable compliance |
|---|---|
| New diagnosis | High-output ileostomy |
| Long-term prescriptions | Codeine phosphate 60 mg 4 times/d (anti-diarrhoeal to reduce stoma output)<br>Loperamide 24 mg 4 times/d (anti-diarrhoeal to reduce stoma output)<br>Omeprazole 40 mg twice/d (anti-secretory to reduce stomach acid production)<br>Potassium-free oral rehydration solution (ORS) (1.5 l K$^+$-free glucose electrolyte mix to aid fluid and salt absorption and prevent dehydration due to diarrhoea)<br>Sodium bicarbonate 1000 mg 4 times/d (to aid fluid absorption and reduce losses from stoma) |
| Follow-up | 3-monthly dietetic follow-up in LGI telephone clinic<br>GP to monitor biochemistry |

## ACKNOWLEDGEMENTS

The authors acknowledge support from Dr Danielle Bear, Consultant Dietitian - Critical Care at Guy's and St Thomas' NHS Foundation Trust. We would like to thank her for her valuable contribution to this chapter.

## REFERENCES

1. Intensive Care National Audit and Research Centre (ICNARC). Our National Audit Programme (NAP). www.icnarc.org/Our-Audit/Audits/Cmp/Reports/SummaryStatistics
2. Findlay, G.P., Goodwin, A.P.L., Protopapa, K. et al. (2011). Knowing the risk: A review of the peri-operative care of surgical patients. London: NCEPOD. https://www.ncepod.org.uk/2011report2/downloads/POC_fullreport.pdf
3. Alazawi, W., Pirmadjid, N., Lahiri, R., and Bhattacharya, S. (2016). Inflammatory and immune responses to surgery and their clinical impact. *Ann. Surg.* 264 (1): 73–80.
4. Weissman, C. (1990). The metabolic response to stress: an overview and update. *J. Am. Soc. Anesthesiolog.* 73 (2): 308–327.
5. Traynor, C. and Hall, G.M. (1981). Endocrine and metabolic changes during surgery: anaesthetic implications. *Br. J. Anaesth.* 53 (2): 153–160.
6. Gillis, C. and Carli, F. (2015). Promoting perioperative metabolic and nutritional care. *Anesthesiology* 123 (6): 1455–1472.
7. Wilmore, D.W. (2000). Metabolic response to severe surgical illness: overview. *World J. Surg.* 24 (6): 705–711.
8. Weimann, A., Braga, M., Carli, F. et al. (2017). ESPEN guideline: clinical nutrition in surgery. *Clin. Nutr.* 36 (3): 623–650.
9. Plank, L.D. and Hill, G.L. (2000). Sequential metabolic changes following induction of systemic inflammatory response in patients with severe sepsis or major blunt trauma. *World J. Surg.* 24 (6): 630–638.
10. Desborough, J.P. (2000). The stress response to trauma and surgery. *Br. J. Anaesth.* 85 (1): 109–117.
11. Ramos, M., Khalpey, Z., Lipsitz, S. et al. (2008). Relationship of perioperative hyperglycemia and postoperative infections in patients who undergo general and vascular surgery. *Ann. Surg.* 248 (4): 585–591.
12. NICE-SUGAR Study Investigators, Finfer, S., Chittock, D.R. et al. (2009). Intensive versus conventional glucose control in critically ill patients. *N. Engl. J. Med.* 360 (13): 1283–1297.
13. Buchleitner, A.M., Martínez-Alonso, M., Hernandez, M. et al. (2012). Perioperative glycaemic control for diabetic patients undergoing surgery. *Cochrane Database of Sys. Rev.* 9, CD007315.
14. van Gassel, R.J., Baggerman, M.R., and van de Poll, M.C. (2020). Metabolic aspects of muscle wasting

during critical illness. *Curr. Opin. Clin. Nutr. Metab. Care* 23 (2): 96.

15. Reid, C.L., Campbell, I.T., and Little, R.A. (2004). Muscle wasting and energy balance in critical illness. *Clin. Nutr.* 23 (2): 273–280.

16. Puthucheary, Z.A., Rawal, J., McPhail, M. et al. (2013). Acute skeletal muscle wasting in critical illness. *JAMA* 310 (15): 1591–1600.

17. Latronico, N., Herridge, M., Hopkins, R.O. et al. (2017). The ICM research agenda on intensive care unit-acquired weakness. *Inten. Care Med.* 43 (9): 1270–1281.

18. Bear, D.E., Wandrag, L., Merriweather, J.L. et al. (2017). The role of nutritional support in the physical and functional recovery of critically ill patients: a narrative review. *Crit. Care.* 21 (1): 226.

19. Hermans, G., Van Aerde, N., Meersseman, P. et al. (2019). Five-year mortality and morbidity impact of prolonged versus brief ICU stay: a propensity score matched cohort study. *Thorax* 74 (11): 1037–1045.

20. Dos Santos, C., Hussain, S.N., Mathur, S. et al. (2016). Mechanisms of chronic muscle wasting and dysfunction after an intensive care unit stay. A pilot study. *Am. J. Resp. Crit. Care Med.* 194 (7): 821–830.

21. National Institute for Health and Clinical Excellence (NICE). (2009). Rehabilitation after critical illness in adults. Clinical guideline [CG83]. www.nice.org.uk/guidance/cg83

22. McClave, S., Martindale, R.G., Rice, T.W., and Heyland, D.K. (2014). Feeding the critically ill patient. *Crit. Care Med.* 42 (12): 2600–2610.

23. Singer, P., Blaser, A.R., Berger, M.M. et al. (2019). ESPEN guideline on clinical nutrition in the intensive care unit. *Clin. Nutr.* 38 (1): 48–79.

24. National Institute for Health and Care Excellence. (2017). Nutrition support for adults: oral nutrition support, enteral tube feeding and parenteral nutrition Clinical Guideline [CG32]. www.nice.org.uk/guidance/cg32.

25. Critical Care Nutrition Systematic Reviews (2021). 2.0 Early vs Delayed Nutrient Intake. www.criticalcarenutrition.com/docs/2.0%20Early%20vs%20Delayed%20EN_12May21.pdf

26. Herbert, G., Perry, R., Anderson, H.K. et al. (2019). Early enteral nutrition within 24 hours of lower GI surgery versus later commencement for length of hospital stay and postoperative complications. *Cochrane Database of Sys. Rev.* (7): CD004080.

27. Barlow, R., Price, P., Reid, T.D. et al. (2011). Prospective multicentre randomised controlled trial of early enteral nutrition for patients undergoing major upper gastrointestinal surgical resection. *Clin. Nutr.* 30 (5): 560–566.

28. Blaser, A.R., Starkopf, J., Alhazzani, W. et al. (2017). Early enteral nutrition in critically ill patients: ESICM clinical practice guidelines. *Inten. Care Med.* 43 (3): 380–398.

29. British National Formulary. (n.d.). Metoclopramide hydrochloride. https://bnf.nice.org.uk/drug/metoclopramide-hydrochloride.html

30. McClave, S.A., Taylor, B.E., Martindale, R.G. et al. (2016). Guidelines for the provision and assessment of nutrition support therapy in the adult critically ill patient: Society of Critical Care Medicine (SCCM) and American Society for Parenteral and Enteral Nutrition (ASPEN). *JPEN. J. Parent. Enter. Nutr.* 40 (2): 159–211.

31. British Association of Parenteral and Enteral Nutrition (BAPEN). (2016). Complication management. www.bapen.org.uk/nutrition-support/parenteral-nutrition/complication-management

32. Harvey, S., Parrott, F., Harrison, D.A. et al. (2014). Trial of the route of early nutritional support in critically ill adults. *N. Engl. J. Med.* 371: 1673–1684.

33. Reignier, J., Boisrame-Helms, J., Brisard, L. et al. (2018). Enteral versus parenteral early nutrition in ventilated adults with shock: a randomised, controlled, multicentre, open-label, parallel-group study (NUTRIREA-2). *Lancet* 391: 133–143.

34. Doig, G.S., Simpson, F., Sweetman, E.A. et al. (2013, 2013). Early PN in critically ill with relative contraindication to early EN: a randomised controlled trial. *JAMA* 309 (20): 2130–2138.

35. Tian, F., Heighes, P.T., Allingstrug, M.J., and Doig, G.S. (2018). Early enteral nutrition provided within 24 hours of ICU admission: a meta-analysis of randomised controlled trials. *Crit. Care Med.* 46 (7): 1049–1056.

36. Alberda, C., Gramlich, L., Jones, N. et al. (2009). The relationship between nutritional intake and clinical outcomes in critically ill patients: results of an international multicentre observational study. *Inten. Care Med.* 35 (10): 1728–1737.

37. Villet, S., Chiolero, R.L., Bollmann, M.D. et al. (2005). Negative impact of hypocaloric feeding and energy balance on clinical outcome in ICU patients. *Clin. Nutr.* 24: 502–509.

38. Elke, G., van Zanten, A.R.H., Lemieux, M. et al. (2016). Enteral versus parenteral nutrition in critically ill patients: an updated systematic review and met-analysis of randomised controlled trials. *Crit. Care* 20 (1): 117.

39. Mittal, R., Bebs, L.H., Patel, A.P. et al. (2017). Neurotransmitters: the critical modulators regulating gut-brain axis. *J. Cell. Physiol.* 232 (9): 2359–2372.

40. Bangash, M., Kong, M., and Pearse, R. (2012). Use of inotropes and vasopressor agents in critically ill patients. *Br. J. Pharmacol.* 165: 2015–2033.

41. Wischmeyer, P.E. (2019). Enteral nutrition can be given to patients on vasopressors. *Crit. Care Med.* 48 (1): 122–125.

42. Caluwaerts, M., Castanares-Zapatero, D., Laterre, P.F., and Hantson, P. (2019). Prognostic factors of acute mesenteric ischaemia in ICU patients. *BMC Gastroenterol.* 19 (1): 80.

43. Bala, M., Kashuk, J., Moore, E.E. et al. (2017). Acute mesenteric ischaemia: guidelines of the world Society of Emergency Surgery. *World J. Emerg. Sur.* 12: 38.

44. Marvin, R.G., McKinley, B.A., McQuiggan, M. et al. (2000). Nonocclusive bowel necrosis occurring in critically ill trauma patients receiving enteral nutrition manifests no reliable clinical signs for early detection. *Am. J. Surg.* 179 (1): 7–12.

45. Mancl, E.E. and Muzevich, K.M. (2013). Tolerability and safety of enteral nutrition in critically ill patients receiving intravenous vasopressor therapy. *JPEN J. Parenter. Enteral. Nutr.* 37 (5): 641–651.

46. Ohbe, H., Jo, T., Matsui, H. et al. (2020). Differences in effect of early enteral nutrition on mortality among ventilated adults with shock requiring low-, medium-, and high-dose noradrenaline: a propensity-matched analysis. *Clin. Nutr.* 39 (2): 460–467.

47. Oritz-Reyes, L., Patel, J.J., Jiang, X. et al. (2022). Early versus delayed enteral nutrition in mechanically ventilated patients with circulatory shock: a nested cohort analysis of an international multicenter, pragmatic clinical trial. *Crit. Care* 26: 173.

48. Rice, T.W., Wheeler, A.P., Thompson, B.T. et al. (2012). Initial trophic vs full enteral feeding in patients with acute lung injury. *JAMA* 307 (8): 795–803.

49. Arabi, Y.M., Aldawood, A.S., Haddad, S.H. et al. (2015). Permissive underfeeding or standard enteral feeding in critically ill adults. *N. Engl. J. Med.* 372 (25): 2398–2408.

50. Arabi, Y.M. and McClave, S.A. (2020). Enteral nutrition should not be given to patients on vasopressor agents. *Crit. Care Med.* 48 (1): 119–121.

51. Merchan, C., Altshuler, D., Aberle, C. et al. (2017). Tolerability of enteral nutrition in mechanically ventilated patients with septic shock who require vasopressors. *J. Intens. Care Med.* 32 (9): 540–546.

52. Melis, M., Fichera, A., and Ferguson, M.K. (2006). Bowel necrosis associated with early jejunal tube feeding: a complication of post-operative enteral nutrition. *Arch. Surg.* 141 (7): 701–704.

53. Moonen, H.P., Beckers, K.J., and van Zanten, A.R. (2021). Energy expenditure and indirect calorimetry in critical illness and convalescence: current evidence and practical considerations. *J. Inten. Care* 9 (1): 1–3.

54. Delsoglio, M., Achamrah, N., Berger, M.M., and Pichard, C. (2019). Indirect calorimetry in clinical practice. *J. Clin. Med.* 8 (9): 1387.

55. Frankenfield, D.C., Coleman, A., Alam, S., and Cooney, R.N. (2009). Analysis of estimation methods for resting metabolic rate in critically ill adults. *JPEN J. Parenter. Enteral. Nutr.* 33 (1): 27–36.

56. Ndahimana, D. and Kim, E.K. (2018). Energy requirements in critically ill patients. *Clin. Nutr. Res.* 7 (2): 81.

57. Reignier, J., Plantefeve, G., Mira, J.P. et al. (2023). Low versus standard calorie and protein feeding in ventilated adults with shock: a randomised, controlled, multicentre, open-label, parallelgroup trial (NUTRI-REA-3). *Lancet Respir. Med.* https://doi.org/10.1016/S2213-2600(23)00092-9.

58. Binnekade, J.M., Tepaske, R., Bruynzeel, P. et al. (2005). Daily enteral feeding practice on the ICU: attainment of goals and interfering factors. *Crit. Care.* 9 (3): 1–8.

59. Hise, M.E., Halterman, K., Gajewski, B.J. et al. (2007). Feeding practices of severely ill intensive care unit patients: an evaluation of energy sources and clinical outcomes. *J. Am. Diet. Assoc.* 107 (3): 458–465.

60. Peev, M.P., Yeh, D.D., Quraishi, S.A. et al. (2015). Causes and consequences of interrupted enteral nutrition: a prospective observational study in critically ill surgical patients. *JPEN J. Parenter. Enteral. Nutr.* 39 (1): 21–27.

61. Kim, M.K., Choi, Y.S., Suh, S.W. et al. (2021). Target calorie intake achievements for patients treated in the surgical intensive care unit. *Clin. Nutr. Res.* 10 (2): 107.

62. Chapple, L.A., Weinel, L., Ridley, E.J. et al. (2020). Clinical sequelae from overfeeding in enterally fed critically ill adults: where is the evidence? *JPEN J. Parenter. Enteral. Nutr.* 44 (6): 980–991.

63. Hoffer, L.J. and Bistrian, B.R. (2012). Appropriate protein provision in critical illness: a systematic and narrative review. *Am. J. Clin. Nutr.* 96 (3): 591–600.

64. Ferrie, S., Allman-Farinelli, M., Daley, M., and Smith, K. (2016). Protein requirements in the critically ill: a randomized controlled trial using parenteral nutrition. *JPEN J. Parenter. Enteral. Nutr.* 40 (6): 795–805.

65. Heyland, D.K., Patel, J., Compher, et al. (2003). The effect of higher protein dosing in critically ill patients with high nutritional risk (EFFORT Protein): an international, multicentre, pragmatic, registry-based randomised trial. *Lancet* 401 (10376): P568–576.

# CHAPTER 9

# Nutritional Management of Patients Undergoing Head and Neck Cancer Surgery

Cathy Skea

*Clinical Lead Dietitian, Department of Nutrition and Dietetics, Royal Victoria Hospital, Belfast, Belfast Health and Social Care Trust, Belfast, Northern Ireland*

---

**KEY POINTS**

- Surgery plays an important role in the management of head and neck cancer.
- The dietitian is an integral part of the multidisciplinary team, providing early nutritional assessment and tailored advice throughout the surgical journey.
- The nutritional impact of life-changing surgery can have both short- and long-term implications affecting quality of life.
- Early identification of nutritional consequences is crucial to improving functional outcomes in this patient group.

---

Cancers that are known collectively as head and neck cancers (HNC) usually begin in the squamous cells that line the moist, mucosal membranes inside the head and neck region known as the upper aerodigestive tract (the mouth, the nose, and the throat). The majority are squamous cell carcinoma (SCC) [1]. Salivary glands in the head and neck (H&N) area can be affected, but this is less common.

SCC of the H&N is the seventh most common cancer worldwide, with an annual incidence of approximately 700 000 and mortality rate estimated at 350 000 in 2018 [2]. There are around 12 200 new HNC cases in the UK every year (2015–2017) [3].

Tobacco exposure and high alcohol intake are two strong risk factors in the development of primary and secondary HNC [4]. Infection with the (carcinogenic) type of human papillomavirus (HPV) type 16 is a risk factor particularly in oropharyngeal cancers in the younger population [1, 5].

## HEAD AND NECK CANCERS

Outcome is affected by the anatomical site, the extent of the disease, the patient's age, and general medical status, including any comorbidities.

*Nutritional Management of the Surgical Patient*, First Edition. Edited by Mary E. Phillips.
© 2023 John Wiley & Sons Ltd. Published 2023 by John Wiley & Sons Ltd.

The Union for International Cancer Control (UICC) Tumour Node Metastasis (TNM) cancer staging manual was updated to take prognostic factors into account to better predict patient survival based on disease stage [5, 6]. This staging takes place prior to any intervention [7].

Management of HNC can be divided into four subsections under the following headings (see Figure Figure 9.1) [8]:

- Laryngeal
- Hypopharyngeal
- Oropharyngeal
- Oral cavity

## Laryngeal Cancer

The larynx (voice box) is a tube-shaped organ (approximately 5–6 cm in length) in the neck that contains the vocal cords, and therefore facilitates speech. It is located at the opening of the trachea (windpipe). It can be felt and seen as the prominence in the front of the neck. Laryngeal cancers include cancers of the supraglottis, glottis, and subglottis. SCC represents 90% of cases [3].

The functions of the larynx are:

- *Producing sound*: Vibration of the two vocal cords contained in the glottis when air passes between them creating sound.
- *Protecting the airway during swallowing*: Acting as a valve, closing to prevent food, liquids, and saliva from entering the trachea during swallowing.
- *Breathing*: Allowing us to breathe by opening the vocal cords to allow air movement.

One of the main symptoms with laryngeal cancer is dysphonia (hoarseness) or a change in the voice.

As the tumour increases in size over time, other symptoms may occur, including pain in the throat, otalgia, headache, dysphagia, odynophagia, or difficulty breathing to the point where the breathing may become noisy (stridor). There may also be a lump in the neck if the tumour has spread to other glands.

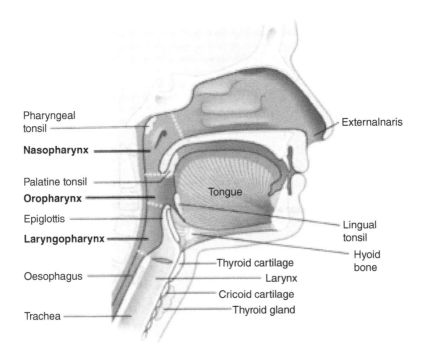

**FIGURE 9.1**    Anatomy of the head and neck. *Source*: Reproduced by permission from Dutton H and Finch J (2018). *Acute and Critical Care Nursing at a Glance*, Chichester: Wiley-Blackwell.

## Hypopharyngeal Cancer

The hypopharynx lies beside and behind the larynx. It is the connection point through which food, water, and air pass, and refers to the point at which the pharynx divides anteriorly into the larynx and posteriorly into the oesophagus [9]. It extends from the level of the hyoid bone to the inferior edge of the cricoid cartilage, corresponding to the C4 through C6 vertebral bodies.

Dysphagia and unexplained weight loss are common symptoms. Hoarseness may also be evident if the larynx is involved.

Hypopharyngeal cancers include tumours of the post-cricoid area, pyriform fossa, and posterior pharyngeal wall.

## Oropharyngeal Cancer

The oropharynx is the middle section of the pharynx (throat) behind the mouth and includes the base of tongue, soft palate (at the back of the roof of mouth), tonsils, and back of the throat. It is situated behind the oral cavity, below the soft palate and above the epiglottis. Oropharyngeal cancer includes tumours of the base of the tongue, tonsil, and soft palate.

The tongue is situated in the floor of the mouth and is attached to the hyoid bone, mandible, and pharynx. It is important in taste, chewing, swallowing, and speech. It is composed of skeletal muscle partly covered by mucous membrane and presents a tip and margin, dorsum, inferior surface, and root. The apex usually rests against the incisors.

Symptoms may include dysphagia and or odynophagia, limited opening of the mouth (trismus), reduced movement of the tongue, unexplained weight loss, ear pain, or a white patch on the tongue or lining of the mouth (leucoplakia).

## Oral Cavity Cancer

The oral cavity is the part of the mouth that is anterior to the soft palate and tonsils. It contains the cheek, tongue, lower jaw, hard palate, and teeth. It is lined with mucous membranes and the main salivary glands, parotid, submandibular, and sublingual, and minor salivary glands open into it.

The oral cavity provides space for food to be ingested; the food is then chewed within the mouth and mixed with saliva, which creates a bolus. This bolus is forced into the oesophagus as the swallowing process is started. The lining of the mouth also creates lubrication along with the salivary glands, making it easier to swallow, speak, and digest food.

Symptoms of cancers of the oral cavity include mouth ulcers that are painful and do not heal within several weeks, or unexplained persistent lumps in the mouth that do not go away, persistent numbness, or an odd feeling on the lip or tongue.

Oral cavity cancer includes tumours of the buccal mucosa, retromolar trigone, alveolus, hard palate, anterior two-thirds of the tongue, floor of the mouth, and mucosal surface of the lip.

## GENERAL NUTRITIONAL IMPLICATIONS FOLLOWING SURGICAL INTERVENTION

Laryngeal and hypopharyngeal cancer can often be successfully treated if detected early. However, preserving the function of the affected organ is equally important as this affects quality of life (QOL), body image, breathing, eating, and drinking.

There is a high risk of malnutrition associated with lifestyle factors, the cancer site, and the disease process, as well as socio-economic factors.

The aims of treatment are to eliminate the disease and achieve long-term survival. However, the five-year mortality rate from HNC has not improved significantly over the last 40 years [10, 11], despite scientific advances in both surgical and oncological treatments.

Considerations of QOL and organ function are crucial in the decision for radical surgical options, as resection may restrict or prevent the patient from consuming oral nutrition [10, 12, 13].

Nutritional status has been recognised as a fundamental long-term prognostic factor [14]. The incidence of weight loss before and after surgery has been used an indicator for specific disease survival [14–16].

There are a number of factors that can affect nutritional status; these include pre-operative fasting for investigations, acute-phase response to the surgery, and anxiety surrounding the reintroduction of oral foods. Patients may experience altered taste and smell or difficulty chewing, which can cause food aversion and limit intake.

Post-operative complications such as poor wound healing, strictures/stenosis, oral and nasal regurgitation, aspiration, dumping syndrome, a chyle leak, or formation of a pharyngeal pouch all have an impact on nutritional status, and dedicated dietetic support, to allow early identification of nutritional factors and intervention, is associated with improved outcomes [11, 17].

## SURGICAL PROCEDURES

Surgical resection is typically offered to those with:

- Early supraglottic or locally advanced laryngeal cancer.
- Hypopharyngeal cancers, especially when there is laryngeal cartilage invasion (T4/stage IV) or a non-functioning larynx.
- Oral cavity tumours, if the patient is considered fit for surgery and reconstruction.

Patients with severe malnutrition should receive nutrition support for 10–14 days prior to major surgery [18].

Consideration of enteral nutrition is indicated regardless of pre-operative undernutrition, as it is usual for patients to be unable to achieve adequate oral intake for some time post-operatively, and as such nutritional interventions have been incorporated into enhanced recovery after surgery (ERAS) programmes (see Chapter 5).

### Glossectomy

Glossectomy is the surgical removal of part or all of the tongue. This is associated with poor QOL in the post-operative setting, but poor prognosis renders assessment of long-term outcomes difficult [19].

### Total Laryngectomy

A laryngectomy is a surgical operation in which all or part of the larynx and all or part of the thyroid gland (which sits in front of the larynx) are removed. Post-operatively, the mouth and lungs will no longer be connected. Lymph glands on either side of the neck are usually removed to ensure that clear margins are achieved. This is called a neck dissection and the extent will vary depending on the magnitude of disease.

Once the voice box has been removed, the top of the trachea is separated in front of the oesophagus and a permanent hole will be created at the front of the neck allowing the patient to breathe. This is called a stoma (permanent neck breather). It may be necessary for the patient to wear a tube through the opening until the size of the stoma can be established. The tube will be held in place by tapes and tied at each side of the neck. A tracheoesophageal puncture may also be created at the time of surgery to enable speech once wounds have healed.

### Pharyngo-Laryngo-Oesophagectomy

Hypopharyngeal cancer accounts for 8% of HNCs. The pyriform fossae, pharyngeal wall, and post-cricoid regions are typically involved. The prognosis with five-year survival rate is particularly poor, ranging from 49% T1 (stage I) to 23% T4 (stage IV) with a prolonged period of rehabilitation [13].

Surgery involves partial or total pharyngo-laryngo-oesophagectomy (PLO) with reconstruction to restore functional continuity of the aerodigestive tract.

The initial surgical procedure is much the same as a laryngectomy. The larynx is separated from the trachea. The end of the trachea is brought forward and a hole created in the neck, which allows a permanent opening for the patient to breathe through. Once the stomach has been released, it can be pulled up through the chest.

The join can then be made between the top of the stomach and the remaining part of the pharynx. The neck and abdominal wounds are then stitched with drains attached. The recovery may take much longer due to the major disruption involved within the chest and abdomen [20].

Post-resection anatomical changes to the pharynx and larynx are associated with significant changes in speech and the swallow function following PLO. Both result in a deterioration in QOL.

## METHODS OF POST-OPERATIVE NUTRITIONAL SUPPORT

### Early Oral Feeding

Patients who have undergone a total laryngectomy (TL)/PLO/glossectomy should receive early nutrition support within 24 hours after surgery [18].

Some centres consider initiation of early oral feeding on day 1 post TL as opposed to delayed feeding until day 5/7, as this may reduce LOS. However, Sousa et al. report that the early oral feeding group failed to meet their caloric and protein needs and required additional nutrition via another route [21]. A randomised multicentre study was conducted including 89 patients subjected to undergoing TL. The participants were allocated to two groups: early oral feeding (n = 44) and late oral feeding (n = 45). The results showed that in the early group, total energy and protein needs were not met through oral feeding alone at any time during the first seven post-operative days. The time to attain 25% and 50% of the energy and protein needs by oral feeding after surgery was four and seven days, respectively.

Currently the evidence available has shown no difference in rates of developing fistulae with early oral feeding compared to delayed feeding [11]. However, there is a lack of appropriate nutritional measures in outcome data [22].

### Enteral Feeding

It is highly likely that patients who have had radiotherapy will be kept nil by mouth (NBM) and fed enterally until at least days 5–7 due to an increased risk of post-operative complications such as fistulae or stomal wound break down.

The delivery route, such as continuous, bolus, or overnight feeding, depends on patients' requirements and preference, in addition to medical interventions [23].

### Route of Delivery

It is likely that nasogastric, radiological inserted gastrostomy, and jejunostomy tubes will be common choices for short- and long-term feeding. The access route chosen will depend on the surgery and reconstruction methods used, as well as the availability of local radiology and gastroenterology services.

If enteral feeding is likely to be required for more than four weeks, then a gastrostomy tube is indicated [17, 23].

At present there are no nationally agreed selection criteria for placement of feeding tubes in HNC patients.

### Choice of Formulae

Polymeric 1.5 kcal/ml feeds are routinely used to meet the patient's nutritional requirements.

Evidence supporting the use of immuno-nutrition remains limited. Howes et al. assessed the effects of immuno-nutrition, compared to standard feeding, on post-operative recovery in adult patients undergoing elective surgery for HNC [24]. Nineteen randomised control trials (RCTs; total of 1099 participants) were identified, with some variation in type and quantity of formulae, but predominantly using immuno-nutrition formulae containing arginine. This study found no difference in the length of hospital stay (−2.5 days, 95% confidence interval [CI] −5.11 to 0.12) or wound infection (risk ratio [RR] 0.94, 95% CI 0.70–1.26), thus further research is required.

### Parenteral Nutrition

Parenteral nutrition is not routinely used in this patient group, but should be considered if enteral nutrition is contraindicated [17, 23, 25].

## POST-OPERATIVE COMPLICATIONS AND THEIR NUTRITIONAL MANAGEMENT

### Fistulae/Wound Breakdown

Typically patients undergo a water-soluble contrast study before progressing onto clear fluids. This is an examination of the oesophagus and stomach, involving swallowing contrast (clear liquid) that shows up in a fluoroscopic image (x-ray), which detects any abnormalities, including leaks.

If no abnormality is identified, and the patient has had a speech and language therapist (SLT) assessment, they may progress onto oral/clear fluids for 24–48 hours. Progress from a liquid to a soft diet is supervised by SLTs and carried out in conjunction with a reduction in enteral nutrition and the use of oral nutritional supplements (ONS). Progressing onto a softer diet is important to enable the muscles and nerves that are involved in the swallowing process to adapt to the new anatomical structure. Monitoring for weight loss during this phase is crucial.

This is a particularly important phase in the rehabilitation process as it promotes self-esteem and confidence, which will help motivate and encourage patients to eat. This will help meet their overall nutritional requirements from oral diet alone, bearing in mind that many patients will experience an altered sense of smell, taste, or change in tongue movement, depending on the type of surgery undertaken.

### Long-Term Management of Fistulae and Wound Breakdown

In some patients, oral feeding remains contraindicated due to poorly healing wounds or dehiscence, development of a pharyngo-cutaneous fistula, or a sustained anastomotic leak.

Long-term feeding tube placement may be indicated in patients who fail to heal following surgery in order to optimise healing and promote rehabilitation.

### Dysphagia Due to Delayed Wound Healing Resulting in Dysphagia

Dysphagia can occur post TL if there has been a significant delay in healing. Propulsion of food and liquids through the neo-pharynx (new post-surgical swallow passage) can also be delayed post-operatively [26].

Advice from an SLT and the dietitian will be required to ensure adherence to modified-consistency food and fluids and to meet individual requirements.

The use of ONS is likely to be required in both the short and long term, depending on the severity and duration of dysphagia.

The overall impact on QOL may contribute to reduced levels of compliance with dietary advice and will be an important consideration at every review.

### Pseudo-epiglottis

Surgical closure used with a TL will be unique to each patient. Some patients may develop a pseudo-epiglottis (pouch), which forms a pocket-like structure at the base of the tongue that collects food or liquid, resulting in an effortful swallow. This may affect motivation to eat as it becomes increasingly tiresome. [26]. It may also restrict the quantity that the patient can consume at each meal and thus their overall nutritional intake. The use of food fortification, low-volume liquids before and after meals, and ONS will help to manage this effectively.

### Nasal Regurgitation/Gastro-oesophageal Reflux

Effortful swallowing may occur because of an overall 'tight' surgical closure. Patients may require significant tissue removal (partial pharyngectomy in addition to the larynx) that creates a tight closure, therefore swallowing may require more forceful effort [26].

In severe cases, the narrowed passage may result in backflow of swallowed material all the way up into the oral cavity or nasal passage, which can cause aspiration. A liquid diet may be necessary in these circumstances.

The use of specific dietary advice such as food-fortification methods with meals, ONS, reducing the volumes of liquids before and after each small meal, or positioning of the chin on eating, alongside the use of certain pharmacological agents such as proton pump inhibitors (PPI) and prokinetics, may help reduce gastro-oesophageal reflux.

## Chylous Fistula (Chyle Leak)

Chyle leaks are a rare but serious complication in patients who have undergone H&N surgery. It is most commonly seen after neck dissection. It is caused by injury to the fragile thoracic duct and occurs in approximately 1–2% of cases [27].

Chyle has a milk-like appearance and is produced following the digestion of food. It is a mixture of chylomicrons and lymph.

Chylomicrons form when long-chain fatty acids are ingested and are triglyceride rich [27, 28].

Lymph is a clear fluid that contains white blood cells (lymphocytes). In addition to chylomicrons and lymph, chyle contains electrolytes, protein, fat-soluble vitamins, trace elements, and glucose, and plays a key role in the absorption of long-chain triglycerides [28].

Chyle leaks are typically determined by the visible presence of a milky white fluid in the surgical drains. Alternatively chyle can be aspirated using a needle from a collection in the neck or surgical wound.

### Definition of a Chyle Leak

A chyle leak is defined by biochemical analysis of the drain fluid showing:

- Triglyceride levels >1.24 mmol/l (110 mg/dl) OR
- Chylomicron level >4%.

If triglyceride levels are <1.2 mmol/l but >0.5 mmol/l, chylomicron levels should be checked [11, 28, 29].

Chyle leaks are rare and unpredictable, therefore there is a lack of RCTs and systematic reviews to support the production of guidelines [29]. However, observational studies report that 80% of cases resolve with nutritional management alone without the use of surgery [30].

### Nutritional Management of a Chyle Leak

Management of chyle leaks is summarised in Table 9.1.

If patients on enteral or parenteral nutrition are allowed fluids, they should consume only clear fluids such as black tea, coffee, squash, or water.

Fat-free ONS can also be offered alongside the enteral feed or if starting to reduce the enteral feed to meet the patient's nutritional requirements.

It must be noted that as these supplements are fat free, they are not nutritionally complete, so a source of essential fatty acids will need to be administered [28].

There are several publications that advocate the use of a medium-chain triglyceride (MCT) supplement alongside the dietary intake. However, this may be unpalatable and compliance may be poor, although it could be considered [11, 27–29].

### Fat-Free Diets

A fat-free diet may be requested in the clinical setting, and is defined as <5 g of fat per serving. It is often unpalatable and the patient is unlikely to adhere to it, which may exacerbate malnutrition [31].

If a patient has a chyle output <500 ml and is allowed to eat and drink, then a low-fat diet should be started.

Suitable foods would include fruit, vegetables, rice, pasta, potatoes, fish, chicken, turkey, beans, lentils, low-fat dairy products, skimmed milk, fat-free yoghurt, and high-protein jellies.

### Long-Term Management of Oesophageal Strictures

Oesophageal strictures are a frequent complication occurring when a benign stricture (scar tissue) develops either from surgery or following oncological

**TABLE 9.1**   Nutritional management of post-operative surgical complications.

| Surgical complication | Nutritional management |
| --- | --- |
| **Fistulae**<br>Can occur in pharynx, larynx, and oral cavity affecting tissue healing and ability to swallow | Requires nil by mouth (NBM) and enteral feeding |
| **Wound dehiscence** | Elevated nutritional requirements<br>Micronutrient supplementation |
| **Aspiration** | NBM<br>Enteral feeding |
| **Dysphagia** | Oral nutritional supplements (ONS; in line with speech and language therapist [SLT] advice)<br>Enteral feeding |
| **Oral regurgitation**<br>Due to reconstruction following pharyngo-laryngo-oesophagectomy (PLO) | Small, frequent meals<br>Remain upright after meals for an hour |
| **Nasal regurgitation**<br>Functional impairment of soft palate and pharynx can be distressing and embarrassing | Small, frequent meals<br>Remain upright after meals for an hour |
| **Chyle leak**<br>Medium-chain triglyceride (MCT) lipids are absorbed via the portal vein and processed in the liver, thus bypassing the lymphatic system and reducing the production of chyle<br>More than 1000 ml/d is considered high volume | >1000 ml chyle output over 24 h<br>Total parenteral nutrition (TPN) should be considered<br>Patient should remain NBM<br><br>500 to <1000 ml chyle output per 24 h<br>If the patient is NBM following surgery – MCT/low-fat feed<br>If eating – very low-fat diet and fat-free ONS<br>If no improvement after 5 days, TPN should be started [31]<br><br><500 ml chyle output per 24 h<br>If patient is NBM following surgery – MCT/low-fat feed<br>If eating – very low-fat diet and fat-free ONS<br><br>Consider essential fatty acid supplement and micronutrient supplementation |
| **Early dumping syndrome after PLO**<br>This can occur 30–60 min after eating and can last 10–60 min<br><br>Rapid delivery of food into the small bowel causes a sensation of fullness, bloating, abdominal cramps, nausea, vomiting, and diarrhoea<br><br>The hyperosmolar effect of early delivery of a chyme into the small bowel draws water from the vascular system into the small bowel. This causes a drop in blood pressure, which may cause palpitations, sweating, and dizziness | Aim for 5–6 small meals per day rather than the usual 3 larger meals, and aim to eat every 2–3 h<br>Limit refined carbohydrate<br>Avoid sugary drinks, breakfast cereals, honeys, and syrups<br>Use sugar replacements<br>Drink fluids slowly between meals rather than with meals (30–45 min after eating)<br><br>Avoid eating sweet foods on empty stomach |

**TABLE 9.1** (Continued)

| Surgical complication | Nutritional management |
|---|---|
| **Late dumping syndrome after PLO**<br>This is caused by rapid delivery of carbohydrates into the small bowel with an early peak in blood glucose. Insulin release is out of synchrony, occurring later than the glucose peak, resulting in a drop in blood glucose levels 1–3 h after meals | Increase complex carbohydrate such as wholegrains, pasta, potatoes, bread, and rice<br>Combine protein foods with fat and sugary foods<br>Increase fibre into the diet to help slow the emptying of the stomach and prevent sugar being released too quickly |
| **Strictures and stenosis**<br>Complete or partial, may require frequent dilatation | Texture modifications<br>Will require the use of ONS and enteral feeding in some cases |

treatment. The stricture creates a narrowing in the swallowing passage. Dysphagia to solids or semi-solids appears to be the initial symptom, particularly with bread and meat. Reduced appetite and further weight loss are also likely if this is not managed quickly and effectively.

Strictures can be resolved temporarily with a balloon or radiological dilatation. However, they may reoccur and require frequent dilatation.

Dietary modification should include the avoidance of tough meats, breads, hard or coarse skins, pips, and seeds. Foods should be mashed to a softer consistency/easy chew, using additional sauces [32]. ONS will also be required.

In severe cases, long-term enteral feeding may be needed to maintain the patient's nutritional status, using a combination of enteral feeding and an oral/liquid diet.

| Routine Case Study | |
|---|---|
| **Patient** | **Mrs A, age 64 yr** |
| Presenting complaint | Ongoing dysphonia (hoarseness for six months) |
| Past medical history | Spinal stenosis, type 2 diabetes |
| Social history | Lives with husband, good family support with daughter |
| Investigations | CT neck and chest – soft tissue in both sides of supraglottic larynx extending into paraglottic spaces. Tumour abuts thyroid cartilage and hyoid on right side without erosion. Extends superiorly to involve epiglottis and pre-epiglottic fat<br>Bilateral necrotic level III lymph nodes<br>No metastases seen elsewhere |
| Oral intake | Consists of three small meals per day:<br>Breakfast: Bacon sandwich, scrambled egg, and toast<br>Lunch: Soup with cup of tea and biscuit<br>Evening meal: Meat/potatoes (2–3 egg sized) and veg<br>Snacks: Chocolate bars 2–3 per day<br>Appetite normal, but taking longer to swallow and manage meals, approx. 45 mins per meal<br>Fluids – 8–10 cups of tea, with milk, no sugar |

| Anthropometrics | Current weight 94.5 kg, BMI 35.6 kg/m$^2$ |
| | No reported weight loss |
| | Handgrip strength 21.0 kg (dominant hand) |
| Bowel function | Regular bowel movement twice daily |
| Diagnosis | T3N2cM0 SCC larynx |
| Surgical plan | Chemotherapy combined with radiotherapy vs laryngectomy and neck dissection |
| | Agreed plan for surgery given reduced vocal cord mobility and likely risk of airway compromise if proceeded with chemo/radiotherapy |
| | Prehab exercise regime |
| | Optimise blood glucose control |
| Nutritional plan | Meet nutritional requirements and prevent significant weight loss prior to surgery |
| | Optimise type 2 diabetes advice |
| | Consider long-term feeding options |
| | Unsuitable for carbohydrate loading |
| Admission 1 | Underwent total laryngectomy with (R) and (L) II–IV neck dissection. Naso-gastric tube (NGT) inserted at time of surgery. Enteral feed started 6 h post-operatively |
| Nutritional support | **Requirements:** |
| | Fed to resting energy expenditure (REE) due to BMI >30 –2200 kcal and 107 g protein provided |
| | (Mifflin St Jeor = 1770 kcals + physical activity level [PAL] 1.2 = 2100 kcal) |
| | Protein (1.2–1.5 g/kg) based on ideal body weight (IBW) – 80–105 g |
| | IBW – 67 kg |
| | **Feed:** |
| | 1.28 kcal/ml polymeric high-protein fibre feed (1700 ml at 100 ml/h × 17 h = 2176 kcal; 107 g protein) |
| | **Management:** |
| | Remained NBM until day 5 |
| | Blood glucose levels 6.5–9.0 mmol/l |
| | Contrast swallow showed no defects. Allowed to progress slowly from fluids and enteral feed onto softer option diet. NGT removed |
| | Patient reported swallow 'tight', but managed to meet nutritional requirements with high-energy/high-protein soft diet and ONS alongside (1.5 kcal/ml; 600 kcal daily) |
| Outcome | Successful recovery from surgery |
| | Discharged on day 12 |
| | Full oral diet with ONS (2100 kcal and 90 g protein) |
| | Blood glucose levels remain stable 7–7.5 mmol/l |
| | Weight reduced – 93.8 kg, BMI 35.3 kg/m$^2$ |
| | Handgrip strength 20 kg (dominant hand) |
| Follow up | Referral on to Oncology for radiotherapy |
| | Ongoing six-monthly diabetes team review |
| | Six-weekly surgical and dietetic follow-up |
| | **Four-month follow-up:** |
| | Weight 84.8 kg, BMI 32 kg/m$^2$ (10% weight loss) |

**Subsequent diagnosis:**
Oesophageal stricture – for regular dilatations
Regurgitation/reflux – long-term PPI

**Nutritional management:**
Low-volume liquids pre and post meals
Liquid/soft options – high-energy/high-protein
Upright position after meals
Ongoing use of ONS
Consider enteral feeding if necessary

## Complex Case Study

| Patient | Mrs B, age 36 yr |
|---|---|
| Presenting complaint | Dysphagia to solids and weight loss for four to six months<br>Choking on food |
| Past medical history | Cervical cancer treated with hysterectomy |
| Social history | Lives with partner and two children<br>Non-smoker<br>Social alcohol intake |
| Investigations | Rigid oesophagoscopy – unable to enter oesophagus at level of cricoid, no lumen evident, biopsies taken<br>CT neck/thorax – nil significant<br>Positron emission tomography (PET) CT – low-grade uptake extending from the oesophagus at the C7 extending superiorly to the post-cricoid region to the level c4/5 disc spaces |
| Oral intake | Typical meal – pot of custard, tin of spaghetti hoops, or mashed potatoes/carrots with gravy<br>Ice cream 2 scoops (×2 per day)<br>Corn-based snacks that melt easily in the mouth<br>Using ONS prescribed by GP 1–2 per day<br>Fluid intake: fizzy drinks 5–6 cans per day and coffee 3–4 mugs with 2 sugars added |
| Anthropometrics | Current weight 59 kg, BMI 21.4 kg/m$^2$<br>13% weight loss in four months<br>Usual weight 68 kg<br>Mean handgrip strength 16.7 kg (dominant hand) |
| Bowel function | Constipation, using laxatives |
| Diagnosis | Post-cricoid upper oesophageal adenocarcinoma – T2N0M0 |
| Surgical plan | Standard approach would be for surgery. However, given age and rare to see adeno-carcinoma, opted for chemo/radiotherapy as preferred option |

| | |
|---|---|
| Nutritional plan | Laparoscopic jejunostomy to improve nutritional status prior to oncological treatment<br>Referral to speech and language therapist<br>High risk of refeeding syndrome given weight loss/reduced oral intake (B vitamin and micronutrient supplements) |
| Admission 1 | Admitted for insertion of jejunostomy tube and training<br>Biochemical refeeding syndrome with phosphate drop down to 0.45 mmol/l (reference range [RR] 0.7–1.2 mmol/l), magnesium 0.5 mmol/l (RR 0.8–1.3 mmol/l), treated with phosphate and magnesium infusions<br>Trained to manage jejunostomy tube independently |
| Nutritional support | **Requirements:**<br>25 kcal/kg + 400 kcal for weight gain = 1875 kcal<br>1.5 g protein/kg = 89 g<br>Fluid 35 ml/kg = 2100 ml<br><br>**Oral intake:**<br>Variable: 300–600 kcal and 12.5–25 g protein<br><br>**Target feed:**<br>1.5 kcal/ml polymeric feed with fibre (history of constipation)<br>1000 ml, 125 ml/h × 8 h overnight = 1500 kcal and 62.7 g protein<br>Overnight feeding used due to practicality with childcare during the day |
| Outcome | Completed chemotherapy and radiotherapy<br>Observational routine biopsy showed recurrent disease four months later<br>Planned for pharyngo-laryngo-oesophagectomy (PLO) as only surgical option remaining |
| New diagnosis | Recurrent adenocarcinoma post-cricoid oesophagus |
| Surgical plan 2 | Admitted three months later for surgical resection and underwent PLO with gastric pull-up, thyroidectomy, and partial parathyroidectomy<br>Admission weight 59 kg, BMI 21.4 kg/m²<br>Hypoglycaemia – blood glucose 2.1 mmol/l<br>Developed anastomotic leak; abdominal cramping and pharyngo-cutaneous fistula at stoma site<br>Calcium supplements for hypocalcaemia due to hypoparathyroidism secondary to surgery – referred to Endocrinology |
| Nutritional plan | NBM<br>Mouth-care regime<br>Continue with full enteral feeding via jejunostomy using 1.5 kcal polymeric feed<br>Discharge weight 60.9 kg, BMI 22.1 kg/m²<br>Handgrip strength –16.0 kg<br>Monitoring for dumping syndrome/hypoglycaemia<br>Regular dietetic follow-up |
| Long-term prescription | Alpha-calcidol 2 µg twice a day<br>Thyroxine 150 µg a day<br>Calcit 500 effervescent 6 tablets four times a day |

# REFERENCES

1. National Cancer Institute (2021). Head and neck cancers. www.cancer.gov/types/head-and-neck/head-neck-fact-sheet. Accessed 24 March 2021.

2. Bray, F., Ferlay, J., Soerjomataram, I. et al. (2018). Global cancer statistics 2018: GLOBOCAN estimates of incidence and mortality worldwide for 36 cancers in 185 countries. *CA Cancer J. Clin.* 68 (6): 394–424.

3. Cancer Research UK (n.d.). Head and neck cancers incidence. www.cancerresearchuk.org/health-professional/cancer-statistics/statistics-by-cancer-type/head-and-neck-cancers#heading-Zero. Accessed 24 May 2021.

4. Marron, M., Boffetta, P., Zhang, Z.F. et al. (2010). Cessation of alcohol drinking, tobacco smoking and the reversal of head and neck cancer risk. *Int. J. Epidemiol.* 39 (1): 182–196.

5. Machiels, J.P., Rene Leemans, C., Golusinski, W. et al. (2020). Squamous cell carcinoma of the oral cavity, larynx, oropharynx and hypopharynx: EHNS-ESMO-ESTRO clinical practice Guidelines for diagnosis, treatment and follow-up. *Ann. Oncol.* 31 (11): 1462–1475.

6. Roland, N., Porter, G., Fish, B., and Makura, Z. (2016). Tumour assessment and staging: United Kingdom National Multidisciplinary Guidelines. *J. Laryngol. Otol.* 130 (S2): S53–S58.

7. O'Sullivan, B., Brierley, J., Byrd, D. et al. (2017). The TNM classification of malignant tumours-towards common understanding and reasonable expectations. *Lancet Oncol.* 18 (7): 849–851.

8. SIGN. (2006). Diagnosis and management of head and neck cancer – SIGN 90. www.scottishdental.org/library/diagnosis-and-management-of-head-and-neck-cancer-sign-90. Accessed 24 May 2021.

9. Bruss, D.M. and Sajjad, H. (2021). *Anatomy, Head and Neck, Laryngopharynx*. Treasure Island, FL.: StatPearls.

10. List, M.A. and Bilir, S.P. (2004). Functional outcomes in head and neck cancer. *Semin. Radiat. Oncol.* 14 (2): 178–189.

11. Talwar, B. (2019). Head and neck cancer. In: *The Manual of Dietetic Practice*, 6e (ed. C. Shaw), 822–831. Oxford: Blackwell Wiley.

12. Homer, J.J. and Fardy, M.J. (2016). Surgery in head and neck cancer: United Kingdom National Multidisciplinary Guidelines. *J. Laryngol. Otol.* 130 (S2): S68–S70.

13. Mahalingam, S., Srinivasan, R., and Spielmann, P. (2016). Quality-of-life and functional outcomes following pharyngolaryngectomy: a systematic review of literature. *Clin. Otolaryngol.* 41 (1): 25–43.

14. Brookes, G.B. (1985). Nutritional status—a prognostic indicator in head and neck cancer. *Otolaryngol. Head Neck Surg.* 93 (1): 69–74.

15. Langius, J.A., Bakker, S., Rietveld, D.H. et al. (2013). Critical weight loss is a major prognostic indicator for disease-specific survival in patients with head and neck cancer receiving radiotherapy. *Br. J. Cancer* 109 (5): 1093–1099.

16. National Institute for Health and Care Excellence. (2004). Improving outcomes in head and neck cancers. Cancer service guideline [CSG6]. www.nice.org.uk/guidance/csg6. Accessed 24 May 2021.

17. Talwar, B., Donnelly, R., Skelly, R., and Donaldson, M. (2016). Nutritional management in head and neck cancer: United Kingdom National Multidisciplinary Guidelines. *J. Laryngol. Otol.* 130 (S2): S32–S40.

18. Weimann, A., Braga, M., Carli, F. et al. (2017). ESPEN guideline: clinical nutrition in surgery. *Clin. Nutr.* 36 (3): 623–650.

19. Lin, D.T., Yarlagadda, B.B., Sethi, R.K. et al. (2015). Long-term functional outcomes of total glossectomy with or without total laryngectomy. *JAMA Otolaryngol. Head Neck Surg.* 141 (9): 797–803.

20. NALC. (2005). PLO - The Operation, October [12-02-2021]. https://www.laryngectomy.org.uk/laryngectomee-info/information-leaflets/. Accessed 24 May 2021.

21. Sousa, A.A., Porcaro-Salles, J.M., Soares, J.M. et al. (2016). Tolerance of early oral feeding in patients subjected to total laryngectomy. *Head Neck* 38 (Suppl 1): E643–E648.

22. Aires, F.T., Dedivitis, R.A., Petrarolha, S.M. et al. (2015). Early oral feeding after total laryngectomy: a systematic review. *Head Neck* 37 (10): 1532–1535.

23. National Institute for Health and Care Excellence. (2017). Nutrition support for adults: oral nutrition support, enteral tube feeding and parenteral nutrition. Clinical guideline [CG32]. www.nice.org.uk/Guidance/CG32.

24. Howes, N., Atkinson, C., Thomas, S., and Lewis, S.J. (2018). Immunonutrition for patients undergoing surgery for head and neck cancer. *Cochrane Database Syst. Rev.* 8 (8): CD010954.

25. Palma-Milla, S., Lopez-Plaza, B., Santamaria, B. et al. (2018). New, immunomodulatory, Oral nutrition formula for use prior to surgery in patients with head and neck cancer: an exploratory study. *JPEN J. Parenteral Enteral Nutr.* 42 (2): 371–379.

26. Gaziano, J. (2020). Dysphagia after Laryngectomy. *Whispers on the Web.* https://webwhispers.org/wp-content/uploads/2020/11/Whispers-on-the-Web-November-2020.pdf. Accessed 24 May 2021.

27. Delaney, S.W., Shi, H., Shokrani, A., and Sinha, U.K. (2017). Management of chyle leak after head and neck surgery: review of current treatment strategies. *Int. J. Otolaryngol.* 2017: 8362874.

28. Sriram, K., Meguid, R.A., and Meguid, M.M. (2016). Nutritional support in adults with chyle leaks. *Nutrition* 32 (2): 281–286.

29. Smoke, A. and Delegge, M.H. (2008). Chyle leaks: consensus on management? *Nutr. Clin. Pract.* 23 (5): 529–532.

30. Smith, R. (2019). Nutritional management of chyle leaks in head and neck surgery patients. *Complete Nutr. (CN)* 19 (3): 30–32.

31. Meyer, C.D., McLeod, I.K., and Gallagher, D.J. (2016). Conservative management of an intraoperative Chyle leak: a case report and literature review. *Mil. Med.* 181 (9): e1180–e1184.

32. Stoner, P.L., Fullerton, A.L., Freeman, A.M. et al. (2019). Endoscopic dilation of refractory postlaryngectomy strictures: a case series and literature review. *Gastroenterol. Res. Pract.* 2019: 8905615.

# CHAPTER 10

# Cardiothoracic Surgery and Nutrition

Rupal Patel[1] and Ann-Marie Nixon[2]

[1] *Department of Nutrition and Dietetics, Royal Brompton and Harefield Hospitals, Guy's and St Thomas' NHS Foundation Trust, London, UK*
[2] *Department of Nutrition and Dietetics, Wythenshawe Hospital, Manchester University NHS Foundation Trust, Manchester, UK*

---

**KEY POINTS**

- Patients undergoing cardiothoracic surgery are a very heterogeneous cohort.
- Systemic inflammation and multiorgan failure are pathophysiological effects of cardiac surgery, with cardiopulmonary bypass being a contributing factor.
- Cardiothoracic transplant can result in multiple long-term nutritional complications.
- There is limited research in the management of chylothorax.
- Mediterranean-style diets and weight management are key in the secondary prevention of further cardiovascular disease.

---

Cardiothoracic (CT) surgery is the speciality of diseases of the thorax, namely the heart and lungs. There are four main subgroups: cardiac, thoracic, transplant (Tx), and congenital surgery. Congenital surgery will not be discussed in this chapter as the surgery is performed in specialist centres. CT transplant (CT Tx) is also performed at specialist centres, however patients are frequently managed in local hospitals pre and post Tx, therefore some key information will be included here.

## OVERVIEW OF SURGICAL PROCEDURES

### Cardiac

Cardiac surgery frequently requires an intensive care unit (ICU) stay, both in the routine post-operative setting and a prolonged ICU stay if post-operative complications occur.

## Cardiopulmonary Bypass

Cardiopulmonary bypass (CPB) is frequently used during cardiac surgery. It is a form of extracorporeal blood oxygenation, along with aortic cross-clamping, which enables systemic and cerebral perfusion during surgery while the heart is stopped. Surgery can be elective, for long-standing heart failure, or emergency, due to a cardiac event. For this reason, the population is very heterogeneous in terms of baseline nutritional status and anthropometry.

## Coronary Artery Bypass Grafting

Coronary artery bypass grafting (CABG) involves surgically bypassing one or more coronary arteries that are either narrowed or completely blocked using venous or arterial grafts as conduits. This is a common procedure used to treat ischaemic heart disease predominantly caused by atherosclerosis. The surgery is carried out under general anaesthesia, typically via a median sternotomy and on CPB. Depending on the target coronary artery, CABG surgery can be carried out 'off pump' without the need for CPB. This is referred to as an 'off-pump coronary bypass'.

## Valve Replacement Surgery

The four heart valves, which keep blood flowing in the correct direction, are the mitral, tricuspid, pulmonary, and aortic valves. Cardiac valve disease covers a range of pathologies that can be classified as those where there is a restriction to valve opening (stenosis) leading to obstruction of flow and an increased pressure gradient; and those where there is insufficient valve closing leading to valvular regurgitation. There are many aetiologies of valve disease, including congenital malformations, degenerative changes relating to age, and rheumatic disease. Depending on the severity of the disease and the resulting dysfunction, it is possible to surgically repair or replace the valves under CPB. There are several different types of valves that can be used in replacement; these are classified as mechanical or biological (tissue). The decision as to which valve is most appropriate will depend on the age of the patient, comorbidities, and personal preference. Mechanical valves are often implanted in younger patients as they last longer and therefore reduce the need for further surgeries. However, lifelong anticoagulation, which carries a risk, is required with mechanical valves, whereas this is not typically needed with biological valves.

## Aortic Surgeries

The aorta is the largest artery in the body. It starts after the aortic valve and passes through the abdomen and chest cavity, taking oxygenated blood all around the body. The main diseases of the aorta are due to atherosclerotic disease or hypertension, which causes damage/changes to the wall of the aorta, for instance aortic aneurysm or dissection. An aortic aneurysm is an abnormal bulge in the artery wall and can occur anywhere along the aorta (abdominal aortic aneurysm or thoracic aortic aneurysm). These can result in tears in the inner layer of the aortic wall, causing blood to split the inner and middle layers of the aorta (aortic dissection), causing a weakening. This can result in rupture of the aorta, which carries a very high mortality. Diseases of the aorta are extremely life-threatening and can present as emergencies. Depending on the site of the aneurysm/dissection, surgical repair will involve a sternotomy, CPB, and resection and replacement with a synthetic tube-shaped graft, as well as potentially reimplantation of the coronary arteries and/or an aortic valve replacement.

## Thoracic Surgery

Thoracic surgery is part of the management of malignancies and infections of the thoracic cavity. This involves operating on pulmonary, pleural, chest wall, or mediastinal structures.

Pulmonary malignancies, infections potentially caused by bronchiectasis and tuberculosis, and acquired or spontaneous pleural disorders are also common causes of thoracic surgery. There are two main approaches for thoracic surgery, a thoracotomy and video-assisted thoracoscopic surgery (VATS).

VATS involves multiple small incisions in the thorax, and the use of a camera (thoroscope) to assist the operation. This is less invasive, there is a potential for a shorter length of stay, less post-operative pain, and quicker return to full function than a thoracotomy [1].

Pulmonary resections are typically named according to the anatomical section of the lung being removed: pneumonectomy – removal of the entire lung; lobectomy or bilobectomy – removal of one or two lobes of the lung; wedge or segmental resection – removal of a wedge position or whole segment of the lung; and sleeve resection – removal of the lobe along with part of the main bronchus.

Pleural surgery is part of the management of recurrent pneumothoraxes, pleural effusions, and empyema (pus in the pleural space). The different surgical options are pleurectomy – partial stripping of the parietal pleura; pleurodesis – use of an irritant (talc or chemical) to adhere the lung to the chest wall; drainage of empyema – drainage of infected plural effusion; and decortication – removal of the thickened fibrous pleural peel.

## Cardiothoracic Transplant

CT Tx is carried out at six regional centres in the UK. Due to the shortage of organs available for transplant, priority is given to those who have the greatest potential for survival. Recipients are assessed against strict eligibility criteria, set by the NHS blood and transplant service.

Tx is carried out when other medical or surgical treatments have failed. HTx, or cardiac transplant, is the surgical replacement of a person's diseased or failing heart, typically due to coronary heart disease, ischaemic heart disease, cardiomyopathy, or congenital heart disease. Lifelong adherence to immunosuppressive therapy is required to prevent organ rejection alongside many other medication and dietary changes.

Lung transplant (LTx) is the removal of one or both diseased lungs and replacement by lungs (double or single) from a donor. Causal factors are chronic obstructive pulmonary disease (COPD), pulmonary hypertension, idiopathic pulmonary fibrosis, alpha 1 antitrypsin deficiency, and cystic fibrosis (CF). (Specialist CF centres should be contacted for advice in managing these patients.)

Contraindications to HTx or LTx are body mass index (BMI) <16 or >35kg/m²; persistent poor glycaemic control (glycated haemoglobin [$HbA_{1c}$] > 58mmol/mol), or diabetes with end-organ damage, excluding retinopathy [2, 3]. In addition, the following are relative contraindications to LTx: BMI 30.0–34.9 kg/m², particularly with truncal (central) obesity; BMI 16–17 kg/m²; severe or symptomatic osteoporosis; poor functional status with limited rehabilitation potential; gastro-oesophageal reflux disease; and gastric dysmotility [2]. Some of these patients may be referred to local hospitals for optimisation prior to CT Tx.

## NUTRITIONAL IMPLICATIONS

### Cardiac Surgery

Nutritional care following cardiac surgery, both in the ICU and in the ward setting, is similar to other post-operative nutritional care. Dietitians apply the same nutritional guidelines and clinical reasoning to treat and assess nutritional needs of patients (Chapter 8). A complex systemic inflammatory response syndrome is triggered after open heart surgery caused by a combination of surgical trauma, CPB, organ reperfusion injury (e.g. heart), and the release of systemic inflammation mediators [4]. This presents as pyrexia, tachycardia, hypotension, oedema, and multi-organ failure [5]. This can result in haemodynamic instability, often requiring inotrope and vasopressor support.

### Fluid Management

Fluid management is a powerful tool in achieving haemodynamic stability [6]. Haemodilution and increase in capillary permeability occur during CPB. This increases the incidence of widespread tissue oedema, which has the potential to prolong post-operative intubation time, ICU stay, and length of hospital stay by causing peri- and post-operative organ dysfunction [7]. Both fluid overload and a very negative fluid balance should be avoided to prevent hypovolaemic-related arrhythmias and acute kidney disease (AKI) [8], with a slightly negative fluid balance being preferable. Dietitians may need to adjust enteral nutrition to meet fluid goals using low-volume/concentrated feeds.

## Thoracic Surgery

Malnutrition is extremely common pre and post thoracic surgery, depending on the severity of the lung disease and surgery required. Patients with lung disease such as COPD and emphysema can have sarcopenia, and this is seen in those with a low BMI and within the obesity paradox spectrum (the latter of which is often overlooked). Patients with cancer often present with cachexia and require aggressive post-operative nutrition support.

Dysphagia can occur in advanced cancer, and tracheoesophageal fistulas can form that require double stenting of the oesophagus and the airway. Dietetic input may involve advice on eating with an oesophageal stent or short- and long-term enteral feeding if there is a risk of aspiration or a fistula.

## Cardiothoracic Transplant

### Body Composition and Weight Management

Chronic use of corticosteroids as used in Tx can result in progressive proximal weakness, sarcopenia, and central adiposity. Sarcopenia often coexists with obesity, and this is associated with higher levels of metabolic disorders and an increased risk of mortality than obesity or sarcopenia alone. Efforts to promote healthy ageing should focus on both preventing obesity and maintaining or increasing muscle mass [9, 10].

Excess weight gain is commonly seen following CT Tx and can result in hypertension, dyslipidaemia, and diabetes mellitus. All are cardiovascular risk factors, and contribute to the risk of post-transplant metabolic syndrome, which has an adverse effect on long-term outcomes. A major therapeutic aim after heart and lung Tx is to prevent and treat any risk factors that might result in new comorbidities. Weight management advice should be individualised based on patient preference, lifestyle, and comorbidities, with the goal of achieving long-term adherence.

### Food Safety

Immunosuppressants increase risk of infection, including food-borne infections. The symptoms can cause dehydration and renal failure, as well as impairing absorption of medications, resulting in rejection and possibly graft failure. Consequently, transplant recipients should be advised to adhere to good food hygiene and handling practices. High-risk foods should be avoided. This is particularly important in the early stages after Tx, after treatment for rejection, or in nutritionally vulnerable patients.

Grapefruit and grapefruit juice should be avoided, as these interact with immunosuppressants.

## COMPLICATIONS

### Gut Ischaemia

Gastrointestinal (GI) complications post cardiac surgery are rare and have an incidence of 0.3–3% [11]. Complications span from GI bleeds, pancreatitis, or ileus, to liver failure and ischaemic bowel [12]. Mesenteric ischaemia and ischaemic colitis can be caused by splanchnic hypoperfusion of the gut. Pathophysiology of poor perfusion is a result of systemic inflammation, hypovolaemia, emboli, or drug interactions as a result of cardiac surgery [13]. The risk of ischaemia is increased with length of time on CBP, use of an intra-aortic balloon pump, pre-existing atherosclerosis, vasopressor usage, post-operative cardiac failure, and being over 70 years of age. The mortality is 75% in mesenteric and stage III ischaemia [14]. Early detection is key, but symptoms can be masked, resulting in delayed diagnosis and higher mortality. Monitoring of biochemical markers such as lactate, serum procalcitonin, aspartate aminotransferase, and myoglobin levels have shown to facilitate early diagnosis [14].

A lower threshold for acceptable gastric residual volumes (GRVs) of less than 300 ml should be maintained if risk factors are present, in place of the more liberal (up to 500 ml) GRVs used in other critical care specialities [15]. If ischaemia is suspected, emergency laparotomies are performed; gut resection can lead to formation of stoma and potentially short bowel syndrome (Chapter 21).

## Vocal Cord Palsy

Vocal cord palsy is the inability of one or both vocal cords to move. It may be caused by intra-operative damage to the vagus nerve, typically the left recurrent laryngeal nerve. The severity may range from mild voice change to life-threatening conditions affecting respiration and swallowing. These occur if the vocal cords can no longer close the entrance to the airway. The patient will require support from the speech and language therapy team and may be nil by mouth until there is spontaneous recovery, or they undergo vocal fold medialisation. This moves the non-functioning vocal cord into a more lateral position to allow the vocal cords to close more effectively. Nasogastric feeding is only safe in the absence of reflux, otherwise jejunal feeding maybe indicated.

## Chylothorax

A chylothorax is an accumulation of lymphatic fluid called chyle in the pleural space. The causes of chylothorax include:

- *Traumatic*: including direct damage to the thoracic duct or one of its contributories (of which thoracic surgery is the most common cause).
- *Non-traumatic*: high pressure in the lymphatic system due to obstruction to the thoracic duct (malignancy being the most common cause) [16, 17].

The incidence of post-operative chylothorax in adults following thoracic surgery is 0.2–1% [16]. Chyle leaks typically consist of a fluid with a milky appearance in about 22–44% of patients, but can also appear serous or bloody [18]. Chylous effusions are composed of chylomicrons, which are lipoproteins (containing triglyceride, phospholipid, cholesterol, and protein), fat-soluble vitamins, lymphocytes, and electrolytes. Pleural fluid losses can be extensive and can cause biochemical, nutritional, and immunological disturbances, and poor wound healing [19].

Management of chylothorax is not well established and while there is no consensus in the literature, case reports and small cohorts of patients suggest management options including dietary fat reduction, octreotide, and surgical and radiological procedures [16, 19]. Patients with chylothorax are at high risk of malnutrition, and dietitians play a key role in mitigating this, as well as reducing the flow of chyle to promote healing, and reduce electrolyte, protein, and fluid losses [16].

## Medium-Chain Triglyceride/Very Low Fat Diet

Dietary fats that are predominantly long-chain fatty acids are absorbed by the lymphatic system and therefore increase the flow of chyle through the thoracic duct [18].

Medium-chain triglycerides (MCTs) bypass the lymphatic system and are absorbed via the portal circulation and therefore only have a minimal effect on chyle flow. A high-protein and very low-fat (VLF) diet (<10 g long-chain triglyceride/day) supplemented with MCTs has been shown to resolve approximately 50% of traumatic chylothorax [16, 20].

The VLF–MCT diet can be administered via food, or enterally by using a fat-free/MCT enteral feed for patients who are unable to meet nutritional requirements orally. Palatability, limited catering provisions, and lack of staff and patient education on the VLF–MCT diet can play a factor in adherence and successful implementation of the diet, especially in the hospital setting [19].

## Essential Fatty Acids and Vitamin Supplementation

Essential fatty acids (EFAs) are not produced by the body and need to be obtained from the diet. Symptoms of EFA deficiency include impaired wound healing, skin lesions, and eczema. Patients who are on a fat-free or VLF–MCT diet for a prolonged period (more than three weeks) will need a source of EFA to avoid deficiency. The daily requirements for EFA can be met by providing 2–4% of total energy intake as linoleic acid, which can be achieved by providing one teaspoon of walnut oil or safflower oil per day [16]. Fat-soluble vitamins A, E, D, and K are also absorbed via the lymphatic system, therefore therapeutic multivitamin with minerals supplementation is advised [16]. If fat-free nutritional supplement drinks are tolerated orally or enterally, additional supplementation may not be required, but this will require dietetic assessment.

## Parenteral Nutrition

If the chyle leak does not resolve/reduce with a fat-free/MCT enteral feed or VLF–MCT diet, parenteral nutrition (PN) is considered. A systematic review found that PN had a slightly lower success rate and increased requirement for surgery compared with VLF–MCT supplementation [21]. However, patients on PN typically had more severe and higher-output chyle leaks than those on VLF–MCT diets and were more likely to require surgery regardless of dietary treatment [21].

## Octreotide

Octreotide, a somatostatin analogue, has been shown to be useful in the conservative treatment of chylothorax [22]. It reduces splanchnic, hepatic, and portal blood flow, thereby decreasing the volume of lymph produced and, ultimately, thoracic duct flow. It inhibits the absorption of triglycerides and decreases acetylcholine release in the gut. Reported side effects include vomiting and other GI issues related to decreased blood flow [23]. At present there are no randomised control trials on the use of octreotide in chylothorax in adults.

## Monitoring

Food record and fluid balance charts, bowel function, body weight, and careful monitoring of electrolytes are required to ensure nutritional, fluid, and electrolyte adequacy.

## Surgical and Radiological Interventions

If conservative management has failed or the tear is presumed to be large, surgical interventions are considered and include the following:

- Ligation of thoracic duct at the base of right chest, adjacent to oesophagus, which may reduce or stop the leak. This can be done surgically or percutaneously through embolisation [18].
- A pleurodesis, in which pleural inflammation is induced with the aim of encouraging the visceral and parietal pleurae to stick together and effectively abolish the pleural space [18].
- Lymphangiography, which allows radiological mapping of the lymphatic system and in some instances the lymphatic leak can be embolised [24].

# LONG-TERM MANAGEMENT POST CARDIAC SURGERY

## Cardioprotective Diet and Weight

Once the initial acute phase of surgery is over and the protein and energy deficit has been reversed, dietary advice should centre on a Mediterranean-style diet. The PREDIMED trial found that the group on the Mediterranean diet supplemented with nuts or olive oil had a 30% reduction in cardiovascular events compared to the group on a low-fat diet [25]. The European Society of Cardiology has set dietary recommendations based on the benefits of a Mediterranean diet; see Table 10.1 [26]. Steps towards weight reduction (if the patient is classed as overweight or obese) are also encouraged. Weight loss of 5–10% has a favourable effect on other cardiovascular disease risk factors – improving lipid profiles, lowering hypertension, and decreasing the risk of developing diabetes [27].

## Cardiac Rehabilitation

Cardiac rehabilitation (CR) is an individually tailored, comprehensive physical activity and educational programme offered to patients after cardiac surgery.

**TABLE 10.1**  Healthy diet characteristics.

- Adopt a more plant- and less animal-based food pattern
- Saturated fatty acids should account for <10% of total energy intake, through replacement by polyunsaturated fatty acids (PUFAs), monounsaturated fatty acids (MUFAs), and carbohydrates from whole grains
- Trans unsaturated fatty acids should be minimized as far as possible, with none from processed foods
- <5 g total salt intake/d
- 30–45 g fibre/d, preferably from whole grains
- >200 g fruit/d (>2–3 servings)
- >200 g vegetables/d (>2–3 servings)
- Red meat should be reduced to a maximum of 350–500 g/wk, in particular processed meat should be minimised
- Fish is recommended 1–2 times/wk, in particular fatty fish
- 30 g unsalted nuts/d
- Consumption of alcohol should be limited to a maximum of 100 g/wk
- Sugar-sweetened beverages, such as soft drinks and fruit juices, must be discouraged

Source: Reproduced from [26] with permission of European Society of Cardiology.

Education on risk factor modification, diet/nutritional counselling (Table 10.1), pharmacology, and vocational and psychosocial support is delivered by the multidisciplinary team [28]. Participation in CR after revascularisation surgery reduces the incidence of myocardial infarction, cardiovascular hospitalisations, cardiovascular mortality, and, in some programmes, all-cause mortality [26]. The National Audit of Cardiac Rehabilitation (NACR) reported that 30% of CR patients start rehabilitation with a BMI >30 kg/m$^2$ and unfortunately this did not reduce over the course of CR. This is hypothesised to be associated with smoking cessation (resulting in weight gain) and overall reduced physical activity and higher levels of depression in this population [29]. Nutritional screening and anthropometry assessments are routinely carried out in CR, and those identified as obese or malnourished are referred on for specialist dietetic input.

## LONG-TERM POST-TRANSPLANT COMPLICATIONS

### Hypertension, Dyslipidaemia, and Diabetes

Corticosteroid-induced fluid retention can be severe enough to cause hypertension, and patients with pre-existing hypertension may develop a worsening of blood pressure control when these drugs are initiated.

The mechanism for hyperlipidaemia post Tx is poorly understood, but may be related to immunosuppressive therapy agents and dose. Some statins are poorly tolerated due to the interaction with immunosuppressive calcineurin inhibitor drugs (CNIs), chronic kidney disease, and liver impairment.

The incidence of diabetes after HTx or LTx has been reported to be 23–44% at one year [30, 31]. Development is largely due to corticosteroids, CNIs, and weight gain. HbA$_{1c}$ is not valid in patients on corticosteroids. As blood glucose levels peak eight hours after taking corticosteroids, morning or fasting blood glucose levels may not be sensitive to glycaemic variability. Achieving good glycaemic control consistently throughout the day is necessary to prevent and slow the progression of vasculopathy.

Lifestyle management should focus on reducing fat mass, increasing lean body mass, and achieving and maintaining a healthy body weight [32]. Dietary intervention is consistent with the non-Tx population: regular exercise, achieving and maintaining a healthy BMI, and the use of healthy eating plant-based diets. The latter are characterised by large consumption of legumes, nuts, olive oil, fruits, and vegetables with a high-fibre content and low glycaemic index. Examples include the Mediterranean, portfolio, or Dietary Approaches to Stop Hypertension (DASH) diets [33–36].

Plant stanols and sterols have also been proven to be beneficial in controlling cholesterol levels [37]; however, they may impair the absorption of CNIs. A two-hour gap before and one hour after CNIs may be beneficial and is recommended.

High glycaemic index foods and drinks should be avoided. Reducing carbohydrate loads and smaller, more frequent meals may have a role in reducing hyperglycaemic peaks for those patients on corticosteroids.

## CHRONIC KIDNEY DISEASE

Impaired kidney function is common post Tx, with both incidence and severity increasing with time [30, 38, 39].

CT Tx recipients may remain on corticosteroids long term; even low doses can induce protein catabolism. Given the importance of protein for the maintenance of lean body mass and optimal immune function, protein requirements of transplant patients should be 1 g/kg body weight [40]. Patients should be carefully assessed regarding corticosteroids dose, protein status, and kidney function prior to applying a restriction of protein intake [35].

## Osteoporosis and Vitamin D

HTx or LTx recipients have an elevated risk for developing osteoporosis due to post-operative immobility, renal dysfunction altering calcium–vitamin D–parathyroid hormone (PTH) equilibrium, and immunosuppressive agents.

Osteoporosis prevention is recommended in patients of any age who have at least three months of anticipated steroid use at a daily dose of prednisolone 5 mg or higher [41, 42]. This includes an optimal intake of 1200 mg/d elemental calcium through diet and supplements combined with 1000 IU/d Vitamin D, with dosages adjusted to maintain vitamin D >75 nmol/l. That is associated with a better outcome in the LTx population [43, 44].

| Routine Case Study | |
|---|---|
| **Patient** | **Mr A, 73-year-old male** |
| Anthropometry | Usual weight 73.0 kg (5 mo ago) |
| | Current weight 65.4 kg, BMI 22.6 kg/m$^2$, 10% weight loss in <6 mo |
| | Handgrip strength 17.2 kg (best) |
| | Visual assessment: loss of lean body mass |
| Biochemistry (reference range [RR]) | Na 134 mmol/l (133–146), K 4.4 mmol/l (3.5–5.3), urea 17.5 mmol/l (2.5–7.8), creatinine 135 µmol/l (64–104), estimated glomerular filtration rate (eGFR) 46 ml/min (>90), alb 21 g/l (35–50), C-reactive protein (CRP) 6 mg/l (<4), blood glucose level (BGL) 5.1–8.2 mmol/l |
| Clinical | Medical history: |
| | Right lower lobectomy for T2aN0M0 squamous cell carcinoma (SCC) 2017 |
| | Dilated cardiomyopathy with severe left ventricular (LV) dysfunction |
| | COPD |
| | CKD stage 3a |
| | Hypertension |
| | Hypercholesterolaemia |
| | Hiatus hernia |
| | No known allergies |
| | |
| | 9 d post left thoracotomy and wedge resection of left upper lobe and biopsy (diagnosed with SCC) |
| | Returned to theatre day 3 with for repair of air leak and resection of 6th rib following left lower lung injury secondary to rib fracture |

| | |
|---|---|
| | Nasogastrically fed on ICU, but multiple tube displacements<br>Transferred to ward on day 6<br>Respiratory: 1 l/min $O_2$ $FiO_2$ 24%, via nasal cannulae<br>Gastro: bowels open 2/7 ago, type 5 stool<br>Swallow assessment: pureed foods (International Dysphagia Diet Standardisation Initiative [IDDSI] level 4), mildly thick fluids (IDDSI level 2)<br>Renal: fluid input 950 ml, urine output 1440 ml<br>Mobility: needs assistance of 2 people to mobilise |
| Social | Retired. Lives alone, independent |
| Dietary | Breakfast: 50% porridge<br>Lunch: 50% chicken casserole, 100% rhubarb fool<br>Dinner: 1/3 cottage pie, 100% custard pot<br>Fluids: 4 cups of tea, 2 sugars, semi-skimmed milk thickened<br>Dislikes plain milk, water, reports food tasting bland |
| Requirements | Requirements 23 kcal/kg with physical activity adjustment: 1.15–1.2 = 1729–1804 kcal/d<br>Protein: 1.2–1.5 g/kg = 78–98 g/d<br>Fluid: 30 ml/kg |
| Evaluation | Given unintentional weight loss and current inadequate intake, decision to minimise nutritional losses by increasing intake via oral route |
| Plan | Trial with oral supplements<br>Prescribed 2.4 kcal/ml low-volume, high-protein supplement three times a day giving 900 kcal, 54 g protein<br>IDDSI level 4 menu<br>Encourage higher-protein, higher-calorie options<br>Encourage frequent meals and snacks<br>Food charts<br>Check vitamin D status |
| Outcome | Vitamin D deficiency identified. Prescribed 40 000 IU cholecalciferol once weekly for 7 wk<br>Upgraded to easy chew (IDDSI level 7) and normal fluid (IDDSI level 0), weight 66.2 kg<br>Oral intake increased<br>Discharged home day 19. Having small, energy-dense ready meals delivered. GP to review vitamin D, bone profile, and PTH on follow-up |

## Complex Case Study

### Reason for Referral

14 days' negligible oral intake. Weight loss 21% in 3/12

| Patient | **Mr B, 70-year-old male** |
|---|---|
| Anthropometry | Height 1.7 m<br>Usual weight 106 kg<br>Weight 2 mo ago 97.6 kg (with gross oedema up to mid-abdomen) |

| | |
|---|---|
| | Estimated dry weight = 87.6 kg, BMI 30.3 kg/m$^2$<br>Current weight 85.5 kg (no oedema), BMI 29.6 kg/m$^2$<br>Visual assessment: loss of tone in limbs<br>Handgrip strength 27.5 kg |
| Biochemistry (RR) | Na 129 mmol/l (133–146), K 5.9 mmol/l (3.5–5.3), urea 19.0 mmol/l (2.5–7.8), creatinine 106 μmol/l (64–104), eGFR 61 ml/min (>90), CRP 103 mg/l (<4), BGL 7.7–14.8 mmol/l, haemoglobin (Hb) 107 g/l (130–180), white cell count (WCC) 11.8 10$^9$/l (4–11) |
| Clinical | Medical history:<br>Type 2 diabetes mellitus<br>Atrial fibrillation<br>Congenital heart disease – coarctation of aorta (2× previous stents)<br>Hypercholesterolaemia<br>Hypertension<br>Cardiovascular accident (CVA)<br>14× dental extractions 2 mo ago<br>Aortic valve replacement and aortic root replacement 1 mo ago, delayed recovery<br>Post-operative complications:<br>Anaemia requiring transfusion<br>AKI<br>Fluid overloaded – treated with diuretics<br>Lower respiratory tract infection<br>2 readmissions due to hyperkalaemia<br><br>Readmitted from wound clinic, cultures sent, and started on co-amoxiclav. Has vacu drain on wound<br>K 6.3 mmol/l, with electrocardiogram (ECG) changes<br>Wound redressed, commenced on 7 d course of tazocin<br>Echocardiogram (ECHO) showed LV ejection fraction 35–40%<br><br>Today:<br>Referred as 14 d negligible oral intake. Weight loss 21% in 3/12<br>Apyrexial<br>Neuro: alert and orientated<br>Respiratory: self-ventilating, oxygen saturations 96–100% on room air<br>Cardiac: sinus rhythm, blood pressure 109/64 mmHg<br>Renal: passing urine – pale yellow, no fluid charts. Hydration chart incomplete – fluid in recorded as three drinks yesterday. No fluid restriction<br>GI: bowels not opened for several days; declining laxatives, had enema this morning<br>Skin: 4 cm × 1 cm sternotomy wound breakdown. Negative-pressure wound therapy<br>Mobility: in hospital spends majority of time in bed. Usually independently mobile. Complaining of fatigue. Normally works and keen to continue |
| Medication | Mixed insulin 50–20 units a.m., 14 units p.m., loop diuretic, bisoprolol, beta blocker, metformin 500 mg twice a day, BGL 4–7 mmol/l |
| Social | Lives alone. Supportive daughter lives nearby |

| | |
|---|---|
| Dietary | Awaiting new dentures – difficulty chewing solids, dry mouth, difficulty swallowing food |
| | Describes himself as 'living off tinned soups' since teeth extracted |
| | Breakfast: small amount of porridge oats made with oat milk |
| | Smoothie (spinach, mango, raspberries, cherries) |
| | Lunch: tinned tomato soup, cheese triangles ×3 |
| | Dinner: tinned mushroom soup, custard pot 150 g |
| | Drinks: milk 250 ml ×3 |
| Requirements | Energy: 20–26 kcals/kg (65+ yr, 1 mo post surgery) plus adjustment for physical activity: 1.1–1.2 ≡ 1881–2668 kcal/d |
| | Protein: 1–1.5 g/kg = 86–128 g/d |
| | Fluid: 30 ml/kg = 2565 ml/d unless fluid restricted |
| | Potassium: 1 mmol/kg = 85 mmol/day or 60 mmol/day |
| Evaluation | Inadequate nutritional intake due to difficulties masticating food and fatigue, with 10% unintentional weight loss in 2 mo. Recurrent hyperkalaemia likely due to medications, hyperglycaemia, and kidney impairment. Likely increased protein demand due to wound healing |
| Plan | Soft/bite-sized/minced and moist menu |
| | Choose high-protein menu options |
| | Food fortification and list of higher-protein, higher-calorie, soft, moist snacks and meal ideas from and for home. Daughter to support with shopping and cooking when goes home |
| | Nourishing fluids – replace oat milk and fruit and vegetable smoothies with cow or soya milk and milky drinks to increase protein intake |
| | Low-potassium, energy-dense supplement drink twice a day commenced while inpatient and reassess prior to discharge |
| | Food charts |
| | Multivitamin and mineral supplement |
| | Daily weights to assess changes in hydration and nutrition status |
| | Refer to diabetes specialist nurse |
| Outcome | Reviewed 4 d later. For discharge home tomorrow. BGL now 5–11 mmol/l. Potassium 5.4 mmol/l. Tolerating minced moist foods well, taking supplements. Provided with prescription for 5 d of supplement drinks on discharge home and copy of meal delivery service booklet with suitable options highlighted. First-line potassium advice provided in case of further episodes of hyperkalaemia. Referred to community dietitian for follow-up |

## FURTHER RESEARCH

- Further comparison of nutritional management of CT surgery patients vs other surgical patients, especially around energy and protein requirements pre and post surgery.
- Randomised control trials are needed to investigate the nutritional management of chylothorax.
- Further research is needed in the early detection of gut ischaemia following CT surgery, and safe GRVs in this population.
- Larger trials to explore the benefits of dietary manipulation with Mediterranean-style and plant-based diets on risk factors of cardiovascular disease.

## REFERENCES

1. RJ, M.K. Jr. and Houck, W.V. (2005). *New approaches to the minimally invasive treatment of lung cancer. Curr. Opin. Pulm. Med.* 11: 282–286.

2. Mehra, M.R., Canter, C.E., Hannan, M.M. et al. *International Society for Heart Lung Transplantation (ISHLT) Infectious Diseases, Pediatric and Heart Failure and Transplantation Councils.(2016). The 2016 International Society for Heart Lung Transplantation listing criteria for heart transplantation: a 10-year update. J. Heart and Lung Transplant.* 35: 1–23.

3. Leard, L.E., Holm, A.M., Valapour, M. et al. (2021). *Consensus document for the selection of lung transplant candidates: an update from the International Society for Heart and Lung Transplantation. J. Heart Lung Transplant.* 40: 1349–1379.

4. Suleiman, M.S., Zacharowski, K., and Angelini, G.D. (2008). *Inflammatory response and cardioprotection during open-heart surgery: the importance of anaesthetics. Br. J. Pharmacol.* 153: 21–33.

5. Hill, A., Nesterova, E., Lomivorotov, V. et al. (2018). *Current evidence about nutrition support in cardiac surgery patients—what do we know? Nutrients* 10: 597.

6. Bignami, E., Guarnieri, M., and Gemma, M. (2017). *Fluid management in cardiac surgery patients: pitfalls, challenges and solutions. Minerva. Anestesiologica.* 83: 638–651.

7. Toraman, F., Evrenkaya, S., Yuce, M. et al. (2004). *Highly positive intraoperative fluid balance during cardiac surgery is associated with adverse outcome. Perfusion* 19: 85–91.

8. Meersch, M., Schmidt, C., Hoffmeier, A. et al. (2017). *Prevention of cardiac surgery-associated AKI by implementing the KDIGO guidelines in high risk patients identified by biomarkers: the PrevAKI randomized controlled trial. Inten. Care Med.* 42: 1551–1561.

9. Wannamethee, S.G. and Atkins, J.L. (2015). *Muscle loss and obesity: the health implication of sarcopenia and sarcopenic obesity. Proc. Nutr. Soc.* 74: 405–412.

10. Menna Barreto, A. et al. (2019). *Sarcopenia and its components in adult renal transplant recipients: prevalence and association with body adiposity. Br. J. Nutr.* 122: 1386–1397.

11. Mangi, A.A., Christison-Lagay, E.R., and Torchiana, D.F. (2005). *Gastrointestinal complications in patients undergoing heart operations: an analysis of 8709 consecutive cardiac surgical patients. Ann. Surg.* 241: 895–904.

12. Chor, C.Y.T. et al. (2020). *Gastrointestinal complications following cardiac surgery. Asian. Cardiovascul. Thor. Ann.* 28: 621–632.

13. Ohri, S.K. and Velissaris, T. (2006). *Gastrointestinal dysfuntion following cardiac surgery. Perfusion* 21: 215–223.

14. Zogheib, E., Cosse, C., Sabbagh, C. et al. (2018). *Biological scoring system foe early prediction of acute bowel ischemia after cardiac surgery: the PALM score. Ann. Intensive Care.* 8: https://doi.org/10.1186/s13613-018-0395-5.

15. Compher, C., Bingham, A.L., and McCall, M. (2022). *Guidelines for the provision of nutrition support therapy in the adult critically ill patient: the American Society for Parenteral and Enteral Nutrition. J. Enter. Parent. Nutr.* 46: 159–211.

16. McGrath, E.E., Blades, Z., and Anderson, P.B. (2010). *Chylothorax: aetilology, diagnosis and therapeutic options. Respir. Med.* 104: 1–8.

17. Pillay, A. and Ataya, E. (2016). *A review of traumatic chylothorax. Injury* 47 (4): 545–550.

18. Riley, E. and Ataya, A. (2019). *Clinical approach and review of causes of a chylothorax. Res. Med.* 157: 7–17.

19. Srinam, K., Meguid, R., and Meguid, M. (2016). *Nutritional support in adults with chyle leaks. Nutrition* 32 (2): 281–286.

20. Schild, H., Strassburg, C., and Kalff, J. (2013). *Treatment options in patients with chylothorax. Deutsch. Arzteblatt. Int.* 110 (48): 819–826.

21. Steven, S. and Carey, B.R. (2015). *Nutritional management in patients with chyle leakage: a systematic review. Eur. J. Clin. Nutr.* 69: 776–780.

22. Maldonado, F., Cartin-Ceba, R., Hawkins, F., and Ryu, J. (2010). *Medical and surgical management of chylothorax and associated outcomes. Am. J. Med. Sci.* 339 (4): 314–318.

23. Ismail, G.J. and Dunning, J. (2015). *The use of octeotride in the treatment of chylothorax following cardiothoracic surgery. Inter. Cardiovascul.Thorac. Surg.* 20 (6): 848–854.

24. Matsumoto, T., Yamagami, T., Kato, T. et al. (2009). *The effectiveness of lymphangiography as a treatment method for various chyle leakages. Bri. J. Radiograph.* 82 (976): 286–290.

25. Musa-Veloso, K., Poon, T.H., Elliot, J.A., and Chung, C. (2011). *A comparison of the LDL-cholesterol lowering efficacy of plant stanols and plant sterols over a continuous dose range: results of a meta-analysis of randomized, placebo-controlled trials. Prostagland. Leukot. Essent. Fatty Acids* 85 (1): 9–28.

26. FLJ, V., Mach, F., Smulders, Y.M. et al. (2021). *ESC guidelines on cardiovascular disease prevention in clinical practice. Eur. Heart J.* 42: 3227–3337.

27. Franz, M.J., Boucher, J.L., Rutten-Ramos, S., and Van Wormer, J.J. (2015). *Lifestyle weight-loss intervention outcomes in overweight and obese adults with type 2 diabetes: a systematic review and meta-analysis of randomized clinical trials. J. Acad. Nutr. Diet.* 115 (9): 1447–1463.

28. Ambrosetti, M., Abreu, A., Corrà, U. et al. (2020). *Secondary prevention through comprehensive rehabilitation: from knowledge to implementation. Eur. J. Prevent. Cardiol.* 28 (5): 460–495.

29. NACR (2019). *The National Audit of Cardiac Rehabilitation Annual Statistical Report 2019.* London: British Heart Foundation.

30. Christie, J.D., Edwards, L.B., Kucheryavaya, A.Y. et al. (2012). The Registry of the International Society for Heart and Lung Transplantation: 29th adult lung and heart-lung transplant report—2012. *J. Heart Lung Transplant.* 31 (10): 1073–1086.

31. Stehlik, J., Edwards, L.B., Kucheryavaya, A.Y. et al. (2012). The Registry of the International Society for Heart and Lung Transplantation: 29th official adult heart transplant report—2012. *J. Heart Lung Transplant.* 31 (10): 1052–1064.

32. Pham, P.T.T., PMT, P., Pham, S.V. et al. (2011). New onset diabetes after transplantation (NODAT): an overview. *Diab. Metab. Synd. Obes.* 4: 175–186.

33. Ndanuko, R.N., Tapsell, L.C., Charlton, K.E. et al. (2016). Dietary patterns and blood pressure in adults: a systematic review and meta-analysis of randomized controlled trials. *Adv. Nutr.* 7 (1): 76–89.

34. Filippou, C.D., Tsioufis, C.P., Thomopoulos, C.G. et al. (2020). Dietary approaches to stop hypertension (DASH) diet and blood pressure reduction in adults with and without hypertensions: a systematic review and meta-analysis of randomized controlled trials. *Adv. Nutr.* 11 (5): 1150–1160.

35. Jomphe, V., Lands, L.C., and Mailhot, G. (2018). Nutritional requirements of lung transplant recipients: challenges and considerations. *Nutrients* 10 (6): 790.

36. Dyson, P.A., Twenefour, D., Breen, C. et al. (2011). Diabetes UK evidence-based nutrition guidelines for the prevention and management of diabetes. *Diab. Med.* 28: 1282–1288.

37. Han, S., Jiao, J., Xu, J. et al. (2016). Effects of plant stanol or sterol-enriched diets on lipid profiles in patients treated with statins: a systematic revie and meta-analysis. *Sci. Rep.* 6: 31337.

38. Banner, N.R. (2009). Chronic kidney disease after heart transplant. *Nephro. Dial. Transplant.* 24 (5): 1655–1662.

39. Roest, S., Hesselink, D.A., Kimczak-Tomaniak, D. et al. (2020). Incidence of end-stage renal disease after heart transplant and effects of its treament on survival. *ESC Heart Fail.* 7: 533–541.

40. Hasse, J.M. and Matarese, L. (2012). Solid organ transplantation. In: *The ASPEN Adult Nutriton Support Core Curriculum*, 2e (ed. C. Mueller, S. McClave, and J.M. Kuhn), 523–557. Silver Spring, MD: American Society for Parenteral and Enteral Nutrition.

41. Early, C., Stuckey, L., and Tisher, S. (2016). Osteoporosis in the adult solid organ transplant population: underlying mechanisms and available treatment options. *Osteoporos. Int.* 27 (4): 1425–1440.

42. Adami, G. and Saag, K.G. (2019). Glucocorticoid-induced osteoporosis. *Osteoporos. Int.* 30 (6): 1145.

43. Lowery, E.M., Bemiss, B., Cascino, T. et al. (2012). Low vitamin D levels are associated with increased rejections and infections after lung transplantation. *J. Heart Lung Transplant.* 31: 700–707.

44. Verleden, S.E., Vos, R., Geenens, R. et al. (2012). Vitamin D deficiency in lung transplant patients: is it important? *Transplantation* 93: 224–229.

# Nutritional Management of the Surgical Patient: Oesophago-gastric Surgery

Charles Rayner[1] and Fiona Huddy[2]

[1] Department of Surgery, Royal Surrey NHS Foundation Trust, Guildford, UK
[2] Department of Nutrition and Dietetics, Royal Surrey NHS Foundation Trust, Guildford, UK

---

**KEY POINTS**

- Patients with oesophago-gastric pathologies are at high risk of malnutrition and require early assessment and nutrition support.
- Surgery-related complications have a significant impact on risk of malnutrition.
- Permanent anatomical changes to the gastro-intestinal tract have significant impacts on post-operative nutritional status in both the short and long term.
- Post-operative deterioration in nutritional status may be a combination of inadequate oral intake and a range of malabsorptive symptoms. Further research is required to evaluate this.
- Regular screening and assessment of nutritional status with appropriate intervention are effective tools in preventing and minimising dietary intolerances and manifestations of nutrient deficiencies.
- A specialist dietitian should be involved throughout the patient's journey.

---

Oesophago-gastric surgery concerns operative procedures, which may include laparotomy, laparoscopy, robotic, or a combination of techniques, for benign and malignant pathology of the oesophagus and stomach. It is well established that poor nutritional status is directly associated with adverse outcomes from surgery and this is particularly pertinent with oesophago-gastric pathologies, where there is a high incidence of nutritional deficit and malnutrition. These surgical procedures permanently change the structure and function of the gastrointestinal system and result in immediate and long-term nutritional complications. Integration of appropriate nutritional care into the overall management of patients undergoing oesophago-gastric surgery is of the utmost value: from diagnosis, through the treatment pathway, and in the longer term. This chapter will cover the more frequently occurring nutritional issues before and after oesophago-gastric surgery and strategies to manage them.

*Nutritional Management of the Surgical Patient*, First Edition. Edited by Mary E. Phillips.
© 2023 John Wiley & Sons Ltd. Published 2023 by John Wiley & Sons Ltd.

## COMMON OPERATIONS AND THEIR ANATOMY

### Oesophagectomy

Oesophagectomy performed for both malignant and benign disease is a complex surgical procedure requiring multiple operating fields, with high levels of peri-operative morbidity and mortality. Benign resection may be required due to caustic injury, recalcitrant strictures from gastro-oesophageal reflux, and benign neoplasm. Oesophagectomy is more commonly performed to treat oesophageal cancer or pre-malignant disease (such as high-grade dysplasia in the context of Barrett's oesophagus). There are two main subtypes of oesophageal cancer, squamous cell cancer (OSCC) and adenocarcinoma (OAC). Risk factors for OSCC include smoking, alcohol consumption, nutritional deficiencies, and low socio-economic status, while for OAC they are obesity, smoking, Barrett's oesophagus, male sex, a diet low in fruit and vegetables, and increasing age [1]. The classic presentation of oesophageal cancer is that of progressive obstructive dysphagia alongside a history of acid reflux for OAC or smoking/alcohol excess for OSCC, often accompanied by weight loss.

Depending on the type, location, and extent of the disease, the procedure may involve total or subtotal resection of the oesophagus, with or without dissection of regional lymph nodes. The surgical approach may involve a two-stage (Ivor Lewis; Figure 11.1), three-stage (McKeown), transhiatal, or left thoraco-abdominal approach with or without left neck anastomosis. Other options include using the small or large bowel as the conduit, but this will not be covered here in detail. The procedure is usually performed through two main incisions: one in the chest (thoracotomy) to mobilise the oesophagus and one in the abdomen (laparotomy) to dissect and prepare the stomach for oesophageal reconstruction. The tubularised stomach is pulled up into the chest to create a neo-oesophagus. The conduit is anastomosed onto the proximal oesophagus using either a stapling device or suture. The procedure may be carried out using an open or laparoscopic technique (minimally invasive oesophagectomy) or a combination of both. Surgical operating time is

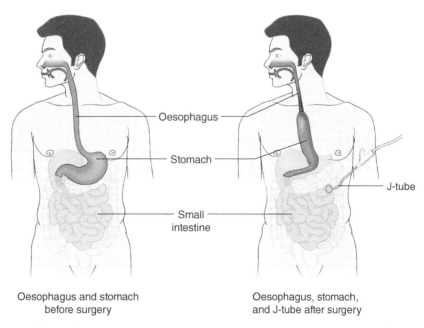

Oesophagus

Stomach

Small intestine

J-tube

Oesophagus and stomach before surgery

Oesophagus, stomach, and J-tube after surgery

**FIGURE 11.1**  Anatomy of an Ivor Lewis oesophagectomy with gastric conduit and insertion of a feeding jejunostomy (J-tube).

approximately seven hours and recovery routinely requires a stay in critical care. Since the adoption of enhanced recovery protocols, median total length of stay has reduced; however, a median of 12 days is reported by most units, for those with an uncomplicated recovery [2]. Reported complication rates after oesophagectomy are approximately 50%, with a 30-day mortality of 2% [1].

Additional procedures can be performed at the time of surgery to aid in nutrition post-operatively. Pyloroplasty increases the diameter of the pylorus to improve gastric emptying, due to the inevitable vagotomy that will have been performed during the operation causing gastric stasis. If this is not performed, patients can suffer from early complications such as aspiration, or experience later issues such as bloating, early satiety, and reflux. Some units also place a feeding jejunostomy or nasojejunal (NJ) tube at the time of oesophagectomy to help with enteral nutrition (EN) post-operatively; the rationale for this is discussed later in this chapter.

## Gastrectomy – Total or Subtotal

Removal of part of or the whole stomach can be performed for both malignant and benign conditions. The major risk factors for gastric cancer are *Helicobacter Pylori* infection, smoking, a diet high in salty or preserved foods, and pernicious anaemia [3]. *H. Pylori* infection can now be treated with antibiotics in conjunction with proton pump inhibitors (PPIs). This has led to a significant decrease in the incidence of gastric cancer in the last 30 years [4].

Total gastrectomy is usually reserved for malignant conditions and reconstruction is performed by anastomosing a Roux limb of jejunum onto the lower oesophagus. As with oesophageal cancer, those with potentially curable gastric cancer will usually undergo neo-adjuvant chemotherapy prior to surgery.

Multiple methods are described for subtotal gastrectomy, which can be performed for cancer, peptic ulcer disease (PUD), and obesity.

In cancer and PUD, the pathology needs to be locally confined for subtotal gastrectomy to be an option. In distal gastrectomy, the resection performed is consistent, but the reconstruction can vary [5]. There

are three main options for reconstruction of the gastrointestinal tract after subtotal distal gastrectomy:

- Anastomosing the duodenum to the stomach, keeping the tract in continuity; this is eponymously named Bilroth I.
- Anastomosing a loop of proximal jejunum onto the remnant stomach; Bilroth II.
- Roux-en-Y reconstruction, which involves a limb of jejunum anastomosed onto the stomach and then back onto the small bowel.

If the cancer is of the proximal stomach, then a proximal gastrectomy can be performed, with reconstruction either being with an oesophago-gastrostomy or interposing a section of jejunum between the oesophagus and the stomach (Merendino procedure) [6].

## Nutritional Optimisation and Prehabilitation

Patients with oesophago-gastric cancer and, perhaps to a slightly lesser extent, benign oesophago-gastric disease frequently present with nutritional deficits [7]. The physical impact of the disease can cause mechanical problems such as obstructive dysphagia and delayed gastric emptying, limiting nutritional intake for some time prior to diagnosis. In addition, patients with oesophago-gastric cancer are routinely referred for neo-adjuvant oncological treatment such as chemotherapy or chemoradiotherapy. Side effects from these treatments, such as nausea, vomiting, diarrhoea, mucositis, and inflammatory dysphagia, can further exacerbate nutritional deficit.

Pre-operative malnutrition is associated with higher rates of morbidity, including infection, delayed wound healing, and pulmonary complications (including acute respiratory distress syndrome and pneumonia), with associated increased mortality [7]. Early nutrition screening, assessment, and support from a specialist oesophago-gastric dietitian are essential to ensure that patients are in the best possible condition.

Strategies to support nutritional status should be tailored to a patient's clinical situation and may include EN support via a feeding tube (such as a NJ tube or jejunostomy), oral nutritional supplements, and/or strategies to optimise oral intake, including texture modification and food fortification. Gastrostomy tubes – percutaneous endoscopic gastrostomy (PEG) or radiologically inserted gastrostomy (RIG) – are generally avoided at this stage of treatment due to the risk that they may render the stomach unusable for the formation of the gastric tube at the time of oesophagectomy.

Pre-operative anaemia is common in oesophago-gastric cancer patients and is a risk factor in itself for a worse clinical outcome [8].

Recent studies have demonstrated that a more formalised prehabilitation programme can be beneficial for those undergoing abdominal surgery [9] and specifically for oesophago-gastric surgical patients [10]. This involves a multi-modal approach incorporating nutritional intervention, medical optimisation (e.g. glycaemic control, blood pressure control, smoking cessation, and alcohol reduction), psychological intervention (e.g. emotional stress reduction), and involvement in a structured and goal-directed exercise programme. Structured pre-operative verbal and written education to prepare the patient for surgery and recovery and manage their expectations has also been shown to accelerate hospital discharge (see Chapter 4).

## Post-operative Nutrition Support

Oesophagectomy, total gastrectomy, and to a lesser extent subtotal gastrectomy are invasive, complex, and long surgical procedures, and the patient's nutritional status deteriorates after surgery, making post-operative nutritional care very important.

Enhanced recovery protocols to provide goal-directed therapy utilising multi-disciplinary care to support and accelerate recovery from surgery are now commonplace in oesophago-gastric surgical units. The Enhanced Recovery After Surgery (ERAS) Society has published guidelines for best care for patients undergoing both oesophageal [11] and gastric resections [12]. Nutritional aspects of this can be summarised as pre-operative optimisation, pre-operative fluid and carbohydrate loading, and early initiation of EN support. Procedure-specific recommendations are summarised in Table 11.1 [1].

**TABLE 11.1**  Summary of enhanced recovery after surgery nutritional recommendations.

| | Gastric resection | Oesophageal resection |
|---|---|---|
| Pre-operative nutrition | Routine use of pre-operative artificial nutrition is not warranted<br>Significantly malnourished patients should be optimised with oral supplements and enteral nutrition before surgery | Nutritional assessment should be undertaken for all patients<br>In high-risk cases enteral support is indicated |
| Pre-operative fasting and carbohydrate loading | Pre-operative fasting should be limited to 2 h for clear fluids and 6 h for solids<br>Pre-operative carbohydrate loading should be given to patients without diabetes | Prolonged fasting should be avoided and clear fluids including pre-operative high-carbohydrate drinks should be allowed until 2 h prior to surgery |
| Early post-operative diet and artificial nutrition | Patients undergoing total gastrectomy should be offered drink and food at will from post-operative day 1. They should be advised to begin cautiously and increase intake according to tolerance<br>Patients clearly malnourished or those unable to meet 60% of daily requirements by post-operative day 6 should be given individualised nutritional support | Early enteral feeding with target nutritional rate on days 3–6 should be considered<br>The ideal route of administration of enteral nutrition in the early post-operative period remains unclear |

Source: Adapted from [1].

Post-operatively, early EN is a cornerstone of the ERAS guidelines. While there is a consensus among oesophago-gastric teams that supporting nutritional intake post-operatively improves outcomes, the most effective route, type, and timing of nutrition support have not been determined and because of this practice differs considerably between units.

In order to protect the surgical anastomosis, because of the potential for delayed gastric emptying and post-operative ileus and as a result of the altered anatomy, patients who have oesophago-gastric surgery often have a delay in recommencing oral intake and a prolonged period without adequate oral intake after surgery. It is generally well accepted therefore that patients require supplementary nutrition support. Options for nutrition support include oral feeding, EN support (via NJ tube or jejunostomy), or parenteral nutrition (PN).

Choice of nutrition support also differs depending on the extent of surgical resection; nutritional needs are greater in oesophagectomy and total gastrectomy. Following subtotal gastrectomy, oral intake generally resumes more quickly and there is less need for more invasive nutrition support strategies such as EN or PN.

EN is considered advantageous over PN for the following reasons: it maintains gut mucosal integrity, inhibits the cytokine response, reduces the secretion of stress hormones, inhibits bacterial translocation, has a decreased risk of complications, and is less expensive [13]. PN, however, avoids placing a strain on the anastomosis and reduces the risk of post-operative impaired gastrointestinal motility. Nutritional requirements are also reached more quickly as there is no delay relating to bowel function. PN is generally reserved for complications when access to the gastrointestinal tract is lost for more than seven days; however, many UK centres continue to use PN as a bridge to establishing oral intake.

Enteral access may be achieved through a surgically placed feeding jejunostomy or an NJ tube. A feeding jejunostomy is a tube that is percutaneously placed 30–40 cm after the ligament of Treitz into the proximal jejunum. Its use post-operatively requires careful management of the flow rate to ensure that patients do not develop diarrhoea or abdominal bloating/discomfort. Jejunostomy-related complications are generally mild, such as tube occlusion, catheter displacement, or local cellulitis at the site of insertion. More severe complications include leakage into the peritoneal cavity resulting in peritonitis, volvulus at the point of fixation to the anterior abdominal wall, or jejunal necrosis at the site of catheter insertion [14]. NJ tubes avoid some of the complications of feeding jejunostomies, but dislodgement can occur and limits the options for longer-term nutrition support in the event of a complication or continued nutrition support on discharge.

## Dietary Reintroduction

Due to concern about anastomotic healing, risk of aspiration pneumonia, and gastric stasis, oral feeding is often delayed during the first post-operative days. Recent research on the safety and impact of early oral feeding is conflicting, however, and has yet to demonstrate the nutritional adequacy of oral intake alone [15]. Most UK centres use a staged dietary reintroduction, starting initially with clear fluids, followed by free fluids then a puréed or soft diet, before building up to normal textures.

All surgical procedures for oesophago-gastric surgery involve permanent anatomical changes, altering the flow of diet through the upper gastrointestinal tract and reducing or removing gastric reserve. Subsequently patients are required to make significant changes to their dietary habits and eating patterns. Education on following a small but frequent meal pattern, using energy-dense foods and fluids, is essential to ensure that patients are able to optimise their oral dietary intake.

## NUTRITIONAL MANAGEMENT OF EARLY COMPLICATIONS

### Anastomotic Leak

Leakage from the oesophago-gastric anastomosis occurs in approximately 10% of patients after oesophagectomy [16]. Anastomotic leak after gastrectomy is a rarer event, but it should always be considered in the unwell patient post total or subtotal gastrectomy [17]. There are a number of factors that can lead to breakdown of the anastomosis [18], but the critical features that are relevant here are that it will result in an inflammatory/infectious insult to the patient who has just undergone major surgery, and lead to the loss of the oral route of feeding. Placement of an NJ tube or feeding jejunostomy allows for continued nutrition of patients and is critical. Therefore, if a feeding tube has not been placed at the time of the initial surgery, one should be placed now. If this is not possible then patients will require total parenteral nutrition (TPN) until the leak has healed and oral nutrition can be resumed.

## Chyle Leak

A critical component of the thoracic stage of oesophagectomy is ligation and transection of the thoracic duct as it travels superiorly, lying between the oesophagus and the aorta. The thoracic duct is the largest lymphatic channel of the body and it conveys lipid-rich lymphatic fluid, known as chyle, from the abdomen and chest back into the main circulation via the left subclavian vein. If the ligation of the duct is unsuccessful, then chyle can flow out of the duct into the chest; clinically this is often detected by the presence of a milky fluid within the chest drain. This is covered in more detail in Chapter 7.

Initial treatment is usually with modification of enteral feed to a product low in fat and where any fat content is medium-chain triglyceride based (MCT) [19], or if this is unsuccessful then PN should be used. In severe cases thoracic duct ligation or embolisation may be carried out in theatre.

## Post-operative Ileus

Post-operative ileus is a common stress response to major oesophago-gastric surgery, leading to abdominal pain, post-operative nausea and vomiting, and delay to oral intake. There is some evidence in abdominal surgery that chewing gum or coffee can reduce post-operative ileus by stimulating early recovery of gastrointestinal function, though most of the evidence exists for patients after caesarean

section or colorectal surgery [20]. Management of post-operative fluid, use of opioid analgesia, early mobilisation, and oral laxatives incorporated within an ERAS pathway are key to limiting the impact of post-operative ileus (see Chapter 20).

## Adjuvant Oncological Treatments

For oesophago-gastric cancer, patients' oncological treatment can continue after surgery, and their nutritional status may have negative impacts on their ability to tolerate this, meaning that treatment can be stopped early or not received. Nutritional issues can also worsen due to the side effects from treatment, including chemotherapy-induced nausea, vomiting, and anorexia.

## NUTRITIONAL MANAGEMENT OF LATE COMPLICATIONS

Permanent anatomical changes after oesophago-gastric surgery can cause symptoms from impaired gastrointestinal function that result in long-term persistent weight loss and malnutrition, with severe implications for quality of life and survival. Severe (>15% of pre-operative weight) and long-lasting weight loss can occur and patients frequently do not return to their pre-operative weight [21].

A key role in the clinician reviewing these patients is to identify the likely cause of these symptoms as they are often multi-factorial, with a number of different disorders contributing to these symptoms.

## Poor Oral Intake and Anorexia

There are many factors that can result in inadequate nutritional intake post oesophago-gastric surgery, including early satiety due to reduced gastric reservoir, altered or complete loss of appetite, changes to taste and smell, and post-prandial abdominal discomfort. The reduction in calorie intake can be drastic and may be the main factor responsible for weight loss.

Many patients report difficulty adapting to the required new eating habits, avoiding social situations that involve food to prevent the embarrassment of not being able to eat as much as their peers, and, without warning, vomiting if they have overeaten. Even at more than 10 years after surgery, some patients still experience symptoms that have impacts on their dietary intake [22].

Intensive dietetic counselling to support changes in dietary habits and making appropriate food choices is fundamental to managing the consequences of oesophago-gastric surgery. Feeding jejunostomy tubes are often used to provide nutrition support after discharge from hospital, and continued to offer supplementary nutrition support for patients undergoing adjuvant therapies. Jejunostomy feeding is of benefit in terms of weight preservation, but there is not yet data to support improved recovery, tolerance of adjuvant treatment, or improvement in quality of life [23]. Further research is required.

## Dysphagia Due to Anastomotic Stricture

Recurrent dysphagia symptoms can be worrying for patients, particularly those who presented with dysphagia prior to a cancer diagnosis. In patients with dysphagia, alongside local recurrence it is important to exclude anastomotic strictures, which affect up to a third of patients after surgery. In general terms the more proximal the anastomosis, the greater the risk of anastomotic stricture [24]. The presence of a stricture can limit dietary intake and patients should be advised to modify the texture of foods, focusing on high-calorie options while being investigated. Anastomotic strictures can be successfully managed by endoscopic dilatation [24].

## Dumping Syndrome

Normal flow of chyme out of the stomach into the duodenum is slow and well controlled. This gradual release allows the cells of the duodenum to sense the contents of the chyme and release hormones to control the release of digestive enzymes and modify absorption to maintain homeostasis. Oesophago-gastric surgery disrupts this process and leads to uncontrolled flow of foods into the small intestine.

This can lead to a constellation of symptoms that are collectively described as 'dumping syndrome' [25]. There are two main symptomatic categories:

- Early dumping syndrome is due to the presence of a large volume of hyperosmolar fluid in the duodenum, causing rapid movement of fluid out of the circulation and into the intestinal lumen. This is characterised by onset of symptoms directly after a meal such as nausea, diarrhoea, sweating, bloating, palpitations, and dizziness.
- Late dumping syndrome usually occurs more than one hour after a meal and is due to the inappropriate management of blood sugar, leading to a reactive hypoglycaemia. Symptoms include sweating, weakness, hypoglycaemia, and hunger.

A diagnosis of dumping syndrome should be clinically suspected following oesophago-gastric surgery with any of these symptoms. However, there are a number of potential causes for the symptoms falling under the umbrella of dumping syndrome that should be considered when investigating a patient.

A modified glucose tolerance test can be performed to definitively diagnose dumping syndrome, in which 75 g of glucose solution is consumed after an overnight fast. Haematocrit, blood pressure, pulse, and blood glucose levels are then checked every 30 min for 3 h. If there is a rise in haematocrit of >3% or elevation of the resting pulse rate by >10 beats per minute at 30 min, then the test should be considered positive for early dumping syndrome. The test is considered positive for late dumping syndrome in case of late (60–180 min after ingestion) hypoglycaemia (<50 mg/dl/2.8 mmol/l) [26].

Treatment of dumping syndrome should initially be attempted with dietary modifications such as eating little and often, with meals spread out across six periods of the day, reducing consumption of simple carbohydrates, and an absence of drinking fluids until at least 30 min after eating.

## Malabsorptive Syndromes

A number of malabsorptive syndromes are thought to cause gastrointestinal symptoms and contribute to macro- and micronutrient deficiencies. Malabsorption is hypothesised to have a complex and multifactorial aetiology in this setting. However, more research is required to fully evaluate the investigation and management of these syndromes and better understand the aetiology and impact on quality of life. The key malabsorptive syndromes seen after oesophago-gastric surgery are now discussed further.

## Pancreatic Exocrine Insufficiency

Pancreatic exocrine insufficiency (PEI) occurs as a result of loss of endogenous neuroendocrine signals that stimulate the release of digestive enzymes by the pancreas. The resultant symptoms include flatulence, diarrhoea, steatorrhoea, vitamin deficiencies (particularly Vitamin A, D, E, and K), and weight loss [26]. The diagnosis of PEI may be achieved by faecal elastase-1 measurement; however, sensitivity and specificity in patients with altered gastrointestinal anatomy are unclear.

PEI following gastrectomy is well recognised [27], although incidence following oesophageal resection is less clear. One study demonstrated that up to 16% of patients after oesophagectomy had faecal elastase-1 levels <200 µg/d, indicating mild to moderate pancreatic insufficiency [28].

Symptoms of PEI can be corrected with pancreatic enzyme replacement therapy along with dietetic counselling and micronutrient supplementation [26].

## Small Intestinal Bacterial Overgrowth

Small intestinal bacterial overgrowth (SIBO) occurs when changes in the bacterial colonisation of the small bowel alter its function and absorption. Development of bacterial overgrowth of the small intestine can occur many years following surgery on the upper gastrointestinal tract [29]. Symptoms include diarrhoea, bloating, pain, and borborygmi. SIBO may occur as a result of anatomical alterations, changes in intestinal motility, and/or diminished gastric acid secretion due to prolonged PPI use. Diagnosis should be considered on the basis of clinical presentation. Investigations to conclusively prove a diagnosis of SIBO can be difficult to achieve. Breath testing and endoscopic sampling of the small intestine can be attempted; however, they may well be inconclusive, especially if the reason for the SIBO is a blind loop of small bowel that is not easily accessible [29]. Treatment of SIBO should be centred on reversal of nutritional deficiencies and can be accompanied by a short course of antibiotics, although this may lead to further issues of dysregulation of the gut microbiome and so should be approached with caution.

## Bile Acid Malabsorption

Bile acid malabsorption (BAM) may result from vagal denervation, but also from disruption of the enterohepatic circulation of bile acids. Diagnosis can be made through the use of 23-seleno-25-homotaurocholic acid (SeHCAT) scan or trial with bile acid sequestrants. Drugs that may be helpful include aluminium hydroxide, budesonide, colesevelam, colestipol, and colestyramine [30].

If dietary intervention is required, advice to reduce dietary fat intake to 20% of total calories can be useful, but requires dietetic expertise, patient education, and supportive literature. Many patients with moderate/severe BAM will be deficient in trace elements and fat-soluble vitamins. These should be checked periodically and supplemented as appropriate [30].

## Micronutrient Deficiencies

Micronutrient deficiencies can develop months to years following resection and can result in deleterious clinical consequences. Nutrient deficiencies can be attributed to malabsorption, rapid gastrointestinal transit time, bacterial overgrowth, and insufficient oral intake [31].

Megaloblastic anaemia due to vitamin B12 deficiency is a common issue following gastric surgery [32]. Parietal cells of the body of the stomach release the glycoprotein intrinsic factor, which binds to vitamin B12 to allow absorption in the terminal ileum. Therefore, all patients who have undergone distal or total gastrectomy require intramuscular injection of vitamin B12 prior to discharge, and this should be continued at three-monthly intervals lifelong.

Malabsorption of dietary iron possibly results from a reduction of gastric acid secretion and bypassing of the duodenum, leading to iron-deficiency anaemia. Reduced gastric acidity impairs the conversion of non-haem iron into the more absorbable ferrous form [33]. In addition, rapid transit of food through the intestine allows for decreased time for absorption of iron. These factors along with decreased intake of foods that are good sources of iron contribute to high incidence of iron deficiency, occurring in 37% of people 48 months after surgery [33].

The prevalence of metabolic bone disease including osteoporosis is also high in oesophago-gastric surgery patients [34]. It is thought to be multifactorial, attributed to decreased intake of calcium, lack of vitamin D, and altered absorption. Therefore, taking calcium-rich foods such as milk, cheese, sardines, and dark leafy greens is encouraged, and surveillance of vitamin D, parathyroid hormone, and bone density assessment should be considered.

Currently, no universal guidelines for vitamin and mineral supplementation are available. Nonetheless, prophylactic supplementation with daily multivitamin and mineral tablets should be considered, along with periodic post-operative monitoring and correction of identified deficiencies.

## Oesophago-gastrectomy Case Study

| Patient | Mr A, age 73 yr |
| --- | --- |
| Presenting complaint | Progressive obstructive dysphagia, phlegm regurgitation, and weight loss |
| Past medical history | Type 2 diabetes mellitus – diet controlled<br>Atrial fibrillation |
| Social history | Lives with wife<br>3 grown-up children – all living locally<br>Retired banker |
| Investigations | Oesophago-gastro-duodenoscopy (OGD) – obstructing oesophageal lesion from 35 to 45 cm<br>Computed tomography (CT) – distal oesophageal thickening with local lymph node involvement<br>Positron emission tomography (PET) CT – fluorodeoxyglucose (FDG) avid distal oesophageal lesion with local lymph nodes, no distant metastasis<br>Endoscopic ultrasound (EUS) – oesophageal lesion including lymph node involvement from 28 to 46 cm uT3N2 (6 lymph nodes) |
| Oral intake | Progressive obstructive dysphagia for 3 mo. Currently managing smooth textures and liquids only<br>Breakfast: 1× low-fat yoghourt<br>Lunch: small bowl of soup<br>Evening meal: small bowl of soup and 1 scoop of ice cream |
| Anthropometrics | Current weight 79 kg, BMI 21.2 kg/m²<br>Pre-morbid weight 88 kg, BMI 23.6 kg/m²<br>Percentage weight loss 10.23% |
| Bowel function | Episodes of constipation, currently taking Laxido® (Galen Ltd., Craigavon, UK) with good effect |

| | |
|---|---|
| Diagnosis | uT3N2 oesophageal cancer. Staged to have operable disease |
| Surgical plan | Refer for neo-adjuvant chemotherapy followed by two-phase oesophago-gastrectomy<br>Nutritional optimisation<br>Refer for prehabilitation plan<br>Diabetic review to optimise diabetic control |
| Nutritional plan | In view of significant dysphagia and weight loss, for placement of feeding jejunostomy as part of staging laparoscopy<br>Dietary education to modify texture of diet and optimise oral dietary intake while limiting episodes of occlusion and regurgitation |
| Admission 1 | Admission for staging laparoscopy and feeding tube placement |
| Nutrition support | Oral intake: patient implementing advice to focus on high-calorie and protein-rich smooth diet and nutritious fluids. Current intake 750–1000 kcal/d<br>Supplementary EN support regimen target:<br>1000 ml Nutrison Energy Multifibre (Nutricia Clinical Care, Trowbridge, UK) with 2× 120 ml flushes<br>Providing 1530 kcal, 60 g protein, 1240 ml fluid |
| Outcome | Discharged home with supplementary nutrition support for monitoring throughout neo-adjuvant treatment |
| New diagnosis | Readmission for surgery. Planned procedure two-phase oesophago-gastrectomy<br>Commenced on standardised recovery pathway with nutrition support via jejunostomy while oral intake re-established |
| Long-term prescriptions | Daily multivitamin and mineral<br>PPI – lansoprazole 30 mg once daily before bed |
| Follow-up | 3-monthly multidisciplinary surgical follow-up for full clinical and dietetic assessment<br>Minimum of annual micronutrient and vitamin screening |

## Caustic Injury Case Study

| Patient | Miss B, age 34 yr |
|---|---|
| Presenting complaint | Caustic injury – intentional ingestion of sulfuric acid |
| Past medical history | Depression<br>No known allergies |
| Social history | No fixed abode. Traumatic childhood. No registered next of kin |
| Investigations | Intubated and emergency OGD – demonstrated significant damage to oesophagus and stomach |
| Oral intake | Currently nil by mouth (NBM) post surgery<br>No known record of pre-admission oral intake, assumed normal pre-admission intake |

| | |
|---|---|
| Anthropometrics | Current weight 85 kg – based on bed scales<br>No known or visible weight loss<br>Ulna length 30 cm giving an estimated height of 1.79 m<br>BMI 26.5 kg/m$^2$ |
| Bowel function | Assumed normal bowel function prior to admission |
| Diagnosis | Caustic injury management |
| Surgical plan | Emergency transhiatal oesophagectomy, total gastrectomy, oesophagostomy, duodenal debridement, and pancreatico-jejunostomy<br>Feeding jejunostomy placed |
| Nutritional plan | To support surgical recovery and meet nutritional requirements while oral intake restricted |
| Admission 1 | Recovering from surgery and stable on the ward<br>Weight reviewed 81.4 kg |
| Nutritional support | Nutrition requirements:<br>Energy (20–25 kcal/kg and 1.25 physical activity level [PAL]): 2035–2544 kcal<br>Protein (1–1.5 g/kg): 81–122 g<br>Fluid: 2442–2849 ml/d<br><br>Oral intake: NBM due to disconnected gastrointestinal tract<br>EN support: jejunostomy regimen to meet full nutritional and fluid requirements<br>Target regimen: 1500 ml Nutrison Energy Multifibre and additional 1100 ml fluid through flushes<br>Providing 2295 kcal, 90 g protein, 2600 ml |
| Outcome | Patient stabilised and discharged to nurse-supported environment while awaiting reconstruction |
| New diagnosis | Readmission for reconstruction: total pharyngo-laryngectomy and substernal colonic interposition<br>EN support via naso-enteric tube while oral intake re-established<br>Post-operative dietary recommendations:<br>Small but frequent meal pattern – aiming for 6 small meals a day<br>High-calorie and protein-rich food and fluid choices |
| Long-term prescriptions | Daily complete multivitamin and mineral |
| Follow-up | 3-monthly multidisciplinary surgical follow-up for full clinical and dietetic assessment<br>Minimum of annual micronutrient and vitamin screening |

## REFERENCES

1. Pennathur, A., Gibson, M.K., Jobe, B.A., and Luketich, J.D. (2013). Oesophageal carcinoma. *Lancet.* 381 (9864): 400–412.

2. NOGCA (2021). *National Oesophago-Gastric Cancer Audit Annual Report 2020.* London: Royal College of Surgeons of England www.nogca.org.uk/reports/2020-annual-report.

3. Van Cutsem, E., Sagaert, X., Topal, B. et al. (2016). Gastric cancer. *Lancet.* 388 (10060): 2654–2664.

4. Crew, K.D. and Neugut, A.I. (2006). Epidemiology of gastric cancer. *World J. Gastroenterol.* 12 (3): 354–362.

5. Weledji, E.P. (2017). The principles of the surgical management of gastric cancer. *Int. J. Surg. Oncol.* 2 (7): e11–e.

6. Gutschow, C., Schröder, W., Wolfgarten, E., and Hölscher, A. (2004). Merendino procedure with

preservation of the vagus for early carcinoma of the gastroesophageal junction. *Zentralblatt. fur. Chirurgie.* 129 (4): 276–281.

7. Mantziari, S., Hübner, M., Demartines, N., and Schäfer, M. (2014). Impact of preoperative risk factors on morbidity after esophagectomy: is there room for improvement? *World J. Surg.* 38 (11): 2882–2890.

8. Bootsma, B.T., Huisman, D.E., Plat, V.D. et al. (2018). Towards optimal intraoperative conditions in esophageal surgery: a review of literature for the prevention of esophageal anastomotic leakage. *Int. J. Surg.* 54 (Pt A): 113–123.

9. Gillis, C., Li, C., Lee, L. et al. (2014). Prehabilitation versus rehabilitation: a randomized control trial in patients undergoing colorectal resection for cancer. *Anesthesiology* 121 (5): 937–947.

10. Akiyama, Y., Sasaki, A., Fujii, Y. et al. (2021). Efficacy of enhanced prehabilitation for patients with esophageal cancer undergoing esophagectomy. *Esophagus* 18 (1): 56–64.

11. Low, D.E., Allum, W., De Manzoni, G. et al. (2019). Guidelines for perioperative care in esophagectomy: enhanced recovery after surgery (ERAS®) society recommendations. *World J. Surg.* 43 (2): 299–330.

12. Mortensen, K., Nilsson, M., Slim, K. et al. (2014). Consensus guidelines for enhanced recovery after gastrectomy: enhanced recovery after surgery (ERAS®) society recommendations. *Br. J. Surg.* 101 (10): 1209–1229.

13. National Institute for Health and Care Excellence (2006). Nutrition support in adults: oral nutritional support, enteral tube feeding and parenteral nutrition. Clinical guideline [CG32]. https://www.nice.org.uk/guidance/cg32. Accessed April 2021.

14. Spalding, D.R., Behranwala, K.A., Straker, P. et al. (2009). Non-occlusive small bowel necrosis in association with feeding jejunostomy after elective upper gastrointestinal surgery. *Ann. Royal Coll. Surg. of Eng.* 91 (6): 477–482.

15. Willcutts, K.F., Chung, M.C., Erenberg, C.L. et al. (2016). Early oral feeding as compared with traditional timing of oral feeding after upper gastrointestinal surgery: a systematic review and meta-analysis. *Ann. Surg.* 264 (1): 54–63.

16. van Workum, F., Verstegen, M.H.P., Klarenbeek, B.R. et al. (2021). Intrathoracic vs cervical anastomosis after totally or hybrid minimally invasive esophagectomy for esophageal cancer: a randomized clinical trial. *JAMA Surg.* 156 (7): 601–610.

17. Kamarajah, S.K., Navidi, M., Griffin, S.M., and Phillips, A.W. (2020). Impact of anastomotic leak on long-term survival in patients undergoing gastrectomy for gastric cancer. *Bri. J. Surg.* 107 (12): 1648–1658.

18. Makuuchi, R., Irino, T., Tanizawa, Y. et al. (2019). Esophagojejunal anastomotic leakage following gastrectomy for gastric cancer. *Surg. Today.* 49 (3): 187–196.

19. Moro, K., Koyama, Y., Kosugi, S.I. et al. (2016). Low fat-containing elemental formula is effective for postoperative recovery and potentially useful for preventing chyle leak during postoperative early enteral nutrition after esophagectomy. *Clin. Nutr.* (6): 35, 1423–1428.

20. Fitzgerald, J.E.F. and Ahmed, I. (2009). Systematic review and meta-analysis of chewing-gum therapy in the reduction of postoperative paralytic ileus following gastrointestinal surgery. *World J. Surg.* 33 (12): 2557–2566.

21. Baker, M., Halliday, V., Williams, R.N., and Bowrey, D.J. (2016). A systematic review of the nutritional consequences of esophagectomy. *Clin. Nutr.* 35 (5): 987–994.

22. Carey, S., Laws, R., Ferrie, S. et al. (2013). Struggling with food and eating–life after major upper gastrointestinal surgery. *Sup. Care Cancer* 21 (10): 2749–2757.

23. Paul, M., Baker, M., Williams, R.N., and Bowrey, D.J. (2017). Nutritional support and dietary interventions following esophagectomy: challenges and solutions. *Nutr. Diet. Suppl.* 9: 9–21.

24. Ahmed, Z., Elliott, J.A., King, S. et al. (2017). Risk factors for anastomotic stricture post-esophagectomy with a standardized sutured anastomosis. *World J. Surg.* 41 (2): 487–497.

25. van Beek, A.P., Emous, M., Laville, M., and Tack, J. (2017). Dumping syndrome after esophageal, gastric or bariatric surgery: pathophysiology, diagnosis, and management. *Obes. Rev.* 18 (1): 68–85.

26. Phillips, M.E., Hopper, A.D., Leeds, J.S. et al. (2021). Consensus for the management of pancreatic exocrine insufficiency: UK practical guidelines. *BMJ Open Gastroenterol.* 8 (1): e000643.

27. Straatman, J., Wiegel, J., van der Wielen, N. et al. (2017). Systematic review of exocrine pancreatic insufficiency after gastrectomy for cancer. *Digest. Surg.* 34 (5): 364–370.

28. Huddy, J.R., Macharg, F.M., Lawn, A.M., and Preston, S.R. (2013). Exocrine pancreatic insufficiency following esophagectomy. *Dis. Esophagus.* 26 (6): 594–597.

29. Brennan, M., Fanning, M., Granahan, A. et al. (2017). Small intestinal bacterial overgrowth in patients post major upper gastrointestinal cancer surgery. *Dis. Esophagus.* 30 (5): 1–7.

30. Gupta, A., Muls, A.C., Lalji, A. et al. (2015). Outcomes from treating bile acid malabsorption using a multidisciplinary approach. *Sup. Care Cancer* 23 (10): 2881–2890.

31. Janssen, H.J.B., Fransen, L.F.C., Ponten, J.E.H. et al. (2020). Micronutrient deficiencies following minimally invasive esophagectomy for cancer. *Nutrients* 12 (3): 778.

32. Hu, Y., Kim, H.I., Hyung, W.J. et al. (2013). Vitamin B(12) deficiency after gastrectomy for gastric cancer: an analysis of clinical patterns and risk factors. *Ann. Surg.* 258 (6): 970–975.

33. Lim, C.H., Kim, S.W., Kim, W.C. et al. (2012). Anemia after gastrectomy for early gastric cancer: long-term follow-up observational study. *World J. Gastroenterol. : WJG.* 18 (42): 6114–6119.

34. Rino, Y., Aoyama, T., Atsumi, Y. et al. (2022). Metabolic bone disorders after gastrectomy: inevitable or preventable? *Surg. Today* 52 (2): 182–188.

# CHAPTER 12

# Endoscopic Procedures and Their Implications for Nutrition

John S. Leeds

*HPB Unit, Freeman Hospital, Newcastle upon Tyne, UK*
*Population Health Sciences Institute, Newcastle University, Newcastle upon Tyne, UK*

---

**KEY POINTS**

- Endoscopic procedures can rapidly improve nutritional status in those with obstruction of the upper gastrointestinal tract.
- Care must be taken in placement of enteral feeding tubes following endoscopic necrosectomy or cyst-gastrostomy.
- Dietary modifications are required in both the short and long term following oesophageal or duodenal stent insertion.

---

Endoscopic procedures are commonly utilised in the management of patients with gastrointestinal diseases, both benign and malignant. Using endoscopy to aid in providing a tissue diagnosis has long been the modality of choice for most gastrointestinal diseases. The increasing use of endoscopy to provide therapy and sometimes curative treatments is perhaps best demonstrated in the area of pancreatico-biliary endoscopy. This chapter will explore both benign and malignant diseases of the upper gastrointestinal tract with respect to endoscopic interventions in patients with pancreatico-biliary diseases, and provide practical tips on the post-procedural management of enteral stenting.

The most commonly employed endoscopic procedures for pancreatico-biliary disorders are endoscopic ultrasound (EUS) and endoscopic retrograde cholangiopancreatography (ERCP). Both of these procedures have developed and progressed over the last few decades from being diagnostic tools to therapeutic interventions.

Well-established techniques surrounding oesophageal and duodenal stent insertion have a significant impact on nutrition, and practical suggestions on managing nutrition in these patients are discussed in this chapter.

While in the medical setting the role of the endoscopist is crucial in the insertion of gastrostomy feeding tubes in patients with neurological or gastrointestinal disease, management of these patients is outside of the scope of this surgical book. However, there are surgical implications of feeding tube placement that are discussed in this chapter.

## ENDOSCOPIC PROCEDURES

### Endoscopic Retrograde Cholangiopancreatography

ERCP is a commonly performed procedure, with most hospitals being able to provide this service [1]. It is now a purely therapeutic intervention, as diagnostic investigations including computed tomography (CT), magnetic resonance imaging (MRI), and EUS are used to identify the therapeutic target. ERCP involves passing an endoscope through the mouth into the duodenum to access the pancreatico-biliary system via the ampulla of Vater. To facilitate the procedure patients are placed in the 'swimmer's' position and sedated using intravenous agents. Once in the duodenum, various types of catheters can be employed to access either the bile duct or pancreatic duct and a guidewire placed. Different instruments are then used over the guidewire to deliver the desired therapy. The majority of therapies delivered via ERCP are for removing gallstones from the common bile duct, usually following ablation of the sphincter muscle by sphincterotomy [2]. This is achieved using balloons or baskets trawled down the bile duct and delivering the stones into the duodenum under direct vision. If the stones cannot be removed, then a plastic stent is inserted to maintain biliary flow and plans made for how the stones will be removed. In the case of malignant obstruction, sampling can be performed using a cytology brush or biopsy forceps and a metal stent inserted to allow longer-term drainage for relief of jaundice. Sometimes, ERCP is used to deliver therapy to the pancreas in the form of stone removal or stent insertion across a symptomatic stricture.

ERCP is not strictly a 'nutritional' intervention; however, treating the underlying pancreatico-biliary disease or relieving obstruction will have some secondary nutritional value. Patients with gallstones in the common bile duct often lose weight due to pain on eating or from episodes of cholangitis that cause acute admission with attendant catabolism. Similarly, patients with biliary obstruction very quickly become depleted in fat-soluble vitamins, as bile is required to facilitate emulsification of fat in the small intestine and subsequent absorption of lipids and the associated vitamins. Treating these pathologies endoscopically leads to improvement in symptoms and normalisation of biliary flow, thus restoring lipid digestion and preventing further electrolyte losses that occur with external biliary drainage (see Chapter 15).

Following gallstone removal at ERCP, the upper intestinal digestive processes should largely normalise. For patients with malignant obstruction, metal stents usually remain patent for six to nine months and can require reintervention [3]. However, for many patients the stent remains patent until their death. There are no specific dietary restrictions after ERCP, although patients who are unfit to undergo definitive treatment for gallstone disease may require a dietary fat restriction to try to reduce the formation of further stones. In this case care should be taken to ensure that adequate dietary energy and protein is achieved, as rapid weight loss may facilitate further stone formation, and fat-soluble vitamin supplementation may be necessary.

### Endoscopic Ultrasound

Ultrasound technology is a well-understood, non-ionising imaging modality that works best when the target is near to the probe. Transabdominal imaging of the retroperitoneal organs is especially difficult, as gas in the overlying intestine obscures the image. By combining ultrasound and endoscopy it is possible to obtain high-quality images of a number of organs in the upper intestinal tract and retroperitoneum. EUS is also useful for assessment of lesions in the mediastinum and has been used to stage oesophageal and gastric cancers. In addition to this, once a target organ or lesion has been identified, sampling can be undertaken in real time using a variety of different needles. EUS is now the modality of choice for sampling mass lesions in the pancreas, biliary tree, and retroperitoneum [4]. It is also possible to sample lesions in the mediastinum if in close proximity to the oesophagus and can obviate the need for surgical exploration or mediastinoscopy. This was originally performed using fine-needle aspiration (FNA), but in recent years adaptation of the needles has improved tissue quality significantly, so that this has been replaced by fine-needle biopsy (FNB) [5]. EUS FNB can also be used for benign indications such as diagnosing autoimmune pancreatitis and taking parenchymal samples from the liver [6, 7].

EUS has good sensitivity and specificity for detecting changes of chronic pancreatitis and is better than cross-sectional imaging in those with earlier stages of the disease [8]. EUS also has a higher sensitivity than MRI scanning for detection of stones in the common bile duct, especially those <6 mm. Essentially, if a structure is within 8 cm of the upper intestinal tract, then EUS is a good modality for assessment and biopsy.

## Cyst Drainage and Necrosectomy

One of the most rapidly expanding areas in endoscopy is therapeutic intervention and nowhere is this more apparent that in the field of EUS. One of the first interventional techniques was drainage of peripancreatic fluid collections, which was conventionally performed using standard endoscopes. EUS has revolutionised this practice by allowing clear visualisation of the cyst and puncture under real-time ultrasound, with the added advantage of using colour Doppler to avoid important vascular structures [9]. Development of fully covered metal stents such as the NAGI™ stent (Instrumed Surgical, Mississauga, ON, Canada) [10] allowed the endoscopist to tackle cysts containing solid material, especially infected walled-off necrosis following acute pancreatitis. Further modifications of these stents led to the development of lumen-apposing metal stents (LAMS). These stents create a wide opening between the stomach or duodenum and the collection,

similar to a surgical anastomosis, to facilitate high-volume drainage of the cavity. These stents are also wide enough to allow passage of a gastroscope through the stent into the cavity to facilitate debridement and irrigation. Since the advent of endoscopic drainage, very few patients now require surgical intervention of these collections [11].

While most patients are able to eat and drink following endoscopic necrosectomy or cyst-gastrectomy, nausea and anorexia are common, and patients may require supplementary enteral nutrition. Care should be taken when feeding tubes are placed to avoid placing the tip of the tube into the cavity. Naso-jejunal (NJ) feeding is typically recommended in this setting, and NJ tubes should be placed under direct vision, ideally before or at the time of endoscopic stenting to ensure appropriate placement.

## Biliary Access and Drainage

Desired duct cannulation is not always possible at ERCP and therefore other alternatives are required. Recent advances in EUS devices including LAMS have led to utilisation of this approach. EUS-guided biliary access can be used to facilitate ERCP by puncturing the bile duct from the duodenum and then passing a wire across the ampulla, which is then caught by the duodenoscope and standard ERCP continues. In some circumstances the ampulla is not accessible from the duodenum, for example in patients with duodenal obstruction due to a tumour, and EUS can then be employed to deliver a stent across the duodenum into the bile duct to allow biliary drainage (choldocho-duodenostomy) [12]. Similar techniques can also be applied from the stomach directly into the liver, either to access the biliary system or to place a stent (hepatico-gastrostomy) [13]. As with necrosectomy and cyst-gastrostomy, care should be taken over the placement of enteral feeding tubes in this setting, and for those with hepatico-gastrostomy, consideration should be given to the change in pH in the stomach due to the presence of bile. This may prevent the use of pH to determine the position of nasogastric feeding tubes.

## Facilitation of Endoscopy in Patients with Surgically Altered Anatomy

Perhaps one of the most novel uses of EUS is in patients who have had previous surgery meaning that their stomach or duodenum is not easily accessible, such as after Roux-en-Y gastric bypass. Using EUS guidance, a LAMS stent can be placed from the lower end of the oesophagus/stomach remnant to the gastric stump, thereby reconstituting the usual anatomical directions. Through this stent, other endoscopes can be passed that then allow performance of procedures such as ERCP to remove gallstones (this is the endoscopic ultrasound-directed transgastric ERCP or EDGE procedure) [13, 14]. Prior to this advance, patients either had to undergo further surgery, surgical-assisted ERCP, or percutaneous procedures [15]. Interestingly, one of the side effects of this procedure is weight gain due to the reversal of the gastric bypass.

## Endoscopic Ultrasound–Guided Gastroenterostomy

Gastric outlet obstruction occurs due to a number of upper intestinal malignancies, but also in pancreatitis. The nutritional deficits due to this condition are severe and it usually requires urgent treatment, which is mainly in the form of a gastro-jejunostomy. This is usually performed surgically (either open or laparoscopically), but such an operation can also take its toll on the patient. With the development of wide-bore LAMS, it is now possible to use EUS to identify a loop of small intestine from the stomach and then connect the two creating a gastro-jejunostomy [16]. This method has several advantages in that it does not involve a surgical insult, can be performed in a short period of time, leads to rapid symptom improvement, and does not have the issue of tumour ingrowth because the stent is not through the tumour. This is currently being evaluated compared to both surgical gastro-jejunostomy and endoscopic duodenal stent insertion [16, 17].

## Oesophageal Stent

Oesophageal stents are typically used in patients with strictures or tumours obstructing the oesophagus. They can be sited endoscopically or radiologically.

After oesophageal stent placement patients are typically nil by mouth for two to four hours and then start on liquids orally. Food must always be chewed well, and patients should avoid stringy vegetables, gristle on meat, hard lumps, or fresh bread (which expands on contact with liquid). Patients should sip fluids while eating to support the passage of food through the stent.

Malnutrition is common prior to oesophageal stenting due to difficulty or pain on swallowing, and liquid oral nutritional supplements are widely used to support patients both before and after stent insertion.

Patients should be counselled to sit upright while eating and to chew their food well. On occasion oesophageal stents can become blocked, and sips of fizzy drinks and walking around can help clear a blockage. If the stent cannot be unblocked at home using these techniques, admission is required for rehydration and endoscopic clearance of the blockage. If the blockage is caused by tumour eroding the stent, then further stenting or insertion of a gastrostomy feeding tube may be required [18]. On rare occasions perforation can occur at the site of stenting (see Chapter 11).

## Endoscopic Insertion of Feeding Tubes

The insertion of enteral feeding tubes using the endoscopic route has evolved over the last 40 years from the insertion of NJ and percutaneous endoscopic gastrostomy (PEG) to now include gastro-jejunostomy (PEG-J) tubes. The complication rate is relatively low, with an overall mortality of around 0.5% [19].

PEG-J tubes consist of the placement of jejunal extension tubes through a wide-bore PEG (typically CH18-20). While they are prone to the jejunal extension tubes migrating back into the stomach and are not considered as effective as surgical placement of a jejunostomy tube [20], they are an option for those considered unfit for surgical intervention.

Typically, the insertion of PEG tubes has been restricted by poor transluminal vision and concern regarding overlying structures (typically the colon or liver). The use of EUS has been demonstrated to support placement in some patients in whom standard placement has failed or is contraindicated [21].

Following PEG placement, patients typically start an infusion of water prior to feeding to ensure there are no immediate complications.

Pain or clinical deterioration after feeding warrants immediate cessation of feeding and CT imaging to ensure there is no evidence of perforation or misplacement. Transhepatic and transcolonic PEG placement is reported in the literature [21–24].

Detailed analysis of the placement and post-procedural care of PEG tubes is outside the remit of this book, but in the surgical patient care should be taken to ensure that percutaneous feeding tubes are not sited in circumstances where there are uncontrolled abdominal collections or where the patient is at risk of developing ascites.

## Duodenal Stent

Following duodenal stent placement, slow reintroduction of food is recommended, initially with liquids only as the stent expands into position. After two to three days the patient can begin to introduce soft, moist foods, working up to a well-chewed normal diet. Duodenal stents can become blocked and as such hard foods such as seeds, nuts, and crispy chips or biscuits and fresh bread (which typically expand on contact with liquid) should be avoided, and patients should ensure that they consume liquids with their meals. In the event of stent blockage, replacement is usually required. Duodenal stents effectively act like the 'overflow' in a bath, allowing emptying of the stomach when it reaches a certain level. The stomach often does not return to its normal level of function, as the degree of distension when it was obstructed can cause a permanent degree of gastroparesis and infiltrative tumours can destroy the nervous plexus that conducts the signal for peristalsis [25].

Many patients will have ongoing symptoms of reflux or delayed gastric emptying. Eating little and often, and sitting upright while eating and for an hour afterwards, can help reduce symptoms [26]. High-dose proton pump inhibitors and pro-kinetic medication play a key role in minimising ongoing symptoms.

Some patients never progress beyond liquids or very moist foods, and for those where disease treatment is planned, placement of an NJ tube at the same time as stent placement may support a more rapid nutritional recovery with less impact on performance status, thus facilitating earlier access to chemotherapy. In those approaching end-of-life care, oral intake to tolerance and for pleasure is usual practice.

## COMPLICATIONS

Most endoscopic procedures come with a degree of risk. Most have been developed to be a lower-risk alternative to major surgery, for which many patients would not be suitable.

EUS has a risk of causing bleeding and perforation at a rate of around 1 in 1000 for diagnostic procedures [27–29]. In those undergoing biopsy this is slightly higher, and for those having sampling of a pancreatic mass there is also a risk of developing post-biopsy acute pancreatitis. The exact rate of this is not known, but is around 1–2% [30–32]. A patient having a sample taken from a pancreatic cyst also has a risk of infection that is less than 1%. Many centres give a single intravenous dose of antibiotic prior to cyst puncture, but the evidence for this is minimal.

Therapeutic EUS comes with a higher risk of complications, mainly in the form of stent maldeployment, failure, and an increased risk of perforation. A recent UK study looking at choledocho-duodenostomy showed a 20% adverse event rate, although most were managed conservatively [12].

ERCP is perhaps the endoscopic procedure with the highest adverse event profile. Bleeding occurs in about 1% and is mainly following sphincterotomy. Perforation occurs in 1 in 500–1000 [33].

Infection (cholangitis) can occur in approximately 2% of patients after ERCP, often due to incomplete drainage of the biliary system.

The main and most feared complication is post-ERCP acute pancreatitis (see Chapter 13). This occurs in 2–10% overall, although some patient groups and types of procedure carry different risk profiles. Younger females with non-dilated bile ducts, patients with suspected sphincter of Oddi dysfunction, those with previous post-ERCP pancreatitis, patients undergoing choledochoscopy, and those having ampullectomy all have a higher risk of developing acute pancreatitis post ERCP [34]. Several measures are available to help mitigate this risk and include prophylactic stenting of the pancreas, rapid intravenous fluid infusion, and use of rectal non-steroidal anti-inflammatory drugs. All three of these interventions have individually been shown to decrease the risk of post-ERCP pancreatitis, but they are not suitable for all patients and the effects have not been shown to be additive [35].

## Managing Duodenal Perforation

If duodenal perforation is identified at the time of endoscopy, closure of the defect with clips can be attempted, but this is not always possible. Where perforation occurs after any upper gastrointestinal endoscopy, patients are placed nil by mouth and should receive parenteral nutrition until contrast studies demonstrate no further evidence of a leak. NJ feeding tube placement is not recommended, as the inflation of the stomach may result in widening of the perforation or tubes may be misplaced into the peritoneal cavity.

## LONG-TERM MANAGEMENT

For patients with benign diseases (particularly gallstones), there is often no long-term management required as the pathology is gone. For those with chronic pancreatitis, reassessment both clinically and endoscopically is required to determine the optimal intervention. Many of these patients are served well with surgical intervention and therefore require discussion in a multidisciplinary forum to offer best care (Chapter 13).

For patients with malignant disease in the pancreas and bile ducts, the prognosis at five years is dire, with many patients not surviving past 18 months. Reassessment is important, particularly to identify symptoms that might indicate stent occlusion, as this often leads to admission and marked morbidity, prevents delivery of chemotherapy, and can be fatal. Endoscopic reintervention to an occluded stent is usually straightforward and leads to rapid resolution of symptoms.

---

**Case Study**

A 53-year-old male presented to a local hospital with abdominal pain and 'coffee-ground' vomiting. No previous medical history, he consumes a moderate alcohol intake, and is a life-long smoker (20 cigarettes/d). Initial blood tests showed a C-reactive protein level of 6 mg/l (<10), a white cell count of $14.4 \times 10^9$ (4–7), and an amylase of 66 (<30). Upper intestinal endoscopy showed a grossly dilated and fluid-filled stomach (2.5 l aspirated) and a dilated first part of the duodenum, with severe narrowing at the D1/2 junction consistent with extrinsic compression. The endoscopist was concerned about some of the appearances in the distal stomach and took some biopsies. An NJ tube was placed to allow enteral

feeding. Biopsies were benign, demonstrating inflammation only. CT scanning showed a dilated stomach and first part of the duodenum due to compression by a 4.2 cm cyst arising from the head of the pancreas (Figure 12.1).

The patient was transferred to the regional pancreatic centre for further management. A further upper intestinal endoscopy was performed confirming a smooth stricture at the D1/2 junction and no other pathology. EUS was performed to assess the duodenum, pancreas, and cystic lesion (Figure 12.2). This showed an abnormal pancreas consistent with underlying chronic pancreatitis and duodenal stricturing secondary to a cyst arising from the head of the pancreas.

The cyst was drained using a LAMS in a transduodenal approach during the EUS procedure. The NJ tube was left in situ. Over the next three days the patient experienced rapid improvement in symptoms of pain and vomiting and underwent a repeat CT scan, showing complete resolution of the cyst with the LAMS in a good position (Figure 12.3). A barium swallow was performed to assess functional gastric emptying, which showed a now widely patent duodenum with transit of contrast into the distal small bowel. The patient continued to increase oral intake over the next few days, allowing for removal of the feeding tube and discharge home. A repeat endoscopy was planned for four weeks later to remove the LAMS.

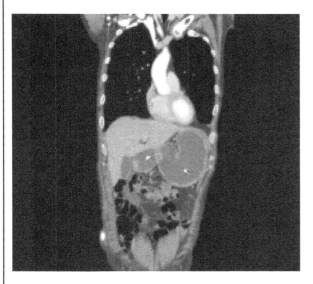

**FIGURE 12.1**  Coronal view computed tomography scan showing dilated stomach and first part of duodenum with previously placed naso-jejunal tube in situ.

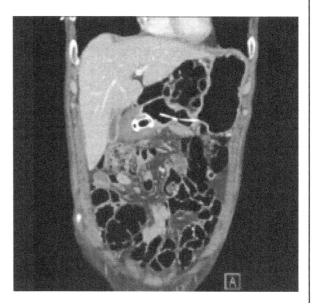

**FIGURE 12.3**  Computed tomography image demonstrating position of lumen-apposing metal stent in situ.

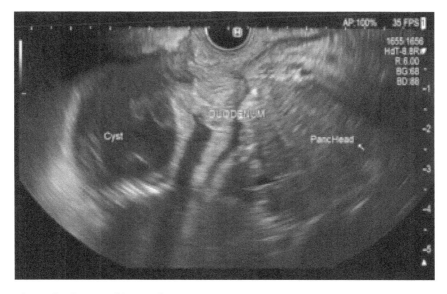

**FIGURE 12.2**  Endoscopic ultrasound image showing cyst.

# REFERENCES

1. Williams, E.J., Taylor, S., Fairclough, P. et al. (2007). Are we meeting the standards set for endoscopy? Results of a large-scale prospective survey of endoscopic retrograde cholangio-pancreatograph practice. *Gut* 56 (6): 821–829.

2. Testoni, P.A., Mariani, A., Aabakken, L. et al. (2016). Papillary cannulation and sphincterotomy techniques at ERCP: European Society of Gastrointestinal Endoscopy (ESGE) Clinical Guideline. *Endoscopy* 48 (7): 657–683.

3. Almadi, M.A., Barkun, A., Martel, M., and Plastic vs. (2017). Self-expandable metal stents for palliation in malignant biliary obstruction: a series of meta-analyses. *Am. J. Gastroenterol.* 112 (2): 260–273.

4. Pouw, R.E., Barret, M., Biermann, K. et al. (2021). Endoscopic tissue sampling – part 1: upper gastrointestinal and hepatopancreatobiliary tracts. European Society of Gastrointestinal Endoscopy (ESGE) Guideline. *Endoscopy* 53 (11): 1174–1188.

5. Oppong, K.W., Bekkali, N.L.H., Leeds, J.S. et al. (2020). Fork-tip needle biopsy versus fine-needle aspiration in endoscopic ultrasound-guided sampling of solid pancreatic masses: a randomized crossover study. *Endoscopy* 52 (6): 454–461.

6. Oppong, K.W., Maheshwari, P., Nayar, M.K. et al. (2020). Utility of endoscopic ultrasound-guided fine-needle biopsy in the diagnosis of type 1 autoimmune pancreatitis. *Endosc. Int. Open.* 8 (12): E1855–E1861.

7. Zeng, K., Jiang, Z., Yang, J. et al. (2022). Role of endoscopic ultrasound-guided liver biopsy: a meta-analysis. *Scand. J. Gastroenterol.* 57 (5): 545–557.

8. Issa, Y., Kempeneers, M.A., van Santvoort, H.C. et al. (2017). Diagnostic performance of imaging modalities in chronic pancreatitis: a systematic review and meta-analysis. *Eur. Radiol.* 27: 3820–3844.

9. Varadarajulu, S., Christein, J.D., Tamhane, A. et al. (2008). Prospective randomized trial comparing EUS and EGD for transmural drainage of pancreatic pseudocysts (with videos). *Gastrointest. Endosc.* 68 (6): 1102–1111.

10. Lakhtakia, S., Basha, J., Talukdar, R. et al. (2017). Endoscopic "step-up approach" using a dedicated biflanged metal stent reduces the need for direct necrosectomy in walled-off necrosis (with videos). *Gastrointest. Endosc.* 85 (6): 1243–1252.

11. Venkatachalapathy, S.V., Bekkali, N., Pereira, S. et al. (2018). Multicenter experience from the UK and Ireland of use of lumen-apposing metal stent for transluminal drainage of pancreatic fluid collections. *Endosc. Int. Open.* 6 (3): E259–E265.

12. On, W., Paranandi, B., Smith, A.M. et al. (2022). EUS-guided choledochoduodenostomy with electrocautery-enhanced lumen-apposing metal stents in patients with malignant distal biliary obstruction: multicenter collaboration from the United Kingdom and Ireland. *Gastrointest. Endosc.* 95 (3): 432–442.

13. van Wanrooij, R.L.J., Bronswijk, M., Kunda, R. et al. (2022). Therapeutic endoscopic ultrasound: European Society of Gastrointestinal Endoscopy (ESGE) technical review. *Endoscopy* 54 (3): 310–332.

14. Kedia, P., Tyberg, A., Kumta, N.A. et al. (2015). EUS-directed transgastric ERCP for Roux-en-Y gastric bypass anatomy: a minimally invasive approach. *Gastrointest. Endosc.* 82 (3): 560–565.

15. Dhindsa, B.S., Dhaliwal, A., Mohan, B.P. et al. (2020). EDGE in Roux-en-Y gastric bypass: how does it compare to laparoscopy-assisted and balloon enteroscopy ERCP: a systematic review and meta-analysis. *Endosc. Int. Open.* 8 (2): E163–E171.

16. Boghossian, M.B., Funari, M.P., De Moura, D.T.H. et al. (2021). EUS-guided gastroenterostomy versus duodenal stent placement and surgical gastrojejunostomy for the palliation of malignant gastric outlet obstruction: a systematic review and meta-analysis. *Langenbeck's Arch. Surg.* 406 (6): 1803–1817.

17. Khashab, M.A., Bukhari, M., Baron, T.H. et al. (2017). International multicenter comparative trial of endoscopic ultrasonography-guided gastroenterostomy versus surgical gastrojejunostomy for the treatment of malignant gastric outlet obstruction. *Endosc. Int. Open.* 5 (4): E275–E281.

18. Cancer Research UK. Oesophageal stent. https://www.cancerresearchuk.org/about-cancer/oesophageal-cancer/treatment/advanced-treatment/making-swallowing-easier/oesophageal-stent.

19. Hitawala, A.A. and Mousa, O.Y. (2022). *Percutaneous Gastrostomy and Jejunostomy*. Treasure Island, FL: StatPearls.

20. Haskins, I.N., Strong, A.T., Baginsky, M. et al. (2018). Comparison of laparoscopic jejunostomy tube to percutaneous endoscopic gastrostomy tube with jejunal extension: long-term durability and nutritional outcomes. *Surg. Endosc.* 32: 2496–2504.

21. Chaves, D.M., Kumar, A., Lera, M.E. et al. (2008). EUS-guided percutaneous endoscopic gastrostomy for enteral feeding tube placement. *Gastrointest. Endosc.* 68: 1168–1172.

22. Alley, J.B., Corneille, M.G., Stewart, R.M. et al. (2007). Pneumoperitoneum after percutaneous endoscopic gastrostomy in patients in the intensive care unit. *Am. Surg.* 73: 765–767.

23. Burke, D.T. and Geller, A.I. (2009). Peritonitis secondary to the migration of a trans-hepatically-placed percutaneous endoscopic gastrostomy tube: a case report. *Arch. Phys. Med. Rehabil.* 90: 354–357.

24. Chhaparia, A., Hammami, M.B., Bassuner, J. et al. (2018). Trans-hepatic percutaneous endoscopic gastrostomy tube placement: a case report of a rare complication and literature review. *Gastroenterology Res.* 11: 145–149.

25. Papanikolaou, I.S. and Siersema, P.D. (2022). Gastric outlet obstruction: current status and future directions. *Gut Liver* 16 (5): 667–675.

26. Pancreatic Cancer Action. (2017). Duodenal Stent. https://pancreaticcanceraction.org/about-pancreatic-cancer/treatment-options-for-pancreatic-cancer/treating-symptoms-of-pancreatic-cancer/duodenal-stent.

27. O'Toole, D., Palazzo, L., Arotcarena, R. et al. (2001). Assessment of complications of EUS-guided fine-needle aspiration. *Gastrointest. Endosc.* 53: 470–474.

28. Gress, F.G., Hawes, R.H., Savides, T.J. et al. (1997). Endoscopic ultrasound-guided fine-needle aspiration biopsy using linear array and radial scanning endosonography. *Gastrointest. Endosc.* 45: 243–250.

29. Eloubeidi, M.A., Chen, V.K., Eltoum, I.A. et al. (2003). Endoscopic ultrasound-guided fine needle aspiration biopsy of patients with suspected pancreatic cancer: diagnostic accuracy and acute and 30-day complications. *Am. J. Gastroenterol.* 98: 2663–2668.

30. Gress, F., Michael, H., Gelrud, D. et al. (2002). EUS-guided fine-needle aspiration of the pancreas: evaluation of pancreatitis as a complication. *Gastrointest. Endosc.* 56: 864–867.

31. Wang, K.X., Sun, S.Y., Sheng, J. et al. (2012). Incidence of hyperamylasemia after endoscopic ultrasound-guided fine needle aspiration of pancreatic lesions: a multicenter study from China. *Pancreas* 41 (5): 712–716.

32. Wang, K.X., Ben, Q.W., Jin, Z.D. et al. (2011). Assessment of morbidity and mortality associated with EUS-guided FNA: a systematic review. *Gastrointest. Endosc.* 73 (2): 283–290.

33. Williams, E.J., Taylor, S., Fairclough, P. et al. (2007). Risk factors for complication following ERCP; results of a large-scale, prospective multicenter study. *Endoscopy* 39 (9): 793–801.

34. Ding, X., Zhang, F., and Wang, Y. (2015). Risk factors for post-ERCP pancreatitis: a systematic review and meta-analysis. *Surgeon* 13 (4): 218–229.

35. Leerhøy, B. and Elmunzer, B.J. (2018). How to avoid post-endoscopic retrograde cholangiopancreatography pancreatitis. *Gastrointest. Endosc. Clin. N. Am.* 28 (4): 439–454.

# CHAPTER 13

# Pancreatitis

Mary E. Phillips

*Department of Nutrition and Dietetics, Royal Surrey NHS Foundation Trust, Guildford, UK*

---

**KEY POINTS**

- Malnutrition is common in severe acute pancreatitis and early enteral feeding is crucial.
- Peptide, medium-chain triglyceride enteral feeds should be first line.
- Multidisciplinary management of chronic pancreatitis is required to ensure all lifestyle factors, malnutrition, and pain control are optimised.
- Pancreatic exocrine insufficiency is common in both acute and chronic pancreatitis and requires treatment with pancreatic enzyme replacement therapy.

---

## TYPES OF PANCREATITIS

Pancreatitis is a benign inflammatory condition. It can be acute or chronic, and both have significant nutritional consequences.

## Acute Pancreatitis

Acute pancreatitis (AP) typically presents with abdominal pain, usually in the epigastric region; it can radiate into the back and usually has a rapid onset. Patients normally present to the emergency department with acute abdominal pain, often requiring opiates. AP may be mild, moderately severe, or severe [1], with predictive scores typically based on the impact pancreatitis has on the other organs of the body and on the severity of the systemic inflammatory response syndrome [1, 2].

Most cases of AP are caused by gallstones or alcohol excess, with less frequent causes including endoscopic retrograde cholangiopancreatiography (ERCP), hypertriglyceridaemia, hypercalcaemia, malignancy, trauma, autoimmune causes, or genetic mutations. In some regions tropical pancreatitis or pancreatitis induced by scorpion bites may occur. It is important that the cause of AP is determined and that treatment, such as laparoscopic

*Nutritional Management of the Surgical Patient*, First Edition. Edited by Mary E. Phillips.

cholecystectomy, is prompt to reduce the risk of recurrent episodes [3].

Most cases are mild, and resolve spontaneously with supportive treatment, but in very severe AP mortality can be as high as 50%. In some cases, patients can have multiple episodes of AP, this is referred to as recurrent acute pancreatitis (RAP).

## Chronic Pancreatitis

Chronic pancreatitis (CP) is progressive fibrosis within the gland. Calcification occurs and this can obstruct the pancreatic duct, causing pain. As the condition evolves, healthy pancreatic tissue is replaced with fibrotic tissue and the function of the pancreas deteriorates. CP is caused by excess alcohol intake in >80% of cases, with other causes include smoking, autoimmune causes, and genetic mutations such as SPINK 1, CFTR, and PRSS [4]. Patients often experience significant and progressive abdominal pain; diabetes and pancreatic exocrine insufficiency (PEI) are common. Patients can develop duodenal stenosis resulting in delayed gastric emptying, recurrent admissions, and malabsorption, and can develop significant malnutrition. Patients with some genetic mutations have a higher risk of developing pancreatic cancer.

## Acute on Chronic Pancreatitis

Patients with CP can develop AP, usually as a result of obstruction of the pancreatic duct, or following consumption of alcohol. In this instance there is likely to be significant underlying malnutrition prior to onset of the acute illness.

## SURGICAL PROCEDURES FOR ACUTE PANCREATITIS

Undertaking a laparotomy is an absolute last resort in AP. Clinical practice has evolved due to the high mortality associated with open procedures. Over the last 20 years practice has developed through the use of minimally invasive procedures and the majority of interventions are now radiological or endoscopic.

## Drainage of Collections/Necrosectomy

Patients with severe acute pancreatitis (SAP) can often develop collections of fluid within the abdomen, which over time can organise into a drainable collection (see Figure 13.1). Large collections can compress the duodenum causing gastric outflow obstruction, compress the bile ducts resulting in jaundice, or in some cases cause portal vein occlusion. These collections can become infected, and can also contain a solid component of necrotic pancreatic tissue. It is important to know that many large fluid collections can take weeks to mature to a point where it is appropriate to drain them, so conservative management in the meantime must include appropriate nutritional intervention.

Management of choice is endoscopic [4], with endoscopists inserting stents from collections into the stomach (see Chapter 12) and carrying out necrosectomy (removal of dead tissue) through stents directly into the stomach. However, these endoscopic procedures are typically only available in specialist centres, and while there is a drive towards remote management of patients with SAP under the supervision of specialist centres, this is not yet in place in every area [5]. Radiological placement of drains, either through the flank or transgastrically, is the second-best option, as this can be associated

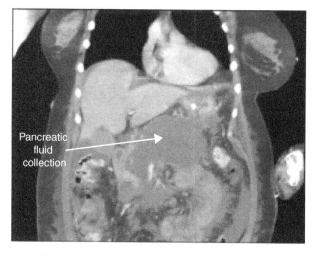

**FIGURE 13.1** Computed tomographic image of extensive pancreatic collection.

with prolonged length of stay and an increased risk of fistula development.

## Embolisation

In some cases pancreatic fluids can erode blood vessels, causing bleeding. This is typically managed with embolisation under the care of an interventional radiologist. The internal bleeding associated with this usually has a rapid onset and this is an emergency procedure.

## Laparoscopic Cholecystectomy

Laparoscopic cholecystectomy is a common operation undertaken by most general surgeons, and should ideally be carried out during the index admission in patients with AP or cholecystitis [5]. In SAP, it is necessary for the patient to recover prior to undertaking surgery. Laparoscopic cholecystectomy means it is less likely that patients will experience a further episode of gallstone pancreatitis, although stones can be retained within the bile duct. If this is suspected an on-table cholangiogram (OTC) may be carried out.

## Other Surgical Procedures

Occasionally SAP can result in damage to other tissues, and in the presence of necrosis of these organs resection may be necessary. This can include the colon or spleen. Occasionally, when patients have had a prolonged episode of pancreatitis adhesions can form, and procedures such as gastro-jejunostomy can be necessary (see Chapter 14).

## SURGICAL PROCEDURES FOR CHRONIC PANCREATITIS

Surgical procedures for chronic pancreatitis fall into two categories: drainage or resection. Drainage procedures such as the Frey procedure or lateral pancreatico-jejunostomy (LPJ) work by allowing the pancreatic duct to drain laterally into a limb of small bowel, and symptoms of ductal obstruction should

resolve. Resection is warranted when it is not possible to drain the gland, or where there is an underlying genetic cause that increases the risk of developing pancreatic cancer, in which case a total pancreatectomy (with or without islet cell transplantation) may be considered [6]. See Chapter 14 for more information on the management of pancreatic resection.

## NUTRITIONAL MANAGEMENT OF ACUTE PANCREATITIS

Patients with mild AP usually have a short hospital stay and with appropriate treatment of the cause (typically laparoscopic cholecystectomy or alcohol cessation) usually resolve without the need for any nutritional intervention. In moderately severe or severe disease, early nutritional intervention is essential.

## Timing of Nutritional Intervention

Meta-analyses have identified that early intervention with enteral nutrition (EN) is associated with reduced morbidity and mortality in SAP [7]. This is thought to be due to the infectious complications of SAP being linked to bacterial translocation, and thus the drive to use EN instead of parenteral nutrition (PN) is well established across all European and international guidelines [1, 4, 8].

## Route of Feeding

Practically, the question has been raised as to the route of EN. Historically patients were managed with PN or naso-jejunal (NJ) feeding [9], but over recent years naso-gastric (NG) feeding has become increasingly popular, as this is less invasive and tubes can be inserted easily at the bedside. Several trials have attempted to compare the outcomes of NG versus NJ feeding, but these are limited by inclusion of patients with mild/moderate pancreatitis and exclusion of those with severe disease, as well as inconsistency in descriptive terms with post-pyloric feeding, including proximal duodenal feeding considered as gastric feeding in some studies and jejunal in others [10–12].

However, these studies were consistent in their conclusion that, where tolerated, NG feeding is safe in AP. The decision over the route of feeding should be a clinical one, with patients who cannot tolerate NG feeding, show signs of developing gastric outflow obstruction, or have significant inflammation in the head of the pancreas, and therefore likely to develop extrinsic duodenal compression, recommended for NJ feeding. The earlier in the disease process NJ tubes are inserted, the less difficult the procedure is.

In some cases it is not possible to insert an NG or NJ feeding tube, such as where patients are receiving non-invasive ventilation or are unable to lie flat without desaturating. Patients with SAP may also develop a paralytic ileus, and in both these instances PN should be used. In this instance there is evidence that intravenous glutamine may improve outcomes [8, 13].

## Formulation of Enteral Feed

Historically peptide/semi-elemental feeding was recommended for patients with SAP as it was assumed that malabsorption would occur [14]. More recent guidelines have suggested that polymeric feeding should be first line [8]. The data used to inform these guidelines compared polymeric feeds with immune-nutrition feeds containing arginine, glutamine, and omega-3 [15], whereas other trials only explored surgical outcomes, without any nutritional considerations [16].

It is vital to consider that these recommendations are based on trials comparing EN with PN, and there is only one small pilot study comparing peptide with polymeric feeding [17]. This study did not demonstrate any change in bowel function, leading to the conclusion that there was no difference between the two study arms. However, stool losses were only assessed over 24 hours, there was significantly less weight loss and a shorter length of stay in patients receiving peptide feeding, suggesting that there is nutritional and functional benefit to peptide feeding [17]. Historically there has been concern that polymeric feeding may stimulate the pancreas, worsening inflammation, but pancreatic stimulation has been found to be associated with the delivery of nutrition into the proximal bowel, rather than with the type of nutrition infused [18].

Current European guidelines state that polymeric feeding should be first line and peptide used if this is not tolerated [8], whereas UK guidelines recommend peptide feeds as first line [19]. Clinically it is difficult to determine if a feed is well tolerated in patients who are acutely unwell with SAP due to the effect of antibiotics, opiates, and oedema on bowel function; the presence of intra-abdominal collections; the influence of peripheral oedema and ascites on body weight; and the effect of prolonged catabolic state, use of paralytics, and sedation on muscle function tests. Therefore, most experienced clinicians feel it is safer to use a peptide feed as first line [20].

## Probiotics

Probiotics are contraindicated in AP. While the evidence base for this is low, a large clinical trial (n = 153) demonstrated increased mortality (relative risk 2.53) in the intervention arm [21], and while there were concerns over the design of this trial, and emerging data to support the use of pro-biotics, Safety data needs to be more consistent before a strong recommendation can be made.

## Oral Diet

Patients with AP should not be restricted from eating unless there is a specific reason for doing so [4]. In some cases there may be a query over a differential diagnosis of a duodenal perforation, or the patient may be vomiting and at risk of aspiration; in these instances it is absolutely appropriate to keep the patient nil by mouth.

Once an oral diet is resumed, there is very limited data to suggest how this should be carried out. Most clinicians believe that low-fat foods should be tried first, but evidence is only available for the introduction of soft foods [8], which appear to be well tolerated. In patients with mild pancreatitis and dyspepsia, there is low-level evidence for a low-fat diet initially [22].

## Pancreatic Exocrine Insufficiency

PEI is common after AP with a prevalence of >60–80% of patients with SAP, and 13–39% in those with mild disease [23, 24]. Due to the complexity of determining the presence of PEI, and the detrimental effect of untreated PEI, all patients with SAP should start pancreatic enzyme replacement therapy (PERT) as soon as they begin eating. This should be continued until they are fully recovered. At this stage a pancreatic function test can be carried out to determine if there is a need to continue with PERT in the long term [19]. PERT should be managed in the same manner as for chronic pancreatitis (see later).

## Diabetes

The incidence of type 3c diabetes is approximately 40% after an episode of AP [25]. Careful blood glucose monitoring is essential during the acute management, as diabetes can develop at any stage in their admission. Erratic oral intake, nil-by-mouth times, inflammation, and infection all contribute to poor glycaemic control, and early involvement of the diabetes team is crucial.

## Lifestyle Advice

People who have recovered from SAP should be advised to avoid alcohol and smoking. Those who have developed diabetes should follow national diabetes recommendations for regular clinical review and optimisation of glycaemic control.

## NUTRITIONAL MANAGEMENT OF CHRONIC PANCREATITIS

There is limited data on the impact of nutritional intervention in the long-term management of CP, except that regardless of whether the intervention is dietary supplementation, enteral feeding, or additional support with PERT, patients who receive an intervention improve, and those who do not deteriorate [26].

## Nutritional Assessment

Nutritional assessment needs to be holistic in patients with CP, taking into account the management of diabetes, malabsorption, and the impact of pain, delayed gastric emptying, and abdominal collections. Micronutrients and bone health also need to be considered, and for these reasons standard nutritional screening tools such as the malnutritional universal screening tool (MUST) are unlikely to detect problems in this cohort (Table 13.1).

**TABLE 13.1** Considerations for nutritional screening in patients with pancreatic disease.

| Anthropometry | Biochemical | Clinical | Diet and lifestyle |
|---|---|---|---|
| Body weight changes Handgrip strength Physical function tests (6-min walk; sit to stand) | Glycaemic control Iron Studies Faecal elastase Fat-soluble vitamins Trace elements Parathyroid hormone C-reactive protein | Presence of:<br>• Calcification<br>• Necrosis<br>• Pseudocyst<br>• Pancreatic atrophy<br>• Obstructed pancreatic duct<br>• Evidence of gastroparesis/ outflow obstruction<br>• Malignancy<br><br>Treatment considerations:<br>• Opioids<br>• Laxatives<br>• Prokinetic<br>• Enzymes<br>• Insulin<br>• Oral hypoglycaemic agents<br>• Proton pump inhibitor/H2 Antagonist | Evidence of food avoidance (fat) Balanced diet Adequate energy and protein Alcohol intake Smoking status Diabetes restrictions Avoidance of fatty liver |

Source: Adapted from [27].

## Oral Diet

There is much debate on the role of dietary restrictions in CP. While high-fat diets are associated with a younger onset of disease [28], they are not associated with worsening symptoms, and in fact a randomised control study examining the outcomes of nutritional supplementation or food fortification in a cohort of patients with CP found that improvements in nutritional status, even though this included the addition of high-fat supplements and fat-containing foods, was associated with improved pain control [29]. Most clinicians support a 'fat to tolerance' approach. Clinically, there is an incidence of bile acid malabsorption in CP that may affect tolerance of dietary fat. It is unknown whether this is due to the CP itself, as there are links in cystic fibrosis [30] and after pancreatic surgery [31], or due to the high prevalence of cholecystectomy in this cohort. Investigation for bile salt malabsorption should take place in patients not tolerating dietary fat, and if confirmed they should be treated with bile acid sequestrants [32].

While normal healthy eating–style dietary composition is recommended in those with CP without malnutrition [8], clinicians should be aware that pancreatic enzymes may be less effective in those taking very high-fibre diets [33].

Where malnutrition is present, a dietary pattern of little and often with high-energy, high-protein foods supplemented with PERT is recommended. There is insufficient evidence to support the use of medium-chain triglyceride (MCT) supplements as first line [8], but if polymeric oral nutritional supplements (taken with high-dose PERT) are not tolerated, then peptide, MCT-based oral nutritional supplements can be tried.

In some cases there may be signs of delayed gastric emptying caused by duodenal stenosis, extrinsic compression, gastric stasis due to high-dose opioids, or poorly controlled diabetes, and in this instance a more liquid diet may be indicated. If this fails, jejunal tube feeding may be required.

## Tube Feeding

Tube feeding is safe and can be effective at reducing pain in patients with CP [34, 35]. In some instances, distal jejunal feeding can be used to ascertain if 'resting' the pancreas is effective at reducing pain. If so, this can help support the decision to undertake pancreatic surgery to try to optimise pain management [35].

## Pancreatic Exocrine Insufficiency

PEI is progressive in patients with CP, in terms of both onset and severity. Patients with symptoms of malabsorption should be treated promptly, with no need for pancreatic function tests. Where the diagnosis is unclear, a faecal elastase test should be performed [19]. Pancreatic enzymes should be taken with all meals, snacks, and oral nutritional supplements. Patients should be consented for the porcine natures of these products and doses escalated until symptoms are under control [19]. PERT should be swallowed with a cold drink, stored below 25 °C, and capsules distributed throughout meals [19].

## Diabetes

Pancreaticogenic (type 3c) diabetes is common in CP and progresses quickly, with 45% of patients on insulin within five years of diagnosis [36]. Type 3c diabetes differs from type 1 and type 2 diabetes, due to the lack of glucagon and the presence of exocrine failure. This results in a form of diabetes that is more brittle, and guidelines recommend that patients with CP are screened every six months, as there is an 80% lifetime risk of developing diabetes [4].

## Lifestyle Advice and Long-Term Follow-Up

Alcohol abstinence and smoking cessation are of vital importance in the long-term management of CP [37], with an increasing recognition that smoking increases the risk of developing diabetes and pancreatic cancer, in addition to worsening pain in patients with CP [38].

Patients with CP are at high risk of developing osteoporosis [39], and thus regular screening with dual-energy x-ray absorptiometry (DEXA) scans is recommended [4].

The prevalence of micronutrient deficiency (aside from vitamin D) is an area for future research, with limited information in the literature [40]. It is

---

### Case Study

A 58-year-old female presented to accident and emergency with acute-onset epigastric pain. On admission her amylase was 2500 U/l (reference range [RR] 30–110).

Her past medical history consisted only of asthma; she did not consume regular alcohol. An ultrasound scan did not demonstrate any evidence of gallstones. Serum triglycerides and calcium levels were within normal ranges.

On day 2 of her admission, she went into type 2 respiratory failure requiring non-invasive ventilation. C-reactive protein (CRP) was 567 mg/l (RR <10). Her nasogastric aspirates were >1500 ml/d, with persistent nausea, and she was unable to tolerate removal of her face mask for long enough for a NJ feeding tube to be inserted. Consequently, she started on PN.

On day 12 she was intubated and at this stage a bedside NJ tube was inserted. Her computed tomography scan demonstrated almost complete necrosis of the pancreas, and on escalating her peptide feed up to 85 ml/h she developed large-volume loose stool. Pancreatic enzymes were added to the feed itself (1.5 kcal/ml peptide formula) and her bowel function improved.

She had a long admission complicated by the development of a large infected collection (walled-off necrosis) that was drained via a flank drain, a bleed into the collection, and several episodes of ileus requiring further episodes of PN.

She was discharged home at month 6 with NJ feeding overnight, pancreatic enzymes, vitamin and mineral supplements, a proton pump inhibitor, and insulin. Despite consistent nutritional support she had lost more than 20% of her body weight during her admission.

Once home she had an endoscopic ultrasound, which detected biliary sludge, and she underwent a cholecystectomy and OTC. After a further 12 months of home NJ feeding, physiotherapy, and psychological support, she was able to return to work.

---

widely accepted that patients require long-term monitoring for micronutrient deficiencies [4], and some micronutrient deficiencies are specifically associated with PEI [41]. While there are consensus statements suggesting the format of this monitoring [19], there is not a robust evidence base for it. However, it is widely accepted that patients with CP require regular review to ensure optimal nutritional support and management of diabetes and exocrine failure [4, 19]. See Chapter 22 for management of micronutrient deficiencies.

## REFERENCES

1. Working Group IAP/APA Acute Pancreatitis Guidelines (2013). IAP/APA evidence-based guidelines for the management of acute pancreatitis. *Pancreatology* 13 (4 Suppl 2): e1–e15.

2. Banks, P.A., Bollen, T.L., Dervenis, C. et al. (2013). Classification of acute pancreatitis – 2012: revision of the Atlanta classification and definitions by international consensus. *Gut* 62 (1): 102–111.

3. O'Reilly, D.A., McPherson, S.J., Sinclair, M.T., and Smith, N. (2017). 'Treat the cause': the NCEPOD report on acute pancreatitis. *Br. J. Hosp. Med. (Lond.)* 78 (1): 6–7.

4. National Institute for Health and Care Excellence (2018). Pancreatitis. NICE guideline [NG104]. https://www.nice.org.uk/guidance/ng104. Accessed 9th September 2022.

5. Findlay, G.P., Goodwin, A.P.L., Protopapa, K. et al. (2011). Knowing the risk: A review of the peri-operative care of surgical patients. London: NCEPOD. https://www.ncepod.org.uk/2011report2/downloads/POC_fullreport.pdf. Accessed 9th September 2022.

6. Behrman, S.W. and Mulloy, M. (2006). Total pancreatectomy for the treatment of chronic pancreatitis: indications, outcomes, and recommendations. *Am. Surg.* 72 (4): 297–302.

7. Petrov, M.S., van Santvoort, H.C., Besselink, M.G. et al. (2008). Enteral nutrition and the risk of mortality and infectious complications in patients with severe acute pancreatitis: a meta-analysis of randomized trials. *Arch. Surg.* 143 (11): 1111–1117.

8. Arvanitakis, M., Ockenga, J., Bezmarevic, M. et al. (2020). ESPEN guideline on clinical nutrition in acute and chronic pancreatitis. *Clin. Nutr.* 39 (3): 612–631.

9. Marik, P.E. and Zaloga, G.P. (2004). Meta-analysis of parenteral nutrition versus enteral nutrition in patients with acute pancreatitis. *BMJ* 328 (7453): 1407.

10. Singh, N., Sharma, B., Sharma, M. et al. (2012). Evaluation of early enteral feeding through nasogastric and nasojejunal tube in severe acute pancreatitis: a noninferiority randomized controlled trial. *Pancreas* 41 (1): 153–159.

11. Piciucchi, M., Merola, E., Marignani, M. et al. (2010). Nasogastric or nasointestinal feeding in severe acute pancreatitis. *World J Gastroenterol* 16 (29): 3692–3696.

12. Eatock, F.C., Chong, P., Menezes, N. et al. (2005). A randomized study of early nasogastric versus nasojejunal feeding in severe acute pancreatitis. *Am. J. Gastroenterol.* 100 (2): 432–439.

13. Asrani, V., Chang, W.K., Dong, Z. et al. (2013). Glutamine supplementation in acute pancreatitis: a meta-analysis of randomized controlled trials. *Pancreatology.* 13 (5): 468–474.

14. Meier, R., Beglinger, C., Layer, P. et al. (2002). ESPEN guidelines on nutrition in acute pancreatitis. European Society of Parenteral and Enteral Nutrition. *Clin. Nutr.* 21 (2): 173–183.

15. Pearce, C.B., Sadek, S.A., Walters, A.M. et al. (2006). A double-blind, randomised, controlled trial to study the effects of an enteral feed supplemented with glutamine, arginine, and omega-3 fatty acid in predicted acute severe pancreatitis. *J. Pancreas* 7 (4): 361–371.

16. Petrov, M.S., Loveday, B.P., Pylypchuk, R.D. et al. (2009). Systematic review and meta-analysis of enteral nutrition formulations in acute pancreatitis. *Br. J. Surg.* 96 (11): 1243–1252.

17. Tiengou, L.E., Gloro, R., Pouzoulet, J. et al. (2006). Semi-elemental formula or polymeric formula: is there a better choice for enteral nutrition in acute pancreatitis? Randomized comparative study. *JPEN.* 30 (1): 1–5.

18. Kaushik, N., Pietraszewski, M., Holst, J.J., and O'Keefe, S.J. (2005). Enteral feeding without pancreatic stimulation. *Pancreas* 31 (4): 353–359.

19. Phillips, M.E., Hopper, A.D., Leeds, J.S. et al. (2021). Consensus for the management of pancreatic exocrine insufficiency: UK practical guidelines. *BMJ Open Gastroenterol.* 8 (1): e000643.

20. Phillips, M.E., Arregui-Fresneda, I., Duggan, S. et al. (2013). Pancreatic disease. In: *A Pocket Guide to Clinical Nutrition*, 4e (ed. V. Todorovic and A. Micklewright); Chapter 20.

21. Besselink, M.G., van Santvoort, H.C., Buskens, E. et al. (2008). Probiotic prophylaxis in predicted severe acute pancreatitis: a randomised, double-blind, placebo-controlled trial. *Lancet* 371 (9613): 651–659.

22. Maruki, J., Sai, J.K., and Watanabe, S. (2013). Efficacy of low-fat diet against dyspepsia associated with nonalcoholic mild pancreatic disease diagnosed using the Rosemont criteria. *Pancreas* 42 (1): 49–52.

23. Boreham, B. and Ammori, B.J. (2003). A prospective evaluation of pancreatic exocrine function in patients with acute pancreatitis: correlation with extent of necrosis and pancreatic endocrine insufficiency. *Pancreatology* 3 (4): 303–308.

24. Xu, Y., Wu, D., Zeng, Y., and Wang, X. (2012). Pancreatic exocrine function and morphology following an episode of acute pancreatitis. *Pancreas* 41 (6): 922–927.

25. Das, S.L., Kennedy, J.I., Murphy, R. et al. (2014). Relationship between the exocrine and endocrine pancreas after acute pancreatitis. *World J Gastroenterol.* 20 (45): 17196–17205.

26. Phillips, M.E., Robertson, M.D., Hart, K. et al. (2021). Long-term changes in nutritional status and body composition in patients with malignant pancreatic disease - A systematic review. *Clin. Nutr. ESPEN* 44: 85–95.

27. Phillips, M.E. (2015). Pancreatic exocrine insufficiency following pancreatic resection. *Pancreatology* 15 (5): 449–455.

28. Castineira-Alvarino, M., Lindkvist, B., Luaces-Regueira, M. et al. (2013). The role of high fat diet in the development of complications of chronic pancreatitis. *Clin. Nutr.* 32 (5): 830–836.

29. Singh, S., Midha, S., Singh, N. et al. (2008). Dietary counseling versus dietary supplements for malnutrition in chronic pancreatitis: a randomized controlled trial. *Clin. Gastroenterol. Hepatol.* 6 (3): 353–359.

30. Weber, A.M., Roy, C.C., Chartrand, L. et al. (1976). Relationship between bile acid malabsorption and pancreatic insufficiency in cystic fibrosis. *Gut* 17 (4): 295–299.

31. Phillips, F., Muls, A.C., Lalji, A., and Andreyev, H.J. (2015). Are bile acid malabsorption and bile acid diarrhoea important causes of loose stool complicating cancer therapy? *Color. Dis.* 17 (8): 730–734.

32. Borghede, M.K., Schlutter, J.M., Agnholt, J.S. et al. (2011). Bile acid malabsorption investigated by selenium-75-homocholic acid taurine ((75)SeHCAT) scans: causes and treatment responses to cholestyramine in 298 patients with chronic watery diarrhoea. *Eur. J. Intern. Med.* 22 (6): e137–e140.

33. Dutta, S.K. and Hlasko, J. (1985). Dietary fiber in pancreatic disease: effect of high fiber diet on fat malabsorption in pancreatic insufficiency and in vitro study of the interaction of dietary fiber with pancreatic enzymes. *Am. J. Clin. Nutr.* 41 (3): 517–525.

34. Stanga, Z., Giger, U., Marx, A., and DeLegge, M.H. (2005). Effect of jejunal long-term feeding in chronic pancreatitis. *JPEN.* 29 (1): 12–20.

35. Lordan, J.T., Phillips, M., Chun, J.Y. et al. (2009). A safe, effective, and cheap method of achieving pancreatic rest in patients with chronic pancreatitis with refractory symptoms and malnutrition. *Pancreas* 38 (6): 689–692.

36. Woodmansey, C., McGovern, A.P., McCullough, K.A. et al. (2017). Incidence, Demographics, and Clinical Characteristics of Diabetes of the Exocrine Pancreas (Type 3c): A Retrospective Cohort Study. *Diabetes Care* 40 (11): 1486–1493.

37. Yadav, D., Hawes, R.H., Brand, R.E. et al. (2009). Alcohol consumption, cigarette smoking, and the risk of recurrent acute and chronic pancreatitis. *Arch. Intern. Med.* 169 (11): 1035–1045.

38. Luaces-Regueira, M., Iglesias-Garcia, J., Lindkvist, B. et al. (2014). Smoking as a risk factor for complications in chronic pancreatitis. *Pancreas* 43 (2): 275–280.

39. Duggan, S.N., Smyth, N.D., Murphy, A. et al. (2014). High prevalence of osteoporosis in patients with chronic pancreatitis: a systematic review and meta-analysis. *Clin. Gastroenterol. Hepatol.* 12 (2): 219–228.

40. Duggan, S.N., Smyth, N.D., O'Sullivan, M. et al. (2014). The prevalence of malnutrition and fat-soluble vitamin deficiencies in chronic pancreatitis. *Nutr. Clin. Pract.* 29 (3): 348–354.

41. Lindkvist, B., Phillips, M.E., and Dominguez-Munoz, J.E. (2015). Clinical, anthropometric and laboratory nutritional markers of pancreatic exocrine insufficiency: Prevalence and diagnostic use. *Pancreatology* 15 (6): 589–597.

# CHAPTER 14

# Pancreatic Resection

Alessandro Parente[1,2], Sarah Powell-Brett[1], and Keith J. Roberts[1,2]

[1] Department of Hepatopancreatobiliary Surgery and Liver Transplantation, University Hospitals Birmingham NHS Foundation Trust, Birmingham, UK
[2] Institute of Immunology and Immunotherapy, University of Birmingham, Birmingham, UK

---

**KEY POINTS**

- Mitigating malnutrition is central to improving outcomes across the patient pathway for pancreatic resection.
- Pancreatic exocrine insufficiency (PEI) is prevalent both before and after pancreatic resection.
- There is no current, acceptable, widely used diagnostic test for reliably assessing PEI after pancreatic resection and thus treating based on suspicion alone is advisable.
- PEI is associated with worse post-operative outcomes, poorer quality of life, and less access to adjuvant therapy, and affects survival.
- Dietitian involvement both pre- and post-operatively is advisable for monitoring of PEI and other nutritional consequences of pancreatic resection.

---

The pancreas is absolutely essential in digestion and glucose regulation and any form of pancreatic resection has consequences for the nutritional well-being of a patient. Before surgery patients often experience significant weight loss, especially with a malignant pathology this is amplified by the effects of surgery on normal physiology. This chapter aims to give an overview of pancreatic resection, the nutritional consequences, and an introduction to their management.

## OVERVIEW OF SURGICAL PROCEDURES

Pancreatic surgery has always been challenging due to the complex anatomy of the pancreas. The anatomical division into head, neck, body, and tail of the pancreas as well as its relationships with the main mesenteric vessels and different structures from right (duodenum, bile duct) to left

*Nutritional Management of the Surgical Patient*, First Edition. Edited by Mary E. Phillips.

(stomach, spleen) are important landmarks for surgical approaches. The main indications for pancreatic surgery are tumours (typically pancreas, ampulla, duodenum, or distal common bile duct), pre-malignant conditions (adenoma and intraductal papillary mucinous neoplasia – IPMN), chronic pancreatitis, and rarely trauma.

## Pancreatico-duodenectomy

The first resections were reported in the early 1900s by Walter Kausch and Allen Whipple, who treated cases of ampullary and duodenal tumours with pancreatic resection, performing the well-known pancreatico-duodenectomy (PD), also called the Kausch–Whipple procedure [1, 2]. This procedure entails the removal of the pancreatic head together with the duodenum, the gallbladder, the distal common bile duct, and the distal stomach. After the resection is completed, reconstruction of gastrointestinal continuity is achieved by three anastomoses: pancreatico-jejunostomy, hepatico-jejunostomy, and gastro-jejunostomy. Complications after classical PD, such as gastritis, bile reflux, and dumping syndrome, relate to removal of the pylorus. Over the years the surgical technique has evolved to include a pylorus-preserving pancreatico-duodenectomy (PPPD) [3, 4]. A recent meta-analysis has concluded that there are no relevant differences in terms of morbidity and mortality between the two operations. However, some peri-operative outcome measures, such as operating time, intraoperative blood loss, and need for blood transfusion, seem to be less frequent in PPPD [5].

The anastomosis of the pancreatic stump is crucial, as it preserves the exocrine and endocrine function of the gland, ensuring a good quality of life after surgical resection. As such, it is considered the most difficult step of PD, as its failure can lead to post-operative pancreatic fistula (POPF). There are several techniques for the reconstruction of the pancreas: pancreatico-jejunostomy (end-to-side or end-to-end, duct-to-mucosa, or dunking) or pancreatico-gastrostomy. So far, no studies have been able to demonstrate clear superiority of any of the available techniques [6–11].

Minimal invasive approaches for PD, such as laparoscopic and robotic surgery, have been pursued during the last decades with good overall outcomes [12–16]. However, there is still insufficient evidence to recommend these types of approaches as gold standard.

## Distal Pancreatectomy

Distal pancreatectomy (DP) entails the resection of the body and tail of the pancreas with or without the spleen, which is often removed for technical reasons. DP has been performed throughout the years for the management of chronic pancreatitis and for tumours localised in the pancreatic body and tail.

In order to avoid the complications of splenectomy, such as overwhelming post-splenectomy infection and thrombocytosis, spleen-preserving procedures have been proposed [17, 18]. During recent years, a laparoscopic approach to DP has become popular with good outcomes [19, 20], but its utility and safety are still under debate [21].

## Total Pancreatectomy

Total pancreatectomy (TP) encompasses the surgical steps of both PD and DP, but without the need for a pancreatic anastomosis. Concurrent splenectomy is common, but its preservation is feasible. Nowadays, indications for TP are neck margin–positive patients during PD, multifocal or R1 IPMN, multifocal neuroendocrine tumour (NET), renal cell metastases, hereditary pancreatic cancer, hereditary chronic pancreatitis, and tumour recurrence or new tumour developing in the remnant pancreas after previous partial pancreatectomy. A minimal invasive approach for TP is feasible, but it has not been widely spread and there are isolated cases reported [22, 23]. In benign disease TP may be carried out with concurrent islet cell transplant to preserve some endocrine function, but this procedure is only carried out in very specific circumstances.

## Central Pancreatectomy

Central pancreatectomy (CP) involves the removal of the neck of the pancreas only. It is considered a parenchyma-sparing surgery that aims to preserve the exocrine and endocrine function of the pancreas. However, it is burdened by a higher rate of complications and has narrowed indications, namely benign or low-grade malignant pancreatic tumours localised in the neck [24, 25].

## Drainage Procedures

Longitudinal pancreatico-jejunostomy (LPJ) and the Frey and Puestow procedures are carried out to relieve obstruction of the main pancreatic duct caused by calcification in chronic pancreatitis. This typically involves creating a Roux limb to the pancreatic duct to allow an alternative route for pancreatic secretions to be drained into the small bowel, thus relieving the pressure within the gland, and in some cases this can be successful in reducing pain and recurrent episodes of acute pancreatitis. Malnutrition is prevalent in the pre-operative setting, with pre-existing PEI and diabetes common in this cohort.

## IMPACT OF PANCREATIC RESECTION ON NUTRITION

While surgical techniques vary, the nutritional management of post-operative complications is consistent.

Nutrition should be a key consideration at all points of care for patients undergoing pancreatic resection. Pre-operatively patients often present with significant weight loss, which is then compounded by resection and reconstruction and, if not promptly addressed, limits post-operative recovery and access to adjuvant treatment.

## Pre-operative Malnutrition and Pancreatic Exocrine Insufficiency

Over 80% of patients with pancreatic cancer have experienced some degree of weight loss by diagnosis [26]. Pre-operatively malnutrition is associated with increased morbidity and mortality [26], and sarcopenia is associated with post-operative complications and mortality [27].

Malnutrition prior to pancreatic surgery is multifactorial and the following should be considered:

- Pancreatic exocrine insufficiency (PEI).
- Duodenal obstruction.
- The Warburg effect (metabolic demands of the tumour).
- Chronic subclinical inflammation as evidenced by raised C-reactive protein (CRP) – a phenomenon present in several solid tumours.
- Tumour-derived islet amyloid polypeptide (a contributor to weight loss that is specific to pancreatic cancer) [28–31].

PEI is common at presentation, with a 2016 systematic review reporting a pre-operative prevalence of 44%, and is likely related to the tumour mass itself, reducing the volume of functioning parenchyma and obstructing the flow of enzymes along the pancreatic duct [32].

Often the pathway to resection is rapid, especially with the advent of 'fast-track' surgery, meaning that nutritional support is frequently overlooked. Early nutritional assessment by an experienced dietitian, and the instigation of pancreatic enzyme replacement therapy (PERT), is recommended in the pre-operative setting [33, 34]. In some cases, pre-operative enteral or parenteral nutrition (PN) may be required, especially in those with duodenal obstruction.

## Post-operative Pancreatic Exocrine Insufficiency

Following resection, malnutrition is associated with increased post-operative complications, poorer survival, reduced quality of life (QoL), and lower access to and tolerance of adjuvant chemotherapy [26, 35, 36]. PEI has a much more complex aetiology following resection, and one must consider the anatomical and physiological alterations that have taken place to appreciate this. Several factors must be considered:

- Removal of pancreatic tissue.
- Hormonal downregulation of pancreatic and biliary secretion (secondary to the removal of duodenum).

- Altered mixing of pancreatic and biliary secretions and gastric emptying (both from the new anatomical arrangement following reconstruction and from the altered innervation following dissection).
- Altered intestinal pH. These factors create a poor environment for the secretion, delivery, activation, and action of pancreatic enzymes. The prevalence of PEI following resection is therefore understandably high.

Where enteral feeding is used post-operatively, peptide medium-chain triglyceride (MCT)–based products should be used.

While many authors have attempted to quantify the incidence of PEI after PD, CP, and DP, the lack of validated function tests and reliance on symptoms mean that this data is likely to under-report the true incidence of PEI. Abdominal symptoms are accepted as an unreliable marker, and steatorrhoea is a very late symptom of PEI and reliant on dietary fat consumption [37]. PEI is also recognised to be progressive following resection, with studies using a significantly longer follow-up period reaching 100% prevalence [38]. Consequently, the routine use of PERT is recommended in those who have undergone drainage procedures, TP, and PD, with regular clinical review recommended following CP and DP [39].

## Consequences of Pancreatic Exocrine Insufficiency and Malnutrition Following Pancreatic Resection

The consequences of PEI are broad and include weight loss, malnutrition, micro/macronutrient deficiencies, increased cardiovascular events, non-alcoholic fatty liver disease (NAFLD), osteoporosis, and sarcopenia [40–43] (Figure 14.1). Of the macronutrients, lipid digestion is the most affected, which in turn affects the absorption of fat-soluble vitamins and essential minerals such as zinc, folic acid, thiamine, magnesium, and calcium. These are essential components of metabolism and failure to absorb them has significant multisystem impacts. PEI is associated with a worse post-operative outcome: longer hospital

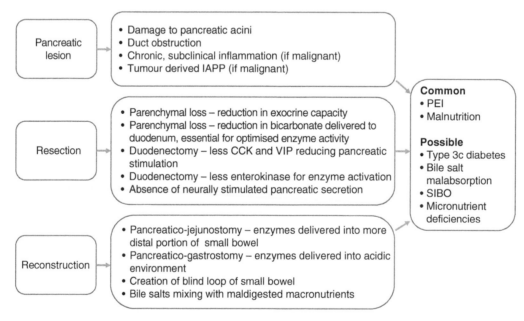

**FIGURE 14.1**    Summary of common factors related to malnutrition and pancreatic exocrine insufficiency among patients undergoing pancreatic surgery. CCK, cholecystokinin; IAPP, islet amyloid polypeptide; PEI, pancreatic exocrine insufficiency; SIBO, small intestine bacterial overgrowth; VIP, vasoactive intestinal peptide.

stays, increased costs, higher rates of post-operative complications, poorer QoL, lower tolerance of adjuvant chemotherapy, and even worse survival [26, 35–37, 44–46].

## Other Nutritional Considerations

Other factors include bile salt malabsorption (resulting from cholecystectomy and binding of bile salts to maldigested macronutrients) and small intestine bacterial overgrowth (SIBO, predisposed to by the creation of a blind loop of bowel during reconstruction). Bile salt malabsorption and SIBO both have significant nutritional implications, display problematic symptoms, and can be confused with PEI. Resection of the duodenum and use of the proximal jejunum in a blind loop after PD and TP results in reduced absorptive capacity for micronutrients. Annual assessment of micronutrients and bone density scanning are recommended to facilitate early detection of deficiencies.

# COMMON POST-OPERATIVE COMPLICATIONS AND THEIR NUTRITIONAL MANAGEMENT

Pancreatic surgery morbidity rates vary from 15 to 40%, depending on the type of resection [47–49]. The most common complications that can develop after pancreatic resection are post-pancreatectomy haemorrhage (PPH), POPF, delayed gastric emptying (DGE), biliary leak, and chyle leak (CL).

## Post-Pancreatectomy Haemorrhage

PPH is defined by time of onset, location, and severity into grades A, B, and C by the International Study Group of Pancreatic Surgery (ISGPS) [50]. In the largest series, it occurs in 6–13% of cases with an overall mortality of 4.8%, which increases to 85% in grade C cases [51–53]. PPH is more frequent in PD and when associated with POPF, the most common pathophysiology is the erosion of the vessels by pancreatic fluid. Treatment depends on severity and if

POPF is concomitant, a combination of interventional endoscopy and angiography suffices for the majority, but operative haemostasis is necessary in around 3.6% of cases [51].

## Delayed Gastric Emptying

DGE is reported to be a frequent complication after pancreatic resection, with rates of 10–30% for PD and up to 24% for DP [54, 55]. It is classified by ISGPS into grades A, B, and C based on nasogastric intubation, type of diet, oral intake, patient's general health condition, the need for prokinetics, and whether diagnostic tests are necessary [56]. DGE is not a life-threatening condition and it is usually self-limiting; however, it can have huge impacts on patients' QoL, length of hospital stay, and hospital readmission [57, 58]. Known risk factors include POPF, biliary leak, post-operative sepsis, and abdominal collections [59, 60].

Management of DGE involves texture modification, with the use of oral nutritional support in those with poor tolerance of solids, or naso-jejunal (NJ) feeding. The reduction in placement of jejunal tubes at the time of operation means that patients often require PN until they are able to re-establish oral intake. Prokinetics [61], such as prucalopride, metoclopramide, domperidone, and erythromycin, are often used. The latter has been shown to reduce the incidence of DGE [62, 63].

## Post-operative Pancreatic Fistula

POPF can be considered the Achilles' heel of PD, being the main contributor to post-operative morbidity and mortality. ISGPF recently updated its 2005 grading system (A, B, and C) to recognise clinically relevant POPF (CR-POPF, grades B and C by the 2005 grading system) as a separate entity to biochemical leak (BL, previously known as grade A POPF) [64, 65]. CR-POPF has a significant impact on post-operative course, lengthening and complicating inpatient stay, being associated with intra-abdominal sepsis and haemorrhage, and carrying a mortality risk of around 1% for all and 25% for those with grade C POPF [66]. Understanding of underlying pathophysiology remains poor, and studies have explored predictive risk scores and preventative strategies (anastomosis technique, somatostatin analogues, omental wrapping, pancreatic duct stents, and drain placement) [67–71].

Despite this, POPF rates remain stubbornly high. Nutrition is a point of contention in the post-operative care of the PD patient. The latest systematic review collated five RCTs and concluded that using the enteral route, even when additional support was required, favoured a shorter length of stay without affecting other outcomes, notably POPF. As it is recognised that enteral nutrition is superior to parenteral following PD, the use of intra-operatively placed NJ or jejunostomy tubes should be considered for those at high risk of POPF. Debate continues as to the necessity for the patient to remain nil by mouth (NBM), thus reducing stimulation of pancreatic secretions. When somatostatin analogues are in use, it seems counterintuitive to allow an oral diet, and patients should be managed with jejunal feeding or PN. Conservatively managed POPF can result in DGE and post-operative ileus, and thus jejunal or PN may be indicated regardless.

### Bile Leak

High-volume leakage at the hepatico-jejunostomy is typically resolved with reoperation, with low-volume leaks managed conservatively. Patients should be kept NBM until reoperation to minimise stimulation of biliary secretions and following reoperation patients should be considered at high risk of post-operative ileus (see Chapter 19).

### Chyle Leak

CL is a less common complication of pancreatic resection [72] and is defined as an 'output of milky coloured fluid from a drain, drain site or wound on or after postoperative day 3, with a triglyceride content $\geq 110\,\mathrm{mg/dl}$'. The same consensus statement delineated severity from grade A (no specific interventions other than oral dietary fat restriction) to grade C

(need for invasive hospital treatment, intensive care unit admission, or mortality) [73]. Risk factors for CL include pre-existing diabetes, long operating times, DP, concomitant POPF, lymph node dissection, and malignant indication for resection [72, 74]. Incidence varies from 4.5 to 10%, dependent on classification [72, 74]. First-line management centres around a low-fat diet, using MCT enteral feeds, non-removal of existing surgical drains (until clinically insignificant volumes with resumption of normal diet), and PN in refractory cases. Operative management is rarely required. The most frequent impact of CL is prolonged hospital stay (for grades B and C), with the associated economic impact [72].

## LONG-TERM MANAGEMENT

Common long-term complications after pancreatic surgery include diabetes, dyspepsia, dumping syndrome (especially in case of classic PD), loss of appetite steatorrhea, and PEI.

### Diabetes after Pancreatic Surgery

Diabetes mellitus (DM) secondary to pancreatic disease is fairly common, with an estimated incidence of 9.2% of all diabetes, and it is commonly referred as type 3c diabetes (T3DM; also known as pancreatogenic diabetes, resulting from loss of pancreatic parenchyma and differing from type 2 diabetes in that peripheral insulin sensitivity is maintained, and there are both insulin and glucagon deficiencies) [75]. The incidence of DM after pancreatic resection, regardless of the underlying pathology, can be up to 54% [76]. There are no specific guidelines regarding its management, but it is highly recommended to refer the patient to a specialised centre with a multidisciplinary team involving dietitians and diabetologists.

### Pancreatic Enzyme Replacement Therapy

Correct management of PEI is key in post-operative recovery. PERT should be given as delayed-release capsules of enteric-coated mini-microspheres and has been shown to improve fat digestion, mitigate weight loss, reduce steathorrhoea, enhance QoL, and even lengthen survival [44, 45, 77–79]. The aim is to deliver the right amount of enzymes to the right place, at the right time, and at the correct pH. This is especially challenging after PD due to the significant anatomical and physiological alterations. The recommended starting dose is 50–75 000 units with meals and 25–50 000 units with snacks or supplements; these should be distributed throughout the meal rather than all before or all after [80–82]. Of note is that pancreatic resection alters the volume of bicarbonate secreted; also, patients may experience a degree of DGE, therefore a proton pump inhibitor (PPI) may need to be considered to ensure an appropriate pH for correct enzyme function [83].

Regular review to monitor compliance and dosing and screen for type 3c diabetes and micronutrient deficiency is imperative; this should preferably be performed by a dietitian experienced in PEI. A detailed explanation of the anthropometric, biochemical, and clinical evaluations required to fully assess PEI and nutritional status after pancreatic resection is beyond the scope of this chapter, but comprehensive overviews are available in the literature [80].

---

## Case Study:   Resectable Pancreatic Cancer

Mr A, aged 75 yr with good performance status, presented with jaundice. Staging investigations demonstrated a mass in the head of the pancreas with biliary and pancreatic duct dilatation. There was no local or metastatic spread of cancer. The patient had lost 5 kg prior to surgery and had symptoms of pancreatic exocrine insufficiency with cramping and bloating after meals, particularly larger meals with a high fat content. He denied steatorrhoea. Faecal elastase testing demonstrated a FE-1 of 57 µg/g.

### Management

Pre-operative work-up included the provision of pancreatic enzymes and exercise targets. Blood glucose levels were assessed and within normal limits (HbA$_{1c}$ 39 mmol/mol).

### Surgery

Pancreatico-duodenectomy. Histology: moderately differentiated pancreatic ductal adenocarcinoma. 2/24 positive lymph nodes.

### Post-operative Care

Mr A followed the enhanced recovery after surgery (ERAS) pathway, starting on sips of water and progressing on to a soft diet by day 3. Drain amylase levels were low at 51 mmol/l and drains were removed on day 3. Epidural was removed on day 3. PERT was recommenced on day 3, and Mr A made good progress and was discharged home on Day 8.

### Discharge Medication

PERT – 50–75 000 units with meals and 25 000 with snacks.

PPI, calcium and vitamin D supplement, multivitamin and mineral.

Oral nutritional supplement (600 kcal, 36 g protein) – each taken with PERT – 25 000 units at the start and a further 25 000 units halfway through, aiming to consume a whole drink in 30 min to optimize mixing of PERT with the supplement.

### Post-operative Review

Week 1 – making steady progress, 1 kg weight loss since discharge.

Week 4 – oral intake returned to normal, PERT increased to 75 000–100 000 units with meals; 50 000 units with snacks due to lose stools. Weight stabilised and oral nutritional supplement discontinued.

Week 8 – commenced adjuvant chemotherapy.

## Case Study:   Resectable Pancreatic Cancer with Post-operative Complications

Mr B, aged 78 yr, presented with jaundice; 7 kg weight loss in 3 months (9%). Imaging confirmed a mass in the head of the pancreas, no metastatic disease. Blood glucose levels were elevated at 21 mmol/l, HbA$_{1c}$ 62 mmol/mol.

### Management

Insulin, PERT, and nutritional support and exercise targets were provided pre-operatively.

### Surgery

Pancreatico-duodenectomy. Histology: poorly differentiated distal cholangiocarcinoma. 1/18 positive lymph nodes.

### Post-operative Care

Mr B commenced sips of water on day 1 and mobilised with the physiotherapists. Blood glucose levels were 4–12 mmol/l on variable-rate insulin. Day 2 – developed nausea. Day 3 – drain amylase was 27 000 and 1200 mmol/l (in each drain). Octreotide had been started on day 1, and this was continued. An NJ tube had been inserted intra-operatively, and low-rate feeding was commenced on day 3: 20 ml/h peptide feed.

NJ feeding was escalated up over the next 2 days and was initially tolerated at 60 ml/h. Day 6 – computed tomographic scan showed pancreatic collection around the pancreatico-jejunostomy, and the surgical drains were manipulated to improve drainage. Day 7 – abdomen distended, no flatus, and poor tolerance of NJ feeding. Day 8 – commenced PN.

PN and octreotide continued until day 12, when inflammatory markers had settled, Mr B had his bowels open, abdomen was soft, and the NJ feed was recommenced. Subcutaneous insulin was commenced. Repeat drain amylase level was 121 mmol/l. Drains were removed on day 13 and Mr B was discharged home on day 18 with NJ feeding due to ongoing poor oral intake.

### Discharge Medication

Peptide enteral feed providing 1500 kcal; 75 g protein.

PERT – 50 000 units with meals and snack (only consuming small meals).

PPI, calcium, and vitamin D; multivitamin and mineral supplements.

Prokinetics and laxatives.

Basal bolus insulin regimen and blood glucose monitoring.

### Follow-Up

Mr B was followed up every week by the dietitian in conjunction with the diabetes team.

Week 1 – ongoing poor intake, food fortification advice reiterated, and patient encouraged to mobilise.

Week 3 – oral intake slowly improving, NJ feed reduced to 1000 kcal, 50 g protein.

Week 5–8 – oral intake continued to improve and NJ was removed 8 weeks after discharge.

Insulin doses were manipulated to achieve good glycaemic control. NJ feeding maintained Mr B's weight and allowed him to progress with his rehabilitation despite poor oral intake and nausea.

11 weeks post-operatively Mr B commenced adjuvant chemotherapy.

# REFERENCES

1. Kausch, W. (2015). Erste operationen berliner chirurgen 1817–1931. In: *Das Carcinom der Papilla duodeni und seine radikale Entfernung* (ed. S. Heinz-Peter, R. Winau, and H. Rudolf), 40–51. Berlin: De Gruyter.

2. Whipple, A.O., Parsons, W.B., and Mullins, C.R. (1935). Treatment of carcinoma of the ampulla of vater. *Ann. Surg.* 102 (4): 763–779.

3. Watson, K. (1944). Carcinoma of ampulla of Vater successful radical resection. *Br. J. Surg.* 31: 366–373.

4. Traverso, L.W. and Longmire, W.P. Jr. (1978). Preservation of the pylorus in pancreaticoduodenectomy. *Surg Gynecol Obstet* 146 (6): 959–962.

5. Hüttner, F.J., Fitzmaurice, C., Schwarzer, G. et al. (2016). Pylorus-preserving pancreaticoduodenectomy (pp Whipple) versus pancreaticoduodenectomy (classic Whipple) for surgical treatment of periampullary and pancreatic carcinoma. *Cochrane Database Syst. Rev.* 2 (2): Cd006053.

6. Yeo, C.J., Cameron, J.L., Maher, M.M. et al. (1995). A prospective randomized trial of pancreaticogastrostomy versus pancreaticojejunostomy after pancreaticoduodenectomy. *Ann. Surg.* 222 (4): 580–588.

7. Bassi, C., Falconi, M., Molinari, E. et al. (2003). Duct-to-mucosa versus end-to-side pancreaticojejunostomy reconstruction after pancreaticoduodenectomy: results of a prospective randomized trial. *Surgery* 134 (5): 766–771.

8. Bai, X., Zhang, Q., Gao, S. et al. (2016). Duct-to-mucosa vs invagination for pancreaticojejunostomy after pancreaticoduodenectomy: a prospective, randomized controlled trial from a single surgeon. *J. Am. Coll. Surg.* 222 (1): 10–18.

9. Berger, A.C., Howard, T.J., Kennedy, E.P. et al. (2009). Does type of pancreaticojejunostomy after pancreaticoduodenectomy decrease rate of pancreatic fistula? A randomized, prospective, dual-institution trial. *J. Am. Coll. Surg.* 208 (5): 738–747.

10. Peng, S.Y., Wang, J.W., Lau, W.Y. et al. (2007). Conventional versus binding pancreaticojejunostomy after pancreaticoduodenectomy: a prospective randomized trial. *Ann. Surg.* 245 (5): 692–698.

11. Shrikhande, S.V., Sivasanker, M., Vollmer, C.M. et al. (2017). Pancreatic anastomosis after pancreatoduodenectomy: a position statement by the International Study Group of Pancreatic Surgery (ISGPS). *Surgery* 161 (5): 1221–1234.

12. Asbun, H.J. and Stauffer, J.A. (2012). Laparoscopic vs open pancreaticoduodenectomy: overall outcomes and severity of complications using the accordion severity grading system. *J. Am. Coll. Surg.* 215 (6): 810–819.

13. Zeh, H.J., Zureikat, A.H., Secrest, A. et al. (2012). Outcomes after robot-assisted pancreaticoduodenectomy for periampullary lesions. *Ann. Surg. Oncol.* 19 (3): 864–870.

14. Croome, K.P., Farnell, M.B., Que, F.G. et al. (2014). Total laparoscopic pancreaticoduodenectomy for pancreatic ductal adenocarcinoma: oncologic advantages over open approaches? *Ann. Surg.* 260 (4): 633–638.

15. Stauffer, J.A., Coppola, A., Villacreses, D. et al. (2017). Laparoscopic versus open pancreaticoduodenectomy for pancreatic adenocarcinoma: long-term results at a single institution. *Surg. Endosc.* 31 (5): 2233–2241.

16. Kornaropoulos, M., Moris, D., Beal, E.W. et al. (2017). Total robotic pancreaticoduodenectomy: a systematic review of the literature. *Surg. Endosc.* 31 (11): 4382–4392.

17. Warshaw, A.L. (1988). Conservation of the spleen with distal pancreatectomy. *Arch. Surg.* 123 (5): 550–553.

18. Kimura, W., Moriya, T., Ma, J. et al. (2007). Spleen-preserving distal pancreatectomy with conservation of the splenic artery and vein. *World J. Gastroenterol.* 13 (10): 1493–1499.

19. Fernández-Cruz, L., Martínez, I., Gilabert, R. et al. (2004). Laparoscopic distal pancreatectomy combined with preservation of the spleen for cystic neoplasms of the pancreas. *J. Gastrointest. Surg.* 8 (4): 493–501.

20. Riviere, D., Gurusamy, K.S., Kooby, D.A. et al. (2016). Laparoscopic versus open distal pancreatectomy for pancreatic cancer. *Cochrane Database Syst. Rev.* 4 (4): CD011391.

21. van Hilst, J., de Rooij, T., Bosscha, K. et al. (2019). Laparoscopic versus open pancreatoduodenectomy for pancreatic or periampullary tumours (LEOPARD-2): a multicentre, patient-blinded, randomised controlled phase 2/3 trial. *Lancet Gastroenterol. Hepatol.* 4 (3): 199–207.

22. Dallemagne, B., de Oliveira, A.T., Lacerda, C.F. et al. (2013). Full laparoscopic total pancreatectomy with and without spleen and pylorus preservation: a feasibility report. *J. Hepatobiliary Pancreat. Sci.* 20 (6): 647–653.

23. Boggi, U., Palladino, S., Massimetti, G. et al. (2015). Laparoscopic robot-assisted versus open total pancreatectomy: a case-matched study. *Surg. Endosc.* 29 (6): 1425–1432.

24. Xiao, W., Zhu, J., Peng, L. et al. (2018). The role of central pancreatectomy in pancreatic surgery: a systematic review and meta-analysis. *HPB (Oxford)* 20 (10): 896–904.

25. Paiella, S., De Pastena, M., Faustini, F. et al. (2019). Central pancreatectomy for benign or low-grade malignant pancreatic lesions – A single-center retrospective analysis of 116 cases. *Eur. J. Surg. Oncol.* 45 (5): 788–792.

26. Gilliland, T.M., Villafane-Ferriol, N., Shah, K.P. et al. (2017). Nutritional and metabolic derangements in pancreatic cancer and pancreatic resection. *Nutrients* 9 (3): 243.

27. Pecorelli, N., Carrara, G., De Cobelli, F. et al. (2016). Effect of sarcopenia and visceral obesity on mortality and pancreatic fistula following pancreatic cancer surgery. *Br. J. Surg.* 103 (4): 434–442.

28. Koppenol, W.H., Bounds, P.L., and Dang, C.V. (2011). Otto Warburg's contributions to current concepts of cancer metabolism. *Nat. Rev. Cancer* 11 (5): 325–337.

29. Tahergorabi, Z., Khazaei, M., Moodi, M., and Chamani, E. (2016). From obesity to cancer: a review on proposed mechanisms. *Cell Biochem. Funct.* 34 (8): 533–545.

30. Miyamoto, R., Oda, T., Hashimoto, S. et al. (2017). Platelet x CRP multiplier value as an indicator of poor prognosis in patients with resectable pancreatic Cancer. *Pancreas* 46 (1): 35–41.

31. Permert, J., Larsson, J., Westermark, G.T. et al. (1994). Islet amyloid polypeptide in patients with pancreatic cancer and diabetes. *N. Engl. J. Med.* 330 (5): 313–318.

32. Tseng, D.S., Molenaar, I.Q., Besselink, M.G. et al. (2016). Pancreatic exocrine insufficiency in patients with pancreatic or periampullary Cancer: a systematic review. *Pancreas* 45 (3): 325–330.

33. Gianotti, L., Besselink, M.G., Sandini, M. et al. (2018). Nutritional support and therapy in pancreatic surgery: a position paper of the International Study Group on Pancreatic Surgery (ISGPS). *Surgery* 164 (5): 1035–1048.

34. National Institute for Health and Care Excellence (2018). Pancreatic cancer in adults: diagnosis and management. NICE guideline [NG85]. https://www.nice.org.uk/guidance/ng85. Accessed 10th January 2022.

35. Basile, D., Corvaja, C., Caccialanza, R., and Aprile, G. (2019). Sarcopenia: looking to muscle mass to better manage pancreatic cancer patients. *Curr. Opin. Support. Palliat. Care* 13 (4): 279–285.

36. Andreyev, H.J., Norman, A.R., Oates, J., and Cunningham, D. (1998). Why do patients with weight loss have a worse outcome when undergoing chemotherapy for gastrointestinal malignancies? *Eur. J. Cancer* 34 (4): 503–509.

37. Moore, J.V., Tom, S., Scoggins, C.R. et al. (2021). Exocrine pancreatic insufficiency after pancreatectomy for malignancy: systematic review and optimal management recommendations. *J. Gastrointest. Surg.* 25 (9): 2317–2327.

38. Nordback, I., Parviainen, M., Piironen, A. et al. (2007). Obstructed pancreaticojejunostomy partly explains exocrine insufficiency after pancreatic head resection. *Scand. J. Gastroenterol.* 42 (2): 263–270.

39. Phillips, M.E., Hopper, A.D., Leeds, J.S. et al. (2021). Consensus for the management of pancreatic exocrine insufficiency: UK practical guidelines. *BMJ Open Gastroenterol.* 8 (1): e000643.

40. Shintakuya, R., Uemura, K., Murakami, Y. et al. (2017). Sarcopenia is closely associated with pancreatic exocrine insufficiency in patients with pancreatic disease. *Pancreatology* 17 (1): 70–75.

41. Centonze, L., Di Sandro, S., Lauterio, A. et al. (2020). The impact of sarcopenia on postoperative course following pancreatoduodenectomy: single-center experience of 110 consecutive cases. *Dig. Surg.* 37 (4): 312–320.

42. Tanaka, N., Horiuchi, A., Yokoyama, T. et al. (2011). Clinical characteristics of de novo nonalcoholic fatty liver disease following pancreaticoduodenectomy. *J. Gastroenterol.* 46 (6): 758–768.

43. Lindkvist, B., Phillips, M.E., and Dominguez-Munoz, J.E. (2015). Clinical, anthropometric and laboratory nutritional markers of pancreatic exocrine insufficiency: prevalence and diagnostic use. *Pancreatology* 15 (6): 589–597.

44. Roberts, K.J., Schrem, H., Hodson, J. et al. (2017). Pancreas exocrine replacement therapy is associated with increased survival following pancreatoduodenectomy for periampullary malignancy. *HPB* 19 (10): 859–867.

45. Roberts, K.J., Bannister, C.A., and Schrem, H. (2019). Enzyme replacement improves survival among patients with pancreatic cancer: Results of a population based study. *Pancreatology* 19 (1): 114–121.

46. Partelli, S., Frulloni, L., Minniti, C. et al. (2012). Faecal elastase-1 is an independent predictor of survival in advanced pancreatic cancer. *Dig. Liver Dis.* 44 (11): 945–951.

47. Cameron, J.L., Riall, T.S., Coleman, J., and Belcher, K.A. (2006). One thousand consecutive pancreaticoduodenectomies. *Ann. Surg.* 244 (1): 10–15.

48. Seeliger, H., Christians, S., Angele, M.K. et al. (2010). Risk factors for surgical complications in distal pancreatectomy. *Am. J. Surg.* 200 (3): 311–317.

49. Sánchez-Velázquez, P., Muller, X., Malleo, G. et al. (2019). Benchmarks in pancreatic surgery: a novel tool for unbiased outcome comparisons. *Ann. Surg.* 270 (2): 211–218.

50. Wente, M.N., Veit, J.A., Bassi, C. et al. (2007). Postpancreatectomy hemorrhage (PPH): an International Study Group of Pancreatic Surgery (ISGPS) definition. *Surgery* 142 (1): 20–25.

51. Wellner, U.F., Kulemann, B., Lapshyn, H. et al. (2014). Postpancreatectomy hemorrhage–incidence, treatment, and risk factors in over 1,000 pancreatic resections. *J. Gastrointest. Surg.* 18 (3): 464–475.

52. Ansari, D., Tingstedt, B., Lindell, G. et al. (2017). Hemorrhage after major pancreatic resection: incidence, risk factors, management, and outcome. *Scand. J. Surg.* 106 (1): 47–53.

53. Duarte Garcés, A.A., Andrianello, S., Marchegiani, G. et al. (2018). Reappraisal of post-pancreatectomy hemorrhage (PPH) classifications: do we need to redefine grades A and B? *HPB* 20 (8): 702–707.

54. Yeo, C.J., Cameron, J.L., Sohn, T.A. et al. (1997). Six hundred fifty consecutive pancreaticoduodenectomies in the 1990s: pathology, complications, and outcomes. *Ann. Surg.* 226 (3): 248–257.

55. Glowka, T.R., von Websky, M., Pantelis, D. et al. (2016). Risk factors for delayed gastric emptying following distal pancreatectomy. *Langenbeck's Arch. Surg.* 401 (2): 161–167.

56. Wente, M.N., Bassi, C., Dervenis, C. et al. (2007). Delayed gastric emptying (DGE) after pancreatic surgery: a suggested definition by the International Study Group of Pancreatic Surgery (ISGPS). *Surgery* 142 (5): 761–768.

57. Tanaka, M. (2005). Gastroparesis after a pylorus-preserving pancreatoduodenectomy. *Surg. Today* 35 (5): 345–350.

58. Ahmad, S.A., Edwards, M.J., Sutton, J.M. et al. (2012). Factors influencing readmission after pancreaticoduodenectomy: a multi-institutional study of 1302 patients. *Ann. Surg.* 256 (3): 529–537.

59. Parmar, A.D., Sheffield, K.M., Vargas, G.M. et al. (2013). Factors associated with delayed gastric emptying after pancreaticoduodenectomy. *HPB* 15 (10): 763–772.

60. Malleo, G., Crippa, S., Butturini, G. et al. (2010). Delayed gastric emptying after pylorus-preserving pancreaticoduodenectomy: validation of International Study Group of Pancreatic Surgery classification and analysis of risk factors. *HPB* 12 (9): 610–618.

61. Parkman, H.P., Hasler, W.L., and Fisher, R.S. (2004). American Gastroenterological Association medical position statement: diagnosis and treatment of gastroparesis. *Gastroenterology* 127 (5): 1589–1591.

62. Yeo, C.J., Barry, M.K., Sauter, P.K. et al. (1993). Erythromycin accelerates gastric emptying after pancreaticoduodenectomy. A prospective, randomized, placebo-controlled trial. *Ann. Surg.* 218 (3): 229–237.

63. Ohwada, S., Satoh, Y., Kawate, S. et al. (2001). Low-dose erythromycin reduces delayed gastric emptying and improves gastric motility after Billroth I pylorus-preserving pancreaticoduodenectomy. *Ann. Surg.* 234 (5): 668–674.

64. Bassi, C., Dervenis, C., Butturini, G. et al. (2005). Postoperative pancreatic fistula: an international study group (ISGPF) definition. *Surgery* 138 (1): 8–13.

65. Bassi, C., Marchegiani, G., Dervenis, C. et al. (2017). The 2016 update of the International Study Group (ISGPS) definition and grading of postoperative pancreatic fistula: 11 years after. *Surgery* 161 (3): 584–591.

66. Pedrazzoli, S. (2017). Pancreatoduodenectomy (PD) and postoperative pancreatic fistula (POPF): A systematic review and analysis of the POPF-related mortality rate in 60,739 patients retrieved from the English literature published between 1990 and 2015. *Medicine (Baltimore)* 96 (19): e6858.

67. Jiang, Y., Chen, Q., Wang, Z. et al. (2021). The prognostic value of external vs internal pancreatic duct stents in CR-POPF after pancreaticoduodenectomy: a systematic review and meta-analysis. *J. Investig. Surg.* 34 (7): 738–746.

68. Schorn, S., Demir, I.E., Vogel, T. et al. (2019). Mortality and postoperative complications after different types of surgical reconstruction following pancreaticoduodenectomy-a systematic review with meta-analysis. *Langenbeck's Arch. Surg.* 404 (2): 141–157.

69. Li, T., D'Cruz, R.T., Lim, S.Y., and Shelat, V.G. (2020). Somatostatin analogues and the risk of post-operative pancreatic fistulas after pancreatic resection – a systematic review & meta-analysis. *Pancreatology* 20 (2): 158–168.

70. Pedrazzoli, S. and Brazzale, A.R. (2020). Systematic review and meta-analysis of surgical drain management after the diagnosis of postoperative pancreatic fistula after pancreaticoduodenectomy: draining-tract-targeted works better than standard management. *Langenbeck's Arch. Surg.* 405 (8): 1219–1231.

71. Roberts, K.J., Hodson, J., Mehrzad, H. et al. (2014). A preoperative predictive score of pancreatic fistula following pancreatoduodenectomy. *HPB* 16 (7): 620–628.

72. Strobel, O., Brangs, S., Hinz, U. et al. (2017). Incidence, risk factors and clinical implications of chyle leak after pancreatic surgery. *Br. J. Surg.* 104 (1): 108–117.

73. Besselink, M.G., van Rijssen, L.B., Bassi, C. et al. (2017). Definition and classification of chyle leak after pancreatic operation: a consensus statement by the International Study Group on Pancreatic Surgery. *Surgery* 161 (2): 365–372.

74. Paiella, S., De Pastena, M., Casciani, F. et al. (2018). Chyle leak after pancreatic surgery: validation of the International Study Group of Pancreatic Surgery classification. *Surgery* 164 (3): 450–454.

75. Ewald, N. and Hardt, P.D. (2013). Diagnosis and treatment of diabetes mellitus in chronic pancreatitis. *World J. Gastroenterol.* 19 (42): 7276–7281.

76. Nguyen, A., Demirjian, A., Yamamoto, M. et al. (2017). Development of postoperative diabetes mellitus in patients undergoing distal pancreatectomy versus whipple procedure. *Am. Surg.* 83 (10): 1050–1053.

77. Whitcomb, D.C., Lehman, G.A., Vasileva, G. et al. (2010). Pancrelipase delayed-release capsules (CREON) for exocrine pancreatic insufficiency due to chronic pancreatitis or pancreatic surgery: A double-blind randomized trial. *Am. J. Gastroenterol.* 105 (10): 2276–2286.

78. Gubergrits, N., Malecka-Panas, E., Lehman, G.A. et al. (2011). A 6-month, open-label clinical trial of pancrelipase delayed-release capsules (Creon) in patients with exocrine pancreatic insufficiency due to chronic pancreatitis or pancreatic surgery. *Aliment. Pharmacol. Ther.* 33 (10): 1152–1161.

79. Landers, A., Brown, H., and Strother, M. (2019). The effectiveness of pancreatic enzyme replacement therapy for malabsorption in advanced pancreatic cancer, a pilot study. *Palliat. Care* 12: 1178224218825270.

80. Phillips, M.E. (2015). Pancreatic exocrine insufficiency following pancreatic resection. *Pancreatology* 15 (5): 449–455.

81. Seiler, C.M., Izbicki, J., Varga-Szabo, L. et al. (2013). Randomised clinical trial: a 1-week, double-blind, placebo-controlled study of pancreatin 25 000 Ph. Eur. minimicrospheres (Creon 25000 MMS) for pancreatic exocrine insufficiency after pancreatic surgery, with a 1-year open-label extension. *Aliment. Pharmacol. Ther.* 37 (7): 691–702.

82. Dominguez-Munoz, J.E., Iglesias-Garcia, J., Iglesias-Rey, M. et al. (2005). Effect of the administration schedule on the therapeutic efficacy of oral pancreatic enzyme supplements in patients with exocrine pancreatic insufficiency: a randomized, three-way crossover study. *Aliment. Pharmacol. Ther.* 21 (8): 993–1000.

83. Dominguez-Munoz, J.E., Iglesias-Garcia, J., Iglesias-Rey, M., and Vilarino-Insua, M. (2006). Optimising the therapy of exocrine pancreatic insufficiency by the association of a proton pump inhibitor to enteric coated pancreatic extracts. *Gut* 55 (7): 1056–1057.

# CHAPTER 15

# Liver Resection

Nabeel Merali and Adam Frampton

*Department of HPB Surgery, Royal Surrey NHS Foundation Trust, Guildford, UK*

---

**KEY POINTS**

- The liver is a highly metabolically active organ.
- Fatty liver is common in obesity and after chemotherapy, and can adversely affect surgical outcome and interpretation of residual liver size.
- In the absence of any clinical research, post-operative liver dysfunction may benefit from the same nutritional management as chronic liver failure.
- Prolonged bile leaks cause electrolyte depletion and fat malabsorption and bile reinfusion may reduce the impact of these.

---

Hepatic (liver) resection is an effective and curative treatment for patients with primary and secondary malignant tumours. Hepatic resections are performed in specialised high-volume centres.

## LIVER PHYSIOLOGY AND ANATOMY

The liver is a fascinating organ that is able to regenerate after a resection. Termed the 'antechamber of the heart', its blood supply is 25% of the resting cardiac output and it is a significant processor of the nutrients absorbed from the gastrointestinal tract, as 75% of its blood supply is from the portal vein. Hepatocytes are the chief functional cells of the liver and perform an astounding number of functions, including maintenance of blood glucose levels, synthesis of clotting factors, production of bile, removal of waste products (metabolites, toxins, hormones), removal of senescent red blood cells, and production of immune factors. The liver lies immediately below, and in contact with, the diaphragm. It is covered with peritoneum except for the gallbladder fossa and the bare area that lies posteriorly. The peritoneum

*Nutritional Management of the Surgical Patient*, First Edition. Edited by Mary E. Phillips.
© 2023 John Wiley & Sons Ltd. Published 2023 by John Wiley & Sons Ltd.

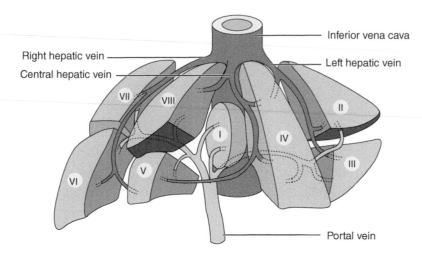

Right hepatic vein

Central hepatic vein

Inferior vena cava

Left hepatic vein

VII    VIII

II

I

IV

III

VI

V

Portal vein

**FIGURE 15.1**    Anatomy of the liver. *Source*: Reproduced from Ellis, H., and Mahadevan, V. (2014). *Clinical Anatomy: Applied Anatomy for Students and Junior Doctors*, 13th ed. Chichester: Wiley.

cover forms folds such as the falciform ligament (anterior superior attachment of the liver to the abdominal wall) and the inferior edge that forms the ligamentum teres. The falciform ligament is an important surface marking that divides the liver into two lobes (right and left). It also extends laterally to form the coronary and left triangular ligament, which attaches the liver to the diaphragm. The liver can be subdivided into eight (Coinaud) segments based on the porta hepatis distribution (branch of the hepatic artery, hepatic vein, and bile duct) (Figure 15.1).

## PRE-OPERATIVE CARE

### Embolisation

Patients with extensive bilobar diseases or major extended right-side resections benefit from pre-operative portal vein embolisation (PVE). This will start hypertrophy of the future liver remnant (FLR). Hepatic vein embolisation (HVE) can facilitate further FLR and create venous collaterals [1]. For large hepatocellular carcinoma (HCC) lesions that are dependent on arterial blood supply, a transarterial chemoembolisation (TACE) can starve the tumour prior to resection.

### Pre-operative Nutrition

Enhanced recovery after surgery (ERAS) is a peri-operative care programme that encourages patients to have early oral intake, mobilise and aims to reduce length of stay. This fast-track method has been shown to be effective and safe in patients undergoing liver resection [2] (see Chapter 5).

Nutritional management in patients undergoing liver resection is paramount, especially as these patients will be in a catabolic state as the liver is regenerating, with electrolyte (phosphate) and glucose dysfunction. Prior to surgery, patients should have a high-protein diet and participate in prehabilitation. Yokoyama et al. stated that patients with low skeletal muscle mass or those with low functional exercise capacity showed a significantly worse post-operative course and poor long-term survival after surgery for liver malignancy [3].

There is an increasing prominence of non-alcoholic fatty liver disease (NAFLD) that is related to HCC. This is directly related to other diseases such as diabetes mellitus and obesity metabolic syndrome [4]. Barth et al. performed a multicentre randomised control trial on the effects of a one-week calorie- and fat-restricted diet in patients undergoing liver surgery, with the aim of reducing steatosis. Results showed a significant reduction in intraoperative blood loss, and surgeons commented that the liver was easier to manipulate [5]. Consequently, patients with high levels of liver steatosis, or those who are obese, should be considered for a calorie-restricted diet prior to undergoing surgery.

## SURGERY

### Indications for Surgery

Indications for hepatic resection can be divided into three categories: malignancy, benign, and trauma related. HCC is the most common primary hepatic malignancy and can occur in the setting of inherited (e.g. hemochromatosis) or acquired (e.g. chronic hepatitis C, alcoholic cirrhosis) pre-existing conditions [6]. Globally, hepatitis B is the most common cause of HCC [7]. The overall survival of patients with HCC is poor at less than 15% at five years [7]. Curative treatment for eligible patients includes ablation (surgical or percutaneous) for small tumours <2 cm, anatomical resection, and orthotopic liver transplantation (OLT). Intrahepatic cholangiocarcinoma (ICC) represents the second most common primary liver cancer [8]. ICC is highly metastatic and has a very poor overall survival rate of 18% within five years [9]. Surgical treatment involves a hemi-hepatectomy or extended hepatectomy to remove the tumour with negative margins. Gallbladder adenocarcinoma has an overall median survival of less than six months and spreads early to distant organs. Surgical management involves an extended cholecystectomy (en bloc resection of the gallbladder and a wedge segmental 4B/5). If the tumour has infiltrated the liver bed, resection of segment 4/5 is recommended.

The liver is a common site for secondary metastasis from solid tumours. Neuroendocrine lesions, primarily from the foregut, are a source of metastases that respond well to liver resection [10]. Resection of tumour metastases from several areas such as breast, sarcoma, genitourinary, and melanoma have also been reported [11]. The prognosis of colorectal cancer patients is in a large part determined by the presence of metastases. The liver is usually the first site of metastatic disease and may be the only site in 30–40% of patients with advanced disease [12]. Safe and effective surgical procedures for treating colorectal cancer patients with liver metastases (CRCLM) have shifted from palliation to prolongation of survival and cure.

Symptomatic benign hepatic lesions (simple cysts, haemangioma, adenoma, focal nodular hyperplasia) that cause pressure effects and pain are considered for resections. Some asymptomatic lesions, such as large or giant haemangiomas and adenomas larger than 5 cm, warrant resection when anatomically feasible [13]. Bacterial or amoebic hepatic abscesses resistant to antibiotic and failed percutaneous drainage treatment may need resection for source control. Interhepatic stone disease that leads to biliary stricture, segmental atrophy, and potential sepsis should be resected. A liver resection may be required for acute haemorrhage control in traumatic injuries, although the majority of cases can be managed conservatively or with interventional radiology.

### Contraindications to Surgery

Contraindications to liver surgery depend on several factors. Patients may be unfit for surgery due to severe underlying liver disease, comorbidities, or frailty. Documented extrahepatic disease is a contraindication for many malignancies, but not for all. Inferior vena cava invasion is generally considered a contraindication to surgical intervention. In the planning stage, the liver is assessed to ensure that there is sufficient healthy liver left (referred to as the remnant). Patients with a predicted FLR <20% are not usually considered suitable for surgery as there is an increased risk of liver failure and death [14, 15].

### Operative Description

The type of resection depends on the location and number of lesions and whether there will be an acceptable FLR.

Small non-anatomical (wedge) resections are not based on interhepatic anatomy (anatomical boundaries of vascular inflow). Segmental resection refers to the anatomical resection of one or more segments of the liver. Removal of several segments is called a sectorectomy. This is performed for tumours that are located at the centre of a segment.

Right hepatectomy involves removing all hepatic parenchyma to the right of the middle hepatic vein (segments 5–8).

Left hepatectomy involves removal of segments 1–4. An extended right hemicolectomy is resection of segments 5–8 with the addition of segment 4 from the left side of the liver, whereas an extended left hepatectomy includes removal of segments 5 and 8 in addition to the left hemi-liver.

Open liver surgery is the standard treatment; however, minimally invasive liver surgery (MILS) is increasingly being used. Benefits include reduced post-operative pain and ileus, shorter length of stay, rapid return to pre-operative activity, and better cosmetic results. The OSLO-COMET randomised control trial was the first of its kind to compare laparoscopic to open liver surgery for patients with CRCLM. A single-centre, double-blinded study randomised 280 patients into two equal groups. The authors concluded that the operative time, blood loss, and R0 resection rates were similar in both groups. However, the length of stay was shorter in the laparoscopic group [16].

Over the last decade, robotic liver surgery has come to the forefront of surgical innovation, with instruments that provide better ergonomics, freedom of movement, and tremor filtering with three-dimensional imaging. A recent multicentre study demonstrated that long-term results for robotic and laparoscopic resection for CRCLM were comparable to open surgery [17].

Patient selection is paramount in deciding the method of surgical liver resection. Minor hepatectomy cases with lesions of ≤5 cm located in one of the peripheral liver segments are mostly performed with MILS [18], whereas difficult hilar, centrally located lesions in close relation to major vessels may be better suited to open surgery [19].

## POST-OPERATIVE CARE

### Post-operative Nutritional Support

If oral feeding can be tolerated, enteral feeding is always preferred over parenteral as it maintains the intestinal integrity and is associated with fewer post-operative complications [20]. Due to the metabolic demands of regeneration, clinicians suspect that patients have high energy requirements following liver resection, but there is no data in the literature.

There is growing evidence that use of branched-chain amino acid (BCAA) supplementation in the peri-operative setting for malnourished patients who undergo liver resection leads to an improved quality of life [21]. BCAAs have shown to increase erythropoietin, which protects hepatocytes from ischaemic injury [22]. European guidelines recommend that the evidence base for this is not yet strong enough for incorporation into clinical practice [23], but it is an area for further research.

### Post-operative Complications

Common post-operative infections are venous catheter related, pleural atelectasis and effusions, incisional surgical site infections, subphrenic collections, and infected ascites.

### Ascites

Ascites is common in patients with underlying liver disease such as cirrhosis who have had a hepatectomy. Paracentesis for treatment of the ascites usually is not recommended; administration of diuretics and albumin is preferred unless the ascites is thought to be infected [24].

### Ileus

Post-operative ileus can occur after liver surgery, as dissecting the porta hepatis and applying a Pringle' manoeuvre can lead to bowel congestion, with a normal physiological surgical stress response and inflammation of intestinal smooth muscle (see Chapter 20).

## Haemorrhage

Post-operative haemorrhage is managed with red blood cell replacement and correction of the coagulopathy profile. A significant haemorrhage is best managed with interventional angiography and embolisation of a bleeding artery. However, if a patient becomes haemodynamically unstable, then laparotomy is obligatory and packing of the liver is advised. Haemobilia implies bleeding into the biliary tree and is indicative of a fistula between vessel and bile duct. The presentation is that of an upper gastrointestinal bleed with haematemesis and melena. An emergency gastroscopy can be diagnostic (bleeding from the ampulla into the duodenum) and therapeutic. Alternatively, an angiogram can distinguish the exact anatomical point of bleeding from the fistula site.

## Bile Leak

The incidence of bile leakage ranges from 4 to 17% [25]. Bile leaking from the biliary tree must be drained. The majority of leaks occur directly after liver surgery and are managed conservatively with an intraoperative abdominal drain, and close spontaneously (small biliary radicle). If a bile leak is suspected, computed tomographic (CT) imaging is recommended to ensure there are no further undrained collections. This will also help define the anatomy of the bile leak and exclude distal biliary obstruction. High-volume persistent bile leaks require an endoscopic retrograde cholangiopancreatography (ERCP) sphincterotomy to reduce biliary pressure. In cases where an obstinate biliary fistula has formed, re-exploration is recommended and a Roux loop can be brought up to secure internal drainage of the fistula into the gastrointestinal tract. Biliary leaks can cause ileus, and in that instance parenteral nutrition is recommended.

## Bile Reinfusion

In the case of a controlled prolonged bile leak, or when reoperation or internalisation needs to be delayed on clinical grounds, reinfusion of bile should be considered. Prolonged bile leaks are associated with change in bacterial flora, sodium depletion, and malnutrition [26], and if the drained bile is not infected it can be reinfused, thus reducing sodium losses and restoring the enterohepatic circulation. Some units reinfuse bile orally, but due to poor tolerance enteral feeding tubes are often used. A naso-gastric tube can be used, but position checks using pH paper are difficult due to the alkaline infusion into the stomach, and physiologically this results in an alkaline stomach that may have an impact on digestion. The use of a naso-jejunal feeding tube to reinfuse bile normalises the pH of the gut, but there is a paucity of data exploring the benefits of each route in clinical practice.

## Liver Failure

Post-operative liver failure is a serious complication and is related to inadequate residual liver tissue and functional capacity [27]. It is associated with high morbidity and mortality. Post-operative liver failure is defined as a rising international normalised ratio (INR) of $\geq 1.5$ and hyperbilirubinaemia (rise in serum bilirubin of 20–40 µmol/l/d) on or after postoperative day 5 [28]. Severity is grades from A (no intervention) to C (requires invasive treatment) [29]. A sudden deterioration and liver decompensation post-surgery may be related to surgical complications such liver ischaemia or necrosis, portal vein thrombosis, or a vascular rotational injury of remnant liver. Therefore, a triple-phase CT liver is recommended. Intensive care management is required with the administration of intravenous acetylcysteine that facilitates oxygen delivery into hepatocytes. Liver function and coagulation profile are closely monitored, with particular attention to the prothrombin time (PT) and haemoglobin. Nutritional management is similar to chronic liver failure with avoidance of periods of starvation; high-energy, high-protein provision; with supplementary enteral nutrition; using naso-jejunal feeding tubes if ascites results in poor tolerance of oral or gastric feeding. Parenteral nutrition is used only if enteral nutrition is not tolerated. Constipation should be avoided and lactulose is often used to promote at least two soft stools per day to reduce ammonia uptake in the bowel, thereby reducing the risk of hepatic encephalopathy. Patients should be started on a prophylactic proton pump inhibitor to reduce the risk of a stress ulcer.

## Small-for-Size Syndrome

Small-for-size syndrome (SFSS) is a recognised complication following major hepatectomy and liver transplantation. SFSS is characterised by persistent hyperbilirubinaemia, coagulopathy, intractable ascites, and encephalopathy. Remnant liver total volume is reduced while the volume of the portal venous return remains the same. This leads to a rise in portal venous pressure (PVP) and portal hypertension [30]. High portal pressures cause direct stress and damage to the endothelial lining of sinusoids, leading to sinusoidal dilatation and hepatocyte swelling [31]. In addition, a reduction in hepatic artery pressures leads to ischaemia [32]. Portal hypertension and intrahepatic portal congestion are the key findings within SFSS after major hepatectomy. Medical treatment consists of somatostatin infusions [32] and non-selective beta-blockers that modulate splanchnic blood flow [33] to reduce PVP in major hepatectomy cases. Future work on SFSS is required to better understand the pathogenesis of SFSS and develop strategies for prevention of liver failure.

There is no data regarding the nutritional management of SFSS in the literature, but European guidelines stress the importance of avoiding malnutrition in the post-operative setting [23]. Clinical practice mirrors the management of chronic liver failure in order to reduce additional metabolic demand on the liver. More holistic management aiming to reduce factors that may contribute to further steatosis should be reinforced. For instance, blood glucose levels should be tightly controlled and patients should completely abstain from alcohol.

## CONCLUSION

In summary, liver resection is the gold-standard curative treatment for several benign and malignant diseases. The liver is a very unforgiving structure and meticulous surgical technique and planning with a multidisciplinary approach are required. While most resections do not result in significant nutritional deficit, post-operative complications can result in complex liver dysfunction needing intensive nutritional support.

---

### Case Study:   Colorectal Liver Metastasis

A 72-year-old man was found to have a solitary liver metastasis in the left lobe of the liver with an associated rise of his carcinoembryonic antigen (CEA). He had an anterior resection 12 months previously following neo-adjuvant chemoradiotherapy for T3 N0 M0 rectal tumour.

CT chest, abdomen, and pelvis showed a 48 mm low attenuation of peripherally enhancing mass in segment 2.

Magnetic resonance imaging (MRI) of the liver with contrast was performed to assess resectability and showed the large lesion was primarily in segment 2 and starting to involve segment 4a.

Nutritional assessment pre-operatively did not identify any evidence of malnutrition, with no change in oral intake, no weight loss, and malnutrition universal screening tool score of 0.

The patient underwent an elective open liver resection (segments 2 and 3 extended to segment 4) plus adhesiolysis. Post-operatively he was managed with the enhanced recovery after surgery (ERAS) protocol, which includes early introduction of an oral diet using three oral nutritional supplements for the first three days until a normal diet was re-established.

His post-operative blood results were unremarkable. He made a full recovery with no post-operative concerns and was discharged on day 4. Follow-up histology revealed fully excised colorectal liver metastasis with clear margins.

## Case Study:    Liver Failure and Bile Leak in a Post-Hepatectomy Patient

A 49-year-old man presented with multiple metastases through all of the lobes of the liver secondary to colorectal cancer. His past medical history consisted of sigmoid colectomy and defunctioning ileostomy for the primary tumour. Initially it was not possible to resect the whole tumour, but following chemotherapy and selective internal radiation therapy (SIRT) his liver was deemed resectable on MRI, CT, and positron emission tomography (PET).

Fluorodeoxyglucose (FDG) PET/CT scan showed a reduction in liver tumour burden with no measurable disease in the left lobe. There are approximately 10 right liver lobe metastases within segments 4a, 8, 7, and 5.

Liver volumes appeared to be adequate and an elective extended right hepatectomy was performed. The operation was successful with no complications, and he was discharged on day 5. However, the patient was readmitted four weeks later with lethargy, increase abdominal distension, and pain.

His blood results showed raised inflammatory markers: C-reactive protein (CRP) 228 g/l (reference range [RR] <4), white cell count $17.8 \times 10^9$/l (RR 4–11), with deranged liver function tests: alkaline phosphatase 170 U/l (RR 30–130); alanine transaminase 48 U/l (RR 10–49); bilirubin 54 μmol/l (RR 0–20); albumin 26 g/l (RR 35–50); sodium 128 mmol/l (RR 133–146).

CT triple phase of liver showed extensive free fluid tracking from the surgical bed and extending throughout the abdomen and pelvis, suspicious of a bile leak (Figure 15.2).

An ultrasound-guided 12 French locking pigtail was inserted into the large biloma and the patient was started on a high-protein oral diet. Bile fluid culture grew *Citrobacter* and antibiotics

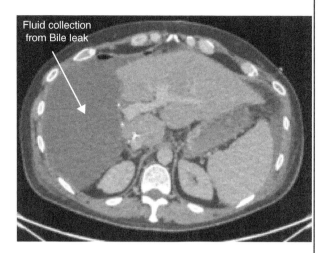

**FIGURE 15.2**    Computed tomographic image of bile leak following liver resection.

commenced. He had a complicated post-operative recovery with small-for-size liver insufficiency, which was likely exacerbated by his pre-operative chemotherapy and chemoembolisation. He was managed with a high-protein diet (30–35 kcal/kg; 1.2–1.5 g protein/g), 50 g carbohydrate bedtime snack to reduce periods of starvation. Blood glucose levels were monitored to ensure they were <10 mmol/l, oral adequacy was assessed using food record charts, and handgrip strength was used to assess functional improvements, as weight was inaccurate due to the presence of ascites.

Due to the presence of ascites he struggled with solid foods, and thus oral nutritional supplements were commenced ($3 \times 125$ ml supplements; 900 kcal; 54 g protein). He was managed with a reducing dose of diuretics (spironolactone), fluid restriction (1500 ml), and was discharged after a month's stay in hospital. His histology showed completely excised metastases from previous colorectal cancer.

# REFERENCES

1. Munene, G., Parker, R.D., Larrigan, J. et al. (2013). Sequential preoperative hepatic vein embolization after portal vein embolization for extended left hepatectomy in colorectal liver metastases. *World J. Surg. Oncol.* 11: 134.

2. van Dam, R.M., Hendry, P.O., Coolsen, M.M. et al. (2008). Initial experience with a multimodal enhanced recovery programme in patients undergoing liver resection. *Br. J. Surg.* 95 (8): 969–975.

3. Yokoyama, Y., Nagino, M., and Ebata, T. (2021). Importance of 'muscle' and 'intestine' training before major HPB surgery: a review. *J. Hepatobiliary Pancreat. Sci.* 28 (7): 545–555.

4. McGlynn, K.A., Petrick, J.L., and London, W.T. (2015). Global epidemiology of hepatocellular carcinoma: an emphasis on demographic and regional variability. *Clin. Liver Dis.* 19 (2): 223–238.

5. Barth, R.J. Jr., Mills, J.B., Suriawinata, A.A. et al. (2019). Short-term preoperative diet decreases bleeding after partial hepatectomy: results from a multi-institutional randomized controlled trial. *Ann. Surg.* 269 (1): 48–52.

6. Bruix, J. and Sherman, M. (2005). Practice Guidelines Committee, American Association for the Study of Liver Diseases. Management of hepatocellular carcinoma. *Hepatology* 42 (5): 1208–1236.

7. El-Serag, H.B. (2011). Hepatocellular carcinoma. *N. Engl. J. Med.* 365 (12): 1118–1127.

8. Balzan, S., Belghiti, J., Farges, O. et al. (2005). The '50-50 criteria' on postoperative day 5: an accurate predictor of liver failure and death after hepatectomy. *Ann. Surg.* 242 (6): 824–828.

9. Brown, K.M., Parmar, A.D., and Geller, D.A. (2014). Intrahepatic cholangiocarcinoma. *Surg. Oncol. Clin. N. Am.* 23 (2): 231–246.

10. Tan, M.C. and Jarnagin, W.R. (2014). Surgical management of non-colorectal hepatic metastasis. *J. Surg. Oncol.* 109 (1): 8–13.

11. Groeschl, R.T., Nachmany, I., Steel, J.L. et al. (2012). Hepatectomy for noncolorectal non-neuroendocrine metastatic cancer: a multi-institutional analysis. *J. Am. Coll. Surg.* 214 (5): 769–777.

12. Weiss, L., Grundmann, E., Torhorst, J. et al. (1986). Haematogenous metastatic patterns in colonic carcinoma: an analysis of 1541 necropsies. *J. Pathol.* 150 (3): 195–203.

13. Cho, S.W., Marsh, J.W., Steel, J. et al. (2008). Surgical management of hepatocellular adenoma: take it or leave it? *Ann. Surg. Oncol.* 15 (10): 2795–2803.

14. Ferrero, A., Vigano, L., Polastri, R. et al. (2007). Postoperative liver dysfunction and future remnant liver: where is the limit? Results of a prospective study. *World J. Surg.* 31 (8): 1643–1651.

15. Kishi, Y., Abdalla, E.K., Chun, Y.S. et al. (2009). Three hundred and one consecutive extended right hepatectomies: evaluation of outcome based on systematic liver volumetry. *Ann. Surg.* 250 (4): 540–548.

16. Fretland, A.A., Dagenborg, V.J., Bjornelv, G.M.W. et al. (2018). Laparoscopic versus open resection for colorectal liver metastases: the OSLO-COMET randomized controlled trial. *Ann. Surg.* 267 (2): 199–207.

17. Beard, R.E., Khan, S., Troisi, R.I. et al. (2020). Long-term and oncologic outcomes of robotic versus laparoscopic liver resection for metastatic colorectal cancer: a multicenter, propensity score matching analysis. *World J. Surg.* 44 (3): 887–895.

18. Buell, J.F., Cherqui, D., Geller, D.A. et al. (2009). The international position on laparoscopic liver surgery: the Louisville Statement, 2008. *Ann. Surg.* 250 (5): 825–830.

19. Shiraiwa, D.K., Carvalho, P., Maeda, C.T. et al. (2020). The role of minimally invasive hepatectomy for hilar and intrahepatic cholangiocarcinoma: a systematic review of the literature. *J. Surg. Oncol.* 121 (5): 863–872.

20. Richter, B., Schmandra, T.C., Golling, M., and Bechstein, W.O. (2006). Nutritional support after open liver resection: a systematic review. *Dig. Surg.* 23 (3): 139–145.

21. Okabayashi, T., Iyoki, M., Sugimoto, T. et al. (2011). Oral supplementation with carbohydrate- and branched-chain amino acid-enriched nutrients improves postoperative quality of life in patients undergoing hepatic resection. *Amino Acids* 40 (4): 1213–1220.

22. Ishikawa, Y., Yoshida, H., Mamada, Y. et al. (2010). Prospective randomized controlled study of short-term perioperative oral nutrition with branched chain amino acids in patients undergoing liver surgery. *Hepato-Gastroenterology* 57 (99-100): 583–590.

23. Bischoff, S.C., Bernal, W., Dasarathy, S. et al. (2020). ESPEN practical guideline: Clinical nutrition in liver disease. *Clin. Nutr.* 39 (12): 3533–3562.

24. Di Carlo, I. and Toro, A. (2012). Correct indication for surgery can prevent postoperative ascites in cirrhotic patients affected by hepatocellular carcinoma. *World J. Surg.* 36 (7): 1719–1720.

25. Bhattacharjya, S., Puleston, J., Davidson, B.R., and Dooley, J.S. (2003). Outcome of early endoscopic biliary drainage in the management of bile leaks after hepatic resection. *Gastrointest. Endosc.* 57 (4): 526–530.

26. Ponsky, J.L. and Aszodi, A. (1982). External biliary-gastric fistula: a simple method for recycling bile. *Am. J. Gastroenterol.* 77 (12): 939–940.

27. Hammond, J.S., Guha, I.N., Beckingham, I.J., and Lobo, D.N. (2011). Prediction, prevention and management of postresection liver failure. *Br. J. Surg.* 98 (9): 1188–1200.

28. Rahbari, N.N., Garden, O.J., Padbury, R. et al. (2011). Posthepatectomy liver failure: a definition and grading by the International Study Group of Liver Surgery (ISGLS). *Surgery* 149 (5): 713–724.

29. Glanemann, M., Eipel, C., Nussler, A.K. et al. (2005). Hyperperfusion syndrome in small-for-size livers. *Eur. Surg. Res.* 37 (6): 335–341.

30. Golriz, M., Majlesara, A., El Sakka, S. et al. (2016). Small for size and flow (SFSF) syndrome: an alternative description for posthepatectomy liver failure. *Clin. Res. Hepatol. Gastroenterol.* 40 (3): 267–275.

31. Bolognesi, M., Sacerdoti, D., Bombonato, G. et al. (2002). Change in portal flow after liver transplantation: effect on hepatic arterial resistance indices and role of spleen size. *Hepatology* 35 (3): 601–608.

32. Rhaiem, R., Piardi, T., Chetboun, M. et al. (2018). Portal inflow modulation by somatostatin after major liver resection: a pilot study. *Ann. Surg.* 267 (6): e101–e103.

33. Gruttadauria, S., Pagano, D., Liotta, R. et al. (2015). Liver volume restoration and hepatic microarchitecture in small-for-size syndrome. *Ann. Transplant.* 20: 381–389.

# CHAPTER 16

# Nutritional Management of the Urological Surgical Patient

Gregory J Nason, Wissam Abou Chedid, Matthew J.A. Perry, and Krishna Patil

*Department of Urology, Royal Surrey NHS Foundation Trust, Guildford, UK*

---

**KEY POINTS**

- Malnutrition is present in 33% of patients prior to radical surgery for bladder cancer.
- Prehabilitation can improve patients' pre-operative nutritional and functional capacity, resulting in improved post-operative outcomes.
- Management of post-operative complications such as prolonged paralytic ileus requires early nutritional input.

---

Bladder cancer is the 11th most common cancer in the UK, with approximately 10 000 new cases per year [1]. The 'two-week rule' referral system is the most common route to diagnosis in the UK, with patients referred to one-stop diagnostic clinics with haematuria (blood in the urine). The majority of patients present with early non-muscle-invasive bladder cancer (NMIBC); however, approximately 30% of patients diagnosed with NMIBC progress to muscle-invasive bladder cancer (MIBC), while a further 25% present upfront as MIBC [2]. Treatment of bladder cancer is based on stage at diagnosis and the current standard of care for MIBC is radical cystectomy (removal of the bladder) [3, 4]. The overall five-year survival rate for MIBC after radical cystectomy is approximately 50%, whereas for untreated MIBC it is near 5% [5].

## OVERVIEW OF SURGICAL PROCEDURE

The majority of urological procedures have limited impact on nutritional status (i.e. vasectomy, transurethral prostatectomy, and simple nephrectomy), therefore for the purposes of this chapter our focus is on radical cystectomy, which is one of the most significant operations in urology. It encompasses the removal of the bladder and prostate in a man and

*Nutritional Management of the Surgical Patient*, First Edition. Edited by Mary E. Phillips.
© 2023 John Wiley & Sons Ltd. Published 2023 by John Wiley & Sons Ltd.

the bladder, uterus, ovaries, and anterior vagina in a woman, a bilateral extended pelvic lymph node dissection, and a urinary diversion. Traditionally this was performed as an open operation, with reported complication rates between 30 and 70% and significant length of stay (LOS) of 10–14 days [6]. Robotic-assisted radical cystectomy use has grown exponentially and has now surpassed open radical cystectomy in Europe and North America [7]. Randomised control trials (RCTs), including the recently reported CORAL trial from the UK, have demonstrated the oncological safety of robotic-assisted radical cystectomy [8, 9]. The procedure has proven benefits in terms of reduced LOS, lower blood loss, and less need for blood transfusion [10].

Following the extirpative part of the procedure, the urinary tract requires reconstruction. An ileal conduit is the choice of diversion in over 75% patients in the UK [11, 12]. This involves harvesting a 20 cm segment of ileum, anastomosing both ureters into the proximal end, and exteriorising the distal end as a spouted incontinent stoma. Alternatively, an orthotopic neobladder can be created. This involves using a 60 cm segment of ileum to form a pouch, anastomosing the distal end to the urethra and the ureters into the proximal part of the pouch. The choice of diversion is multifactorial based on disease factors, patient preference, and surgeon experience. Health-related quality of life scores are near equivalent between ileal conduits and neobladders, with younger and fitter patients more likely to choose a neobladder [13, 14]. Pre-operative counselling is of paramount importance in understanding the risks and benefits associated with diversion type [15].

Radical cystectomies are predominantly performed in an older comorbid cohort. The 30-day mortality rate for radical cystectomy is reported at 4% and the peri-operative complication rate was 40–50%, with a Clavien Dindo 3b–4 complication rate of 3–4% [16]. The high complication rate is multifactorial based on patients' pre-operative condition, and the length and complexity of the procedure. Long term, patients undergo oncological surveillance, but also surveillance of their renal function and urinary diversion.

One of the key recommendations from the NHS Cancer Plan and the 'Improving Outcomes Guidelines' was the centralisation of major surgical procedures such as radical cystectomy to high-volume centres. The guidelines recommended that radical surgery for prostate and bladder cancer should be provided by teams serving populations of one million or more, and carrying out a cumulative total of ≥50 operations per annum [17]. The volume–outcome relationship for radical cystectomy is well recognised. The European Association of Urology recommends that hospitals perform 10, preferably 20, radical cystectomies per year or refer patients to centres that achieve this number [18]. In a systematic review, Bruins et al. demonstrated improved 30- and 90-day mortality and quality indicators (nodal yield and neobladder rates) as well as decreased complications, positive surgical margins, LOS, and blood loss when radical cystectomy was performed at higher-volume centres [18]. For complex procedures such as radical cystectomy, hospital volume appears to be more important than surgeon volume [19]. Radical cystectomy is a multidisciplinary effort involving urology, anaesthesia, intensive care, nursing, physiotherapy, and dietetic support.

## ENHANCED RECOVERY AFTER SURGERY AND PREHABILITATION

Enhanced recovery after surgery (ERAS) is a multimodal approach with a focus on optimising and standardising the peri-operative care of patients following major surgery. After radical cystectomy, ERAS programmes have demonstrated decreased hospital LOS, time to return of bowel function, readmissions, and overall complication rate after surgery [20]. The implementation of ERAS programmes has also been shown to be at least cost neutral, if not cost effective, based on reduced LOS [20] (see Chapter 5).

An area of ERAS that has become more topical is prehabilitation. A randomised control trial exploring multimodal home-based prehabilitation before open radical cystectomy showed that it can mitigate the negative impact of surgery on functional status.

The prehabilitation programme involved a home-based exercise regimen three times a week, a dietary intervention involving protein supplementation, as well as an anxiety-reducing education programme [21] (see Chapter 4).

Up to 20% of patients have difficulty being discharged home following radical cystectomy and require step-down or transitional care for rehabilitation [22]. The combination of major surgery and neo-adjuvant chemotherapy has a significant negative effect on patients, hence any pre-operative conditioning intervention based on improving baseline function and reducing post-operative decline is welcomed [23]. Specialist nurses are ideally placed to ensure that individual holistic care needs are addressed, and appropriate care and support are provided. Nurses can trigger timely referrals to members of the wider multidisciplinary team to coordinate an integrated, person-centred approach to prehabilitation service provision to address the unmet needs of people undergoing treatment for MIBC [24].

## IMPACT ON NUTRITION

### Pre-operative Nutritional Support

The prevalence of malnutrition in bladder cancer patients is reported to be as high as 50%, but this varies widely, likely due to the variety of definitions used [25]. In the pre-operative setting European guidelines suggest that the prevalence of malnutrition is 33% [26]. The catabolic effect of bladder cancer, the pre-existing comorbid status, and the physiological stress of major surgery contribute to the patient's outcome. It is well recognised that malnourished (both under- and over-nourished) surgical patients have more complicated courses – with higher post-operative mortality, morbidity, LOS, readmission rates, and healthcare costs. Nutritional assessment is covered in Chapter 2.

It is important to identify patients with bladder cancer at risk of malnutrition pre-operatively, as a radical cystectomy is associated with significant catabolic changes, including net fat oxidation and lean tissue loss. Malnutrition is a potentially modifiable risk factor for complications following major surgery, and thus early detection and intervention are crucial.

Cancer-related malnutrition can lead to calorie starvation, stress-related catabolic activity, cachexia, unregulated inflammation, and suppression of the immune system. Cancer can lead to an inflammatory state characterised by immunosuppressive macrophages and dendritic cells via secretion of high levels of interleukin (IL)-6, IL-1B, IL-4, and IL-10, and direct tumour progression via high levels of IL-6 [27]. There are some reports that supplementation of immuno-nutrition [28] may be beneficial. Arginine, fish oil, vitamin A, and nucleotides were taken orally pre-operatively, and associated with a reduction in post-operative complications (40% in prospective cohort vs 77% in retrospective controls, P= 0.008) and infection rate (23% vs 60%, P = 0.008) [28].

Ornaghi et al. performed a systemic review highlighting the impact of pre-operative nutritional status on outcomes following radical cystectomy [29]. In the post-operative period, a high body mass index (BMI) is associated with more complications. Patients with a BMI $25–29.9\,kg/m^2$ had a 1.5-fold increased risk of 30-day overall complications (odds ratio [OR] 1.55, 95% confidence interval [CI] 1.14–2.07, P <0.05), whereas patients with BMI $\geq 30\,kg/m^2$ had almost a twofold increased risk (OR 1.73, 95% CI 1.29–2.40, P <0.05). Moreover, the 90-day overall complication rate increased for every one-unit increase in BMI with an OR of 1.05 (95% CI 1.02–1.09, P <0.05) [29]. Swalarz et al. highlighted a significant association between BMI $<18.5\,kg/m^2$ and BMI $>30\,kg/m^2$ and the degree of Clavien Dindo complications ($\chi^2 = 24.8512$; P = 0.03): obese patients were associated with Clavien Dindo complications grade 3, normal-weight patients and overweight ones with Clavien Dindo complications grade 2, and underweight patients with Clavien Dindo complications grade 4 [30]. An increased BMI was related to a higher rate of unplanned readmission within 30 days after radical cystectomy, with increased rates of infection (surgical site infections, urinary tract infections), hernias, wound dehiscence, renal impairment, paralytic ileus, pulmonary complications, and uretero-ileal anastomotic strictures [30]. There is less data pertaining to BMI and complications following robotic-assisted radical cystectomy – further studies are required to ascertain if minimally invasive surgery is a factor. Furthermore, the assessment of nutritional status using BMI alone does not take into account the presence of sarcopenia.

Sarcopenia index, an alternative measure of nutrition as measured by skeletal muscle index on cross-sectional imaging, has been used to distinguish sarcopenic and non-sarcopenic patients. Sarcopenic patients had a twofold risk of major complications after radical cystectomy (Clavien Dindo grade $\geq$3b: OR 2.05, 95% CI 1.20–3.49, P = 0.009) and experienced significantly more severe complications (Clavien Dindo grade 4a–5: OR 2.84, 95% CI 1.33–6.01, P <0.01) compared to non-sarcopenic patients [31].

Patients with pre-operative hypoalbuminemia had a 2.3-fold increased risk of 30-day mortality compared to patients with normal albumin levels (OR 2.33, 95% CI 1.10–4.95, P = 0.03) [32].

Pre-operative weight loss has been shown to have significantly worse complications and mortality rates in patients undergoing surgery. Weight loss of >3 kg prior to radical cystectomy was associated with 90-day high-grade complication rate and wound complication rate [33].

Long term, the pre-operative nutritional index (PNI) has been shown to be an independent predictor of survival following radical cystectomy. PNI combines two biochemical markers: nutritional (serum albumin) and inflammatory (lymphocyte count). Among 516 patients who underwent radical cystectomy for MIBC, PNI independently predicted overall survival (hazard ratio [HR] 0.668, 95% CI 1.147–2.425, P = 0.007) and progression-free survival (HR 1.680, 95% CI 1.092–2.005, P = 0.015). Low PNI predicted worse overall survival for all pathological stages [34]. PNI has also been associated with post-operative complications. Pulmonary complications occurred in 13% of patients following radical cystectomy. The incidence of pulmonary complications was significantly higher based on PNI (20.8% vs 6.8%; P <0.001). The rates of intensive care unit admission and prolonged (>2-day) stay were higher in patients with a low PNI [35].

## Post-operative Nutrition

It is anticipated that patients will lose weight and muscle mass while recovering from major surgery such as radical cystectomy. McDonald et al. reported that mean cumulative post-operative weight loss at two weeks was 9.5 lb (4.3 kg; −5.2%), 14.3 lb (6.5 kg; −7.8%) at one month, 16.9 lbs (7.6 kg; −9.0%) at two months, 12.6 lb (5.7 kg; −6.9%) at three months, and 8.9 lb (4 kg; −4.6%) at four months, demonstrating a persistent weight loss in the first two months after surgery, followed by a slow regain of body weight. There was a significant decrease in five-year survival in patients with $\geq$10% weight loss [36]. Similarly, patients with significant weight loss (defined as $\geq$7.5% at one month) had higher-grade complications within one month and significantly shorter overall survival than those with weight loss of <7.5% [37].

## COMMON POST-OPERATIVE COMPLICATIONS AND THEIR NUTRITIONAL MANAGEMENT

### Ileus

One of the most common complications following radical cystectomy is paralytic ileus (up to 25%) [38]. The rates of paralytic ileus are significantly reduced with ERAS protocols [39]. Protocols often incorporate early instigation of fluids, the use of chewing gum [40], and early progress onto a solid diet. Historically, feeding was postponed until patients started passing flatus and, in some centres, parenteral nutrition (PN) was routine; however, this has been proven to be ineffective [41]. PN is now only considered in cases of prolonged ileus (see Chapter 20).

### Metabolic Acidosis

The formation of an ileal conduit or neobladders can result in hyperchloraemic metabolic acidosis and electrolyte disturbances due to absorption of ammonia through the intestinal mucosa used in the reconstruction. In some cases, patients are not able to compensate and metabolic acidosis may occur. An observational trial described an incidence of 31% in patients following formation of a neobladder and 14.8% after ileal conduit (n = 95); this was sustained with metabolic acidosis still present at 12-month follow-up in 22.9% and 10%, respectively (n = 68) [42]. This is relevant for patients receiving PN, where there is often a high chloride and free amino acid content, which also predisposes patients to metabolic acidosis. Furthermore, lactic acidosis has been linked to thiamine deficiency and the use of PN [43]. Careful acid–base monitoring should take place in patients with post-operative complications, requiring PN following neobladder or ileal conduit formation.

## AREAS FOR FUTURE RESEARCH

The peri-operative nutritional status of a patient undergoing radical cystectomy is of great importance. However, there remains a paucity of data regarding robotic-assisted radical cystectomy, nutritional status, and outcomes. The physiological stress associated with robotic surgery is less than with the traditional open approach [44] and as a result the nutritional status may be less affected.

## REFERENCES

1. Cancer Research UK. Bladder cancer statistics. https://www.cancerresearchuk.org/health-professional/cancer-statistics/statistics-by-cancer-type/bladder-cancer. Accessed 25th May 2023.

2. Antoni, S., Ferlay, J., Soerjomataram, I. et al. (2017). Bladder Cancer incidence and mortality: a global overview and recent trends. *Eur. Urol.* 71 (1): 96–108.

3. National Institute for Health and Care Excellence (2015). Bladder cancer: diagnosis and management. NICE guideline [NG2]. https://www.nice.org.uk/guidance/ng2. Accessed 25th May 2023.

4. Alfred Witjes, J., Lebret, T., Comperat, E.M. et al. (2017). Updated 2016 EAU guidelines on muscle-invasive and metastatic bladder Cancer. *Eur. Urol.* 71 (3): 462–475.

5. Martini, A., Sfakianos, J.P., Renstrom-Koskela, L. et al. (2020). The natural history of untreated muscle-invasive bladder cancer. *BJU Int.* 125 (2): 270–275.

6. Shabsigh, A., Korets, R., Vora, K.C. et al. (2009). Defining early morbidity of radical cystectomy for patients with bladder cancer using a standardized reporting methodology. *Eur. Urol.* 55 (1): 164–174.

7. Zamboni, S., Soria, F., Mathieu, R. et al. (2019). Differences in trends in the use of robot-assisted and open radical cystectomy and changes over time in perioperative outcomes among selected centres in North America and Europe: an international multicentre collaboration. *BJU Int.* 124 (4): 656–664.

8. Venkatramani, V., Reis, I.M., Castle, E.P. et al. (2020). Predictors of recurrence, and progression-free and overall survival following open versus robotic radical cystectomy: analysis from the RAZOR trial with a 3-year followup. *J. Urol.* 203 (3): 522–529.

9. Khan, M.S., Omar, K., Ahmed, K. et al. (2020). Long-term oncological outcomes from an early phase randomised controlled three-arm trial of open, robotic, and laparoscopic radical cystectomy (CORAL). *Eur. Urol.* 77 (1): 110–118.

10. Nason, G.J., Ajib, K., Tan, G.H., and Kulkarni, G.S. (2020). Radical cystectomy-what is the optimal surgical approach? *Transl. Androl. Urol.* 9 (5): 2308–2312.

11. Bachour, K., Faiena, I., Salmasi, A. et al. (2018). Trends in urinary diversion after radical cystectomy for urothelial carcinoma. *World J. Urol.* 36 (3): 409–416.

12. Lin-Brande, M., Nazemi, A., Pearce, S.M. et al. (2019). Assessing trends in urinary diversion after radical cystectomy for bladder cancer in the United States. *Urol. Oncol.* 37 (3): 180 e1–e9.

13. Dutta, S.C., Chang, S.C., Coffey, C.S. et al. (2002). Health related quality of life assessment after radical cystectomy: comparison of ileal conduit with continent orthotopic neobladder. *J. Urol.* 168 (1): 164–167.

14. Ali, A.S., Hayes, M.C., Birch, B. et al. (2015). Health related quality of life (HRQoL) after cystectomy: comparison between orthotopic neobladder and ileal conduit diversion. *Eur. J. Surg. Oncol.* 41 (3): 295–299.

15. Kern, S.Q., Speir, R.W., Tong, Y. et al. (2021). Longitudinal health related quality of life after open adical cystectomy: comparison of ileal conduit, Indiana Pouch, and orthotopic neobladder. *Urology* 152: 184–189.

16. Moschini, M., Simone, G., Stenzl, A. et al. (2016). Critical review of outcomes from radical cystectomy: can complications from radical cystectomy be reduced by surgical volume and robotic surgery? *Eur. Urol. Focus* 2 (1): 19–29.

17. National Institute for Health and Care Excellence (2002). Improving outcomes in urological cancers. Cancer service guideline [CSG2]. https://www.nice.org.uk/guidance/csg2. Accessed 25th May 2023.

18. Bruins, H.M., Veskimae, E., Hernandez, V. et al. (2020). The importance of hospital and surgeon volume as major determinants of morbidity and mortality after radical cystectomy for bladder Cancer: a systematic review and recommendations by the European Association of Urology Muscle-invasive and Metastatic Bladder Cancer Guideline Panel. *Eur. Urol. Oncol.* 3 (2): 131–144.

19. Mayer, E.K., Bottle, A., Darzi, A.W. et al. (2010). The volume-mortality relation for radical cystectomy in England: retrospective analysis of hospital episode statistics. *BMJ* 340: c1128.

20. Brooks, N.A., Kokorovic, A., McGrath, J.S. et al. (2022). Critical analysis of quality of life and cost-effectiveness of enhanced recovery after surgery (ERAS) for patient's undergoing urologic oncology surgery: a systematic review. *World J. Urol.* 40 (6): 1325–1342.

21. Minnella, E.M., Awasthi, R., Bousquet-Dion, G. et al. (2021). Multimodal prehabilitation to enhance functional capacity following radical cystectomy: a randomized controlled trial. *Eur. Urol. Focus* 7 (1): 132–138.

22. Nayak, J.G., Gore, J.L., Holt, S.K. et al. (2016). Patient-centered risk stratification of disposition outcomes following radical cystectomy. *Urol. Oncol.* 34 (5): 235.e17–235.e23.

23. Minnella, E.M., Carli, F., and Kassouf, W. (2022). Role of prehabilitation following major uro-oncologic surgery: a narrative review. *World J. Urol.* 40 (6): 1289–1298.

24. Nahon, I., Paterson, C., and Sayner, A. (2020). The impact of exercise and nutrition as part of a person-centered approach to prehabilitation in patients with bladder cancer. *Semin. Oncol. Nurs.* 36 (5): 151072.

25. Cerantola, Y., Valerio, M., Hubner, M. et al. (2013). Are patients at nutritional risk more prone to complications after major urological surgery? *J. Urol.* 190 (6): 2126–2132.

26. Cerantola, Y., Valerio, M., Persson, B. et al. (2013). Guidelines for perioperative care after radical cystectomy for bladder cancer: Enhanced Recovery After Surgery (ERAS(R®)) society recommendations. *Clin. Nutr.* 32 (6): 879–887.

27. Diakos, C.I., Charles, K.A., McMillan, D.C., and Clarke, S.J. (2014). Cancer-related inflammation and treatment effectiveness. *Lancet Oncol.* 15 (11): e493–e503.

28. Bertrand, J., Siegler, N., Murez, T. et al. (2014). Impact of preoperative immunonutrition on morbidity following cystectomy for bladder cancer: a case-control pilot study. *World J. Urol.* 32 (1): 233–237.

29. Ornaghi, P.I., Afferi, L., Antonelli, A. et al. (2021). The impact of preoperative nutritional status on post-surgical complication and mortality rates in patients undergoing radical cystectomy for bladder cancer: a systematic review of the literature. *World J. Urol.* 39 (4): 1045–1081.

30. Swalarz, M., Swalarz, G., Juszczak, K. et al. (2018). Correlation between malnutrition, body mass index and complications in patients with urinary bladder cancer who underwent radical cystectomy. *Adv. Clin. Exp. Med.* 27 (8): 1141–1147.

31. Mayr, R., Fritsche, H.M., Zeman, F. et al. (2018). Sarcopenia predicts 90-day mortality and postoperative complications after radical cystectomy for bladder cancer. *World J. Urol.* 36 (8): 1201–1207.

32. Arora, K., Hanson, K.T., Habermann, E.B. et al. (2018). Early complications and mortality following radical cystectomy: associations with malnutrition and obesity. *Bladder Cancer* 4 (4): 377–388.

33. Allaire, J., Leger, C., Ben-Zvi, T. et al. (2017). Prospective evaluation of nutritional factors to predict the risk of complications for patients undergoing radical cystectomy: a cohort study. *Nutr. Cancer* 69 (8): 1196–1204.

34. Peng, D., Gong, Y.Q., Hao, H. et al. (2017). Preoperative prognostic nutritional index is a significant predictor of survival with bladder Cancer after radical cystectomy: a retrospective study. *BMC Cancer* 17 (1): 391.

35. Yu, J., Hong, B., Park, J.Y. et al. (2021). Impact of prognostic nutritional index on postoperative pulmonary complications in radical cystectomy: a propensity score-matched analysis. *Ann. Surg. Oncol.* 28 (3): 1859–1869.

36. McDonald, M.L., Liss, M.A., Nseyo, U.U. et al. (2017). Weight loss following radical cystectomy for bladder cancer: characterization and effect on survival. *Clin. Genitourin. Cancer* 15 (1): 86–92.

37. Okita, K., Hatakeyama, S., Fujita, N. et al. (2018). Postoperative weight loss followed by radical cystectomy predicts poor prognosis in patients with muscle-invasive bladder cancer. *Med. Oncol.* 36 (1): 7.

38. Ramirez, J.A., McIntosh, A.G., Strehlow, R. et al. (2013). Definition, incidence, risk factors, and prevention of paralytic ileus following radical cystectomy: a systematic review. *Eur. Urol.* 64 (4): 588–597.

39. Bazargani, S.T., Djaladat, H., Ahmadi, H. et al. (2018). Gastrointestinal complications following radical cystectomy using enhanced recovery protocol. *Eur. Urol. Focus* 4 (6): 889–894.

40. Choi, H., Kang, S.H., Yoon, D.K. et al. (2011). Chewing gum has a stimulatory effect on bowel motility in patients after open or robotic radical cystectomy for

bladder cancer: a prospective randomized comparative study. *Urology* 77 (4): 884–890.

41. Roth, B., Birkhauser, F.D., Zehnder, P. et al. (2013). Parenteral nutrition does not improve postoperative recovery from radical cystectomy: results of a prospective randomised trial. *Eur. Urol.* 63 (3): 475–482.

42. Cho, A., Lee, S.M., Noh, J.W. et al. (2017). Acid-base disorders after orthotopic bladder replacement: comparison of an ileal neobladder and an ileal conduit. *Ren. Fail.* 39 (1): 379–384.

43. Kato, K., Sugiura, S., Yano, K. et al. (2009). The latent risk of acidosis in commercially available total parenteral nutrition (TPN) products: a randomized clinical trial in postoperative patients. *J. Clin. Biochem. Nutr.* 45 (1): 68–73.

44. Porcaro, A.B., Molinari, A., Terrin, A. et al. (2015). Robotic-assisted radical prostatectomy is less stressful than the open approach: results of a contemporary prospective study evaluating pathophysiology of cortisol stress-related kinetics in prostate cancer surgery. *J. Robot. Surg.* 9 (3): 249–255.

# CHAPTER 17

# Colorectal Surgery

Mary E. Phillips[1] and Jeremy R. Huddy[2]

[1] Department of Nutrition and Dietetics, Royal Surrey NHS Foundation Trust, Guildford, UK
[2] Department of Surgery, Frimley Health NHS Trust, Camberley, UK

---

**KEY POINTS**

- Malnutrition has an adverse effect on colorectal surgical outcomes.
- Enhanced recovery after surgery (ERAS) programmes play an important role in patients' recovery from colorectal surgery.
- Patients with inflammatory bowel disease are at particular risk of malnutrition and require multiprofessional team involvement.
- There may be a role for Immuno-nutrition within an enhanced recovery pathway for patients undergoing colorectal surgery.
- Patients with high-output stoma require individualised advice regarding dietary and fluid manipulation.

---

Colorectal surgery includes a wide range of emergency and elective operations to manage diseases of the colon, rectum, and anus, including conditions such as cancer, inflammatory bowel disease (IBD), diverticulitis, mechanical obstruction, and trauma. Proctology for peri-anal disease such as haemorrhoids, abscess-fistula disease, and anal fissure is also widely performed. Common colorectal conditions and operations will be discussed in this chapter, as well as there being an overview of some related small bowel conditions.

## PRESENTATION AND AETIOLOGY

Patients with colorectal disease can present with a wide range of symptoms, including abdominal pain, change in bowel habit, rectal bleeding, iron-deficiency

*Nutritional Management of the Surgical Patient*, First Edition. Edited by Mary E. Phillips.
© 2023 John Wiley & Sons Ltd. Published 2023 by John Wiley & Sons Ltd.

anaemia, or unexplained weight loss [1]. Initial investigations usually include endoscopy (colonoscopy or flexible sigmoidoscopy), computerised tomography (CT) scans, magnetic resonance imaging (MRI), faecal calprotectin, and faecal immunochemical tests (FIT).

Many colorectal patients will present as emergencies with bowel obstruction, bleeding, or perforation. Most small bowel obstructions are caused by adhesions or hernia. Other causes include Crohn's disease, intussusception, gallstone ileus, food bolus, and malignancy. In comparison the majority of large bowel obstructions are caused by malignancy, diverticular stricture, or volvulus.

## Colorectal Cancer

Colorectal cancer is the fourth most common cancer in the UK [2]. Tumours in the bowel may be benign or malignant, and can present with rectal bleeding, sometimes resulting in anaemia, change in bowel habit, abdominal mass, weight loss, or obstruction.

The main treatment for localised colorectal cancer is surgical resection with or without chemotherapy. In rectal cancer radiotherapy may be used, usually prior to surgery. Some metastatic disease to the liver or lungs can also be surgically treated.

Patients may require surgery for non-cancerous polyps. This is because there is a risk that cancerous cells may already be present in the polyp or that there is a chance of the polyp turning into a cancer in the future. There are genetic conditions that increase the risk of a patient developing a colorectal cancer, such as familiar adenomatous polyposis (FAP) or Lynch syndrome. These patients may often be completely asymptomatic prior to their diagnosis.

## Inflammatory Bowel Disease

IBD refers to the conditions of Crohn's disease and ulcerative colitis. Patients may have experienced symptoms for many years, may be on medications including steroids, and many will have previously undergone surgery. Typical symptoms at presentation are diarrhoea, loss of appetite, weight loss,

abdominal pain, obstruction, intra-abdominal abscess, or bleeding of the bowel. Patients may also have extraintestinal manifestations of IBD including conditions of the skin, joints, and eyes. Symptoms of IBD often have periods of remission and relapse. These patients are at high risk of malnutrition for many reasons, including diarrhoea, reduced food intake, nutrient deficiency, malabsorption, and the side effects of medications [3].

Crohn's disease is a non-specific inflammatory disease that can occur anywhere in the digestive tract from the mouth to the anus. It typically occurs in young adults (age 20–40 years), but can occur at any age. It is classified based on its location (ileocolic disease being the most common) and its behaviour; that is, whether the disease predominantly causes fistulae or strictures [4]. These patients are also at risk of B12 deficiency and peri-anal manifestations including fistulae and abscesses.

Ulcerative colitis is a condition that causes chronic mucosal inflammation that starts in the rectum and continues proximally. It only affects the colon and rectum. The symptoms can occur at any age, but often present between the ages of 15 and 25 years. Patients are at increased risk of primary sclerosing cholangitis and colorectal cancer.

It can sometimes be difficult to differentiate between the two forms of IBD. Treatment should be provided by a multidisciplinary team. Medical therapy includes anti-inflammatory drugs, steroids, immunomodulators, and biologic therapies. However, despite optimal medical and nutritional management, many patients will ultimately require surgery for their disease and quality of life. In ulcerative colitis the whole colon and rectum can be removed, leaving the patient with a permanent ileostomy or ileal pouch (see Table 17.1). However, in Crohn's disease measures are taken to reduce bowel resection, as recurrent operations can lead to short bowel syndrome.

Diet and nutrition are a critical part of a patient's management. A poor nutritional status or loss of greater than 10% body mass in six months prior to surgery is associated with poorer outcomes [3, 6]. Patients with IBD should be routinely screened for malnutrition. Guidelines recommend that if

**TABLE 17.1**   Colorectal and small bowel operations.

| Name of the procedure | Resection | Reconstruction | Additional notes/nutritional impact |
| --- | --- | --- | --- |
| Small bowel resection | Non-specific term used to describe any length of jejunum or ileum removed | Usually an anastomosis. Occasionally an ileostomy may be formed | When undergoing small bowel resection, particularly when multiple resections are or have been undertaken in a patient, surgeons often measure the remaining small bowel, as this will support decision making regarding long-term management. Patients with <200 cm of small bowel are likely to develop short bowel syndrome [5] (see Chapter 22) |
| Stricturoplasty | No bowel resected | Various techniques described | This operation is used to manage small bowel strictures, usually in the context of Crohn's disease. It widens the lumen at the site of the stricture without the need for bowel resection |
| Right hemi-colectomy | Distal terminal ileum, caecum, appendix, and right side (ascending) colon resected | Small bowel anastomosed to transverse colon | Can include resection of some or all of terminal ileum (predisposing patients to bile salt malabsorption) |
| Extended right hemi-colectomy | Distal terminal ileum, right side (ascending), and some of transverse colon resected | Small bowel anastomosed to remaining transverse or descending colon | Can include resection of some or all of terminal ileum (predisposing patients to bile salt malabsorption) |
| Left hemi-colectomy | Splenic flexure, left side (descending) colon removed | Transverse colon reconnected to upper rectum | |
| Subtotal colectomy | Removal of colon usually up to distal sigmoid | Either (i) end ileostomy with or without mucus fistula; or (ii) Ileorectal anastomosis | This operation usually procedure of choice for acute colitis |
| Total colectomy (Lane's operation) | All of colon | Ileum reconnected to rectum (ileorectal anastomosis) | Some patients may have ileostomy formed rather than ileal-rectal anastomosis. Can include resection of some or all of terminal ileum |
| Sigmoid colectomy | Sigmoid colon resected | Descending colon reconnected to rectum | |
| High anterior resection | Resection of sigmoid colon and part of rectum | Descending colon anastomosed to remaining remnant rectum | |

(Continued)

**TABLE 17.1**    (Continued)

| Name of the procedure | Resection | Reconstruction | Additional notes/nutritional impact |
|---|---|---|---|
| Low anterior resection | Sigmoid colon and majority of rectum resected | Descending colon reconnected to remaining rectum | Low anterior resection removes more of rectum than high anterior resection. Anastomosis will usually be below peritoneal reflection. This results in increased risk of anastomotic leak; this anastomosis will often be 'protected' while it heals with defunctioning loop ileostomy |
| Proctosigmoidectomy with end colostomy (Hartmann's procedure) | Resection of sigmoid colon and sometimes rectum | Remnant of rectum is sealed (Hartmann's pouch) and end colostomy is formed | This operation often used for emergency procedures undertaken for conditions such as perforated diverticulitis or obstructing sigmoid cancers. Colostomy can be reversed to remove colostomy and utilise rectum again |
| Abdomino-perineal resection (Miles procedure) | Resection of sigmoid colon, rectum, and anus | Formation of permanent colostomy | |
| Pan procto-colectomy | Resection of all of colon and rectum | Formation of permanent ileostomy | |
| Ileal pouch anal anastomosis | This type of anastomosis may be created during procto-colectomy or completion proctectomy (if subtotal colectomy has been previously performed) | Creation of reservoir (pouch) using segment of ileum attached to anus | More commonly used in patients with familiar adenomatous polyposis or ulcerative colitis. Various pouch techniques have been described, but J-pouch is most commonly used |
| Loop ileostomy | Stoma formed to defunction distal bowel. This may be temporary stoma to 'protect' distal anastomosis or to defunction distal disease such as peri-anal Crohn's or obstructing cancer | Ileum is bought up to abdominal wall and opened, leaving two adjacent stomas, one through which faecal matter excreted (efferent limb) and second referred to as afferent limb | Typically reversed when more distal anastomosis (usually ileo-rectal) anastomosis has healed |
| Proctectomy | Resection of all or part of rectum | May require either formation of colostomy, or loop ileostomy to allow an anastomosis to heal | This operation may be carried out after patient has previously had subtotal colectomy. In this setting it is referred to as completion proctectomy |

**TABLE 17.1** (Continued)

| Name of the procedure | Resection | Reconstruction | Additional notes/nutritional impact |
| --- | --- | --- | --- |
| Pelvic exenteration | Involved resection of other pelvic organs – such as uterus, bladder, or prostate | May require colostomy, sometimes in addition to urostomy/ileal conduit | This operation performed in specialist centres for advanced malignancy |

malnutrition is diagnosed then surgery should be postponed, if possible, to allow for nutritional opti-misation. There is evidence to support the use of enteral nutrition in this setting for 4–12 weeks pre-operatively. Although the precise mechanism of action is unclear, several studies have demonstrated decreased rates of infectious and non-infectious complications post-operatively [7]. Parenteral nutri-tion (PN) is an alternative approach for patients where enteral nutrition is not possible due to short bowel, obstruction, or fistulae.

## Other Colorectal Conditions

Diverticular disease is the formation of sacs that pro-trude from the lumen of the bowel. They are typically associated with increasing age, low-fibre diets, and conditions that have impacts on the structure of the bowel (e.g. Ehlers–Danlos syndrome or Marfan syn-drome). When patients are asymptomatic it is referred to as diverticulosis. Patients should be encouraged to eat a healthy, balanced, high-fibre diet including whole grains, fruit, and vegetables. Patients with a low-fibre diet should increase their fibre intake gradu-ally to minimise flatulence and bloating. There is no evidence that patients need to avoid seeds, nuts, pop-corn, or fruit skins, which were previously thought to lodge in diverticula and cause diverticulitis [8]. Diver-ticulitis is inflammation and infection within these diverticula. This can cause pain, diarrhoea, obstruc-tive symptoms, and sepsis. Diverticulitis is usually treated at home with antibiotics and analgesia. The majority of patients are managed without surgery. There is no evidence that fibre reduction is helpful in treating uncomplicated diverticulitis [9]. Patients may experience decreased dietary intake as a result of acute illness and should be encouraged to eat small, fre-quent, nutritious meals, and to drink fluids. This is no evidence that probiotics are helpful in treating epi-sodes of diverticulitis. In recurrent or complicated dis-ease, the affected area of the colon may be removed.

Volvulus occurs when a loop of bowel twists around a blood vessel, causing both an obstruction and a reduction in the blood flow to the gut. The most common site of volvulus in the colon is sig-moid volvulus. This is usually managed with a sig-moidoscopy and sometimes the insertion of a flatus tube. However, if endoscopic decompression fails or complications such as perforation or ischaemia occur, then surgery is required. Surgery is also some-times undertaken for recurrent cases. Caecal volvu-lus is less common and the treatment is surgery.

## Small Bowel Conditions

Intussusception refers to a loop of bowel that has prolapsed into a proximal loop. This commonly occurs in babies and small children. However, intus-susception can occur in adults and is usually pre-cipitated by a colonic lesion such as a cancer.

Gallstone ileus is a rare form of small bowel obstruction, caused when a chronically inflamed gallbladder adheres to the bowel wall. Over time gallstones can erode through the wall, causing a cholecysto-enteral fistula. Gallstones become embedded in the bowel wall, resulting in obstruc-tion. This may occur in the duodenum, stomach, small bowel, or colon [10].

Adhesions are scar-like tissue that form inside the abdomen between tissues and organs. Adhesions are more common in people who have had previous surgery, and typically cause obstruction of the small bowel. Adhesions sometime cause symptoms many years after surgery. When patients present with adhesional small bowel obstruction, in the absence of high-risk features such as pain, sepsis, ischaemia, or internal hernia, a trial of conservative management is often used, historically referred to as 'drip and suck' – meaning the patient is placed nil by mouth (NBM) with intravenous fluids and a wide-bore nasogastric tube placed to drain the stomach. The water-soluble radiology contrast agent Gastrografin (Bayer plc, Reading, UK) may be administered [9]. Electrolyte abnormalities are common in small bowel obstruction. If the obstruction resolves, then no further treatment may be required. However, if this fails or the adhesions recur, surgical adhesiolysis may be required. Small bowel resection may also be required where dense adhesions have led to bowel injury or there is ischaemia. The treatment of small bowel obstruction may take several days and PN may be required.

Ischaemic bowel is the term used to describe a section of bowel where there is insufficient blood flow. It may affect the small bowel or colon and can be acute or chronic. If left untreated this can lead to necrosis, infection, sepsis, and ultimately death. The diagnosis can sometime be challenging, but it should be suspected clinically when patients develop distended abdomen, abdominal pain out of proportion with other clinical findings, or raised lactate. Risk factors include old age, smoking, hypercoagulable states, and atrial fibrillation. There are also case reports linking feeding jejunostomies to small bowel necrosis [11].

## SURGICAL PROCEDURES

Table 17.1 describes the various operations that are performed for colorectal and small bowel disease.

## NUTRITIONAL MANAGEMENT IN THE PERI-OPERATIVE SETTING

Colorectal surgery can be performed open, laparoscopically, or with a surgical robot. Minimal access surgery is associated with reduced pain, a faster recovery, earlier return of bowel function, shorter hospital stay, fewer scars, and reduced adhesion formation. After colorectal surgery patients will often be managed according to an enhanced recovery after surgery (ERAS) pathway (see Chapter 5). These programmes aim to ensure that patients are prepared for their operation, receive optimal peri-operative care, reduce complications in their recovery, and prevent ileus.

There are many elements to a successful enhanced recovery pathway [12]. From a nutritional perspective, current ERAS Society guidelines recommend that patients at risk of malnutrition should receive nutrition support, preferably oral, for at least 7–10 days [12]. Many patients have evidence of malnutrition when they present for colorectal cancer surgery. One study investigated 176 patients undergoing surgery for colorectal cancer and demonstrated that 25.2% were malnourished based on a patient-generated subjective global assessment (PG-SGA) (score ≥4) and radiological evidence of sarcopenia was found in 14% [13]. A smaller study found that malnutrition was associated with worsening mobility, difficulty eating, and low fluid intake [14]. Pre-operative prolonged fasting should be avoided and anaemia should also be corrected prior to surgery (Chapter 7).

Post-operatively most patients can be recommenced on an oral diet from the day of surgery (see Chapter 5). Practice varies by surgeon and institution, with differing use of clear fluids, free fluids, and a low-residue diet [15]. There is also some evidence to support the use of peri-operative immunonutrition in this setting to reduce infectious complications, length of stay, and surgical site infection [16, 17].

### Stoma Management

Many colorectal operations result in the creation of an ileostomy or colostomy as either a temporary or permanent stoma. Stomas may be end or loop (see Table 17.1). Ileostomies are usually spouted and protrude from the abdominal wall to prevent skin irritation from small bowel contents. As the role of the colon is to absorb water and electrolytes, newly formed ileostomies often go through a period of adaptation, where fluid losses can be high initially, but settle after a period of a few days to a few weeks. During this initial period patients may benefit from additional salt in their diet to replace losses and it is important to replace fluid losses. This is less likely to be problematic in those with a colostomy.

Appetite may be reduced following stoma formation. Patients should be encouraged to take small, frequent, energy-dense meals and fluids to meet nutritional requirements [18].

In the long term, those with either an ileal pouch or ileostomy should be advised as follows [19]:

- Follow normal healthy eating advice.
- Chew their food well and do not rush meals.
- Ensure adequate hydration.
- Eat regularly.
- Eat little and often if poor appetite.
- Avoid eating late at night if this causes their stoma to be very active/pouch to fill overnight.

Most stoma patients do not need to follow a restricted diet long term, but may associate some foods with adverse symptoms. For example, changes in smell (eggs, brussels sprouts, baked beans, broccoli, cauliflower, cabbage, onions, and garlic), consistency (alcoholic beverages, fruit juice, some fruits and vegetables), or increased flatulence (fizzy drinks, beans, onion, garlic). In these cases, these foods should be reduced, and care should be taken to ensure that the diet does not become too restrictive, low in energy, protein, or missing specific nutrients [19].

Patients should also be made aware that some foods might change the colour of the stoma output. Beetroot, for instance, can turn the stoma output red and may be confused with bleeding. Managing the effects of different foods on stoma output is variable and advice must be individualised. Unfortunately, patients feel that there is a lack of consistent information provided in this setting [20].

## High-Output Stoma

In some cases, the stoma output does not adapt, and if stoma output volumes continue to exceed 1000 ml/d, the patient becomes at increased risk of dehydration, acute kidney injury, and electrolyte abnormalities. Less than 200 cm of residual small bowel, young age, and high post-operative white cell count were associated with higher output [21]. The use of anti-diarrhoeal medication (loperamide and codeine), oral rehydration solutions, and gelatinous sweets such as marshmallows can help thicken the stoma output and reduce fluid losses [20]. Additional sodium may be required and a restriction of 'normal' fluids in combination with the use of oral rehydration solution can help prevent dehydration. Optimising fluid absorption is vital to managing a high-output stoma. Renal function and serum electrolyte levels, especially magnesium, should be monitored regularly, and magnesium replacement may be required.

## Low-Residue Diet

This diet reduces the consumption of foods most likely to retain their bulk in the small bowel and therefore most likely to cause obstruction. It can be used initially in the conservative management of bowel obstruction and in the long-term management of those with intermittent adhesional bowel obstruction (Chapter 20). High-residue foods are typically fibrous foods such as fruits and vegetables with pith, skins, seeds, or very high-fibre contents such as oranges, grapefruit, tomatoes, peas, beans, sweetcorn, pineapple, celery, nuts, and lentils.

## Ileus

An ileus is a temporary decrease or stoppage in the movement of the intestine and its contents. Ileus is common after colorectal surgery, but is usually self-limiting. The initial management is nasogastric tube drainage and intravenous fluids with electrolyte replacement. If it is prolonged, PN may be required (see Chapter 20).

## Short Bowel Syndrome

Extensive resection of the small bowel can result in short bowel syndrome. This complex syndrome results in the need for life-changing management such as long-term intravenous fluids, regular electrolyte monitoring or replacement, and in severe case home intravenous nutrition (see Chapter 21).

## LONG-TERM COMPLICATIONS

### Kidney Stones

Patients with an ileostomy or ileal pouch are at greater risk of forming uric acid stones due to their reduced urine volume and pH.

### Bile Acid Malabsorption

Patients who have had a resection of their terminal ileum may experience symptoms of bile acid malabsorption due to failure of the enterohepatic circulation. Bile is excreted from the liver, and acts as an emulsifier within the small bowel before being reabsorbed at the terminal ileum. Failure to reabsorb bile due to resection of the terminal ileum can cause bloating, flatulence, and diarrhoea due to the osmotic effects of bile within the colon. Initial treatment with a low-fat diet (to reduce the production of bile) can be complemented with the use of a bile acid sequestrant.

### Low Anterior Resection Syndrome

Low anterior resection syndrome describes a collection of symptoms that patients experience after having their rectum removed. The nature and severity of symptoms each patient experiences are variable and unpredictable. Patients may experience clustering of stools, urgency, incontinence, or leakage of stool or tenesmus. These symptoms can have a detrimental effect on quality of life after surgery. Management includes dietary fibre modification, anti-diarrhoea medications, or pelvic floor physiotherapy.

### Pouchitis

Many patients with an ileal pouch may develop increased frequency, urgency, and more liquid stool. Where there is inflammation within the pouch, antibiotics may help resolve symptoms. There is evidence to support the use of probiotics (VSL#3, De Simone Formulation) in reducing flare-ups of pouchitis [18, 22]. Overall multidisciplinary management using a low-fibre/low-FODMAP diet, probiotics, and medications such as loperamide and mebeverine have been associated with improved outcomes [23]. Some patients may require further biologic therapy to control their symptoms.

## CONCLUSION

The nutritional impact of colorectal surgery varies depending on the extent of surgery and the specific section of bowel removed. Dietitians play a key role in the management of complicated patients, particularly in IBD.

## REFERENCES

1. National Institute for Health and Care Excellence (2021). Suspected cancer: recognition and referral. NICE guideline [NG12]. https://www.nice.org.uk/guidance/ng12. Accessed 3rd June 2022.
2. Cancer Research UK (n.d.). Bowel cancer incidence. https://www.cancerresearchuk.org/health-professional/cancer-statistics/statistics-by-cancer-type/bowel-cancer#heading-Zero. Accessed 3rd June 2022.
3. Lin, A. and Micic, D. (2021). Nutrition considerations in inflammatory bowel disease. *Nutr. Clin. Pract.* 36 (2): 298–311.
4. Silverberg, M.S., Satsangi, J., Ahmad, T. et al. (2005). Toward an integrated clinical, molecular and serological classification of inflammatory bowel disease: report of a Working Party of the 2005 Montreal World Congress of Gastroenterology. *Can. J. Gastroenterol.*; 19 Suppl A: 5A–36A.
5. Pironi, L. (2016). Definitions of intestinal failure and the short bowel syndrome. *Best Pract. Res. Clin. Gastroenterol.* 30 (2): 173–185.
6. Adamina, M., Gerasimidis, K., Sigall-Boneh, R. et al. (2020). Perioperative dietary therapy in inflammatory bowel disease. *J. Crohns Colitis* 14 (4): 431–444.
7. Heerasing, N., Thompson, B., Hendy, P. et al. (2017). Exclusive enteral nutrition provides an effective bridge to safer interval elective surgery for adults with Crohn's disease. *Aliment. Pharmacol. Ther.* 45 (5): 660–669.

8. National Institute for Health and Care Excellence (2019). Diverticular disease: diagnosis and management. NICE guideline [NG 147]. https://www.nice.org.uk/guidance/ng147. Accessed 3rd June 2022.

9. Dahl, C., Crichton, M., Jenkins, J. et al. (2018). Evidence for dietary fibre modification in the recovery and prevention of reoccurrence of acute, uncomplicated diverticulitis: a systematic literature review. *Nutrients* 10 (2): 137.

10. Nuno-Guzman, C.M., Marin-Contreras, M.E., Figueroa-Sanchez, M., and Corona, J.L. (2016). Gallstone ileus, clinical presentation, diagnostic and treatment approach. *World J. Gastrointest Surg.* 8 (1): 65–76.

11. Spalding, D.R., Behranwala, K.A., Straker, P. et al. (2009). Non-occlusive small bowel necrosis in association with feeding jejunostomy after elective upper gastrointestinal surgery. *Ann. R. Coll. Surg. Engl.* 91 (6): 477–482.

12. Gustafsson, U.O., Scott, M.J., Hubner, M. et al. (2019). Guidelines for perioperative care in elective colorectal surgery: enhanced recovery after surgery (ERAS((R))) society recommendations: 2018. *World J. Surg.* 43 (3): 659–695.

13. Klassen, P., Baracos, V., Gramlich, L. et al. (2020). Computed-tomography body composition analysis complements pre-operative nutrition screening in colorectal Cancer patients on an enhanced recovery after surgery pathway. *Nutrients* 12 (12): 3745.

14. Vasilopoulos, G., Makrigianni, P., Polikandrioti, M. et al. (2020). Pre- and post-operative nutrition assessment in patients with colon Cancer undergoing ileostomy. *Int. J. Environ. Res. Public Health* 17 (17): 6124.

15. Rattray, M., Roberts, S., Desbrow, B. et al. (2019). A qualitative exploration of factors influencing medical staffs' decision-making around nutrition prescription after colorectal surgery. *BMC Health Serv. Res.* 19 (1): 178.

16. Achilli, P., Mazzola, M., Bertoglio, C.L. et al. (2020). Preoperative immunonutrition in frail patients with colorectal cancer: an intervention to improve postoperative outcomes. *Int. J. Color. Dis.* 35 (1): 19–27.

17. Xu, J., Sun, X., Xin, Q. et al. (2018). Effect of immunonutrition on colorectal cancer patients undergoing surgery: a meta-analysis. *Int. J. Color. Dis.* 33 (3): 273–283.

18. Lomer, M.C.E., Wilson, B., and Wall, C.L. (2023). British Dietetic Association consensus guidelines on the nutritional assessment and dietary management of patients with inflammatory bowel disease. *J. Hum. Nutr. Diet.* 36 (1): 336–377.

19. Culkin, A. (2019). Intestinal failure and intestinal resection. In: *Manual of Dietetic Practice*, 6e (ed. J. Gandy). Wiley Blackwell, ch. 7.4.9.

20. Mitchell, A., Perry, R., England, C. et al. (2019). Dietary management in people with an ileostomy: a scoping review protocol. *JBI Database System Rev. Implement. Rep.* 17 (2): 129–136.

21. Fujino, S., Miyoshi, N., Ohue, M. et al. (2017). Prediction model and treatment of high-output ileostomy in colorectal cancer surgery. *Mol. Clin. Oncol.* 7 (3): 468–472.

22. Dong, J., Teng, G., Wei, T. et al. (2016). Methodological quality assessment of meta-analyses and systematic reviews of probiotics in inflammatory bowel disease and pouchitis. *PLoS One* 11 (12): e0168785.

23. Gilad, O., Rosner, G., Brazowski, E. et al. (2021). Management of pouch related symptoms in patients who underwent ileal pouch anal anastomosis surgery for adenomatous polyposis. *World J. Clin. Cases* 9 (32): 9847–9856.

# CHAPTER 18

# Nutritional Management of Gynaecological Cancer Patients

Thanuya Mahendran[1], Maria Ashworth[1], Mary E. Phillips[2], and Jayanta Chatterjee[1]

[1] Academic Department of Gynae-oncology, Royal Surrey NHS Foundation Trust, Guildford, UK
[2] Department of Nutrition and Dietetics, Royal Surrey NHS Foundation Trust, Guildford, UK

---

**KEY POINTS**

- Patients with ovarian cancer are at high risk of malnutrition.
- Pelvic tumours can exert a significant mass effect, resulting in bowel obstruction, early satiety, and malnutrition.
- Malnutrition, sarcopenia, and obesity all have impacts on surgical outcomes.
- Radical surgery may result in short bowel syndrome.

---

Patients undergoing surgery for gynaecological (GO) malignancies are at risk of malnutrition due to the mass effect of the tumour, elevated nutritional requirements, and cancer cachexia [1]. Cancer cachexia, unlike simple malnutrition, results from the negative energy balance and skeletal muscle loss caused by a combination of reduced food intake and metabolic derangements. Elevated resting metabolic rate, insulin resistance, lipolysis, and proteolysis that aggravate weight loss are provoked by systemic inflammation and catabolic factors, which may be host or tumour derived. Due to the presence of these metabolic changes, cancer-associated malnutrition can only be partially reversed by conventional nutritional support [2]. (See Chapter 3.)

## DIETARY CONTRIBUTION TO GYNAECOLOGICAL MALIGNANCIES

There are many contributing factors to the development of cervical, ovarian, or endometrial cancers. These are summarised in Table 18.1. Obesity is well associated with both increased prevalence of GO malignancies and worse outcomes [4–6]. Studies exploring patients' knowledge of the relationship

**TABLE 18.1**   Dietary contributions to gynaecological malignancies.

| Type of malignancy | Dietary risk factors | Other risk factors | Beneficial dietary factors |
|---|---|---|---|
| Cervical cancer | | Persistent infection with high-risk oncogenic human papilloma virus (hrHPV) | Potential for antioxidants, beneficial effect of fruit and vegetables [3] |
| | | | Potential benefit of vitamin D supplementation [4] |
| Endometrial cancer | Obesity [5] | Insulin resistance [5] | |
| Ovarian cancer | Saturated fats | Poorly understood | |

between obesity and endometrial cancer suggest that there is acceptance of the need for weight loss as an integral part of the management of endometrial cancer, including the potential use of bariatric surgery [7].

## PRE-OPERATIVE MALNUTRITION

Within cervical cancer patients rates of malnutrition vary considerably: up to 60% of patients with stage IV disease are malnourished, while this rate is only 4% in those with stage I disease [8].

Ovarian cancer patients often present with non-specific early symptoms, including dyspepsia, nausea, lack of appetite, fatigue, and abdominal pain. Patients are often found to have advanced disease with a wide intra-abdominal spread of neoplasms at the time of diagnosis, with 28–67% demonstrating signs of malnutrition on presentation [9], compared to 6% in endometrial cancer using patient-generated subjective global assessment (PG-SGA) [10]. The mass effect of the tumour can be significant (see Figure 18.1).

## PRE-OPERATIVE NUTRITIONAL SUPPORT

Enhanced recovery programmes should not focus only on the immediate pre-operative period of a patient's cancer journey, but should also be embarked on at the time of diagnosis [11]. Bisch et al.'s review

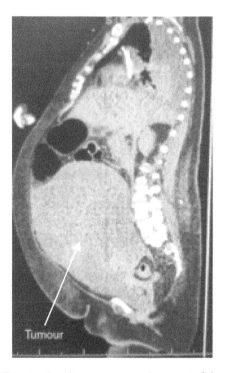

**FIGURE 18.1**   Ovarian mass occupying most of the abdomen and pelvis and compressing the bowel.

explores the evidence for pre- and post-operative nutritional support, using a combination of data specific to GO surgery and extrapolated data from other surgical specialties to highlight the important role that nutritional assessment plays in enhanced recovery, and support the recommendation that nutritional therapies, when needed, should be implemented at least 7–14 days pre-operatively [12].

Pre-operative malnutrition is multifactorial (Table 18.2) and associated with higher morbidity, with malnourished patients undergoing GO surgery being seven times more likely to be readmitted to intensive care in the post-operative period (P = 0.022) [13]. Therefore, nutritional intervention as early as possible prior to the surgery is particularly relevant.

Large heterogeneous cohort studies exploring outcomes of abdominal surgery (including for gynaecological malignancies) associate malnutrition with a higher complication rate (P = 0.018) [14]. In this study malnutrition was defined as those with one of these three criteria: body mass index (BMI) <18.5 kg/m², albumin level <3.0 mg/l, or >20% weight loss in the last six months. There was a correlation of the number of these nutritional markers with serious complications, with an odds ratio of 5.47 of experiencing a Clavien Dindo grade >3 complication in those who had all three criteria present [14]. Conversely baseline BMI was not associated with outcomes, but significant changes in BMI, both increases and decreases, were associated with lower survival [15], highlighting the need for serial monitoring of nutritional status.

In endometrial malignancy, obesity is associated with adverse outcomes, especially with regard to

**TABLE 18.2** Factors contributing to pre-operative malnutrition in gynaecological malignancies.

| Tumour effects | Treatment effects |
| --- | --- |
| Cancer cachexia | Side effects of chemo-radiotherapy: nausea/anorexia/change in bowel habit affecting oral intake |
| Mass effect resulting in early satiety, reflux, nausea/vomiting, constipation resulting in impaired oral intake | Psychological/social/logistical impact of treatment: change in family dynamics, financial difficulties, time-consuming treatments resulting in difficulty in provision of adequate nutrition |
| Tumour mass masking weight loss | Nil-by-mouth times for investigations for diagnosis/staging |

wound infection [6]. These outcomes were based on body weight assessment alone and, since we appreciate that malnutrition assessed purely on body weight is inadequate, research has shifted to explore the role of sarcopenia. A meta-analysis identified that normal muscle attenuation was associated with improved survival at three and five years (both P <0.001) after surgery for ovarian malignancy [16]. This data was reproduced in patients with stage 3 epithelial ovarian cancer [17], and muscle loss during debulking surgery and adjuvant treatment was independently associated with poor overall survival (P = 0.002) [18]. However, these studies only include radiological assessment of sarcopenia, rather than a combined assessment incorporating functional testing (see Chapter 2).

Nutritional interventions in a mixed cohort of lower gastrointestinal and pelvic cancers with structured dietetic assessment demonstrate improvements in nutrient intake and body weight (P = 0.08), but in this small cohort of 40 patients there was no difference in length of stay (P = 0.71) [19].

## Immuno-nutrition

Short-term studies with immuno-nutrition administered five days prior to pelvic exenteration surgery demonstrated a difference in uptake of nutritional supplements in those who were well nourished compared to those who were poorly nourished (P = 0.016) [20], thought to be associated with poor appetite in those with pre-existing malnutrition. There was no difference in surgical complications or length of hospital stay [20]. Of note was the absence of control group in this study, so it is not possible to confirm if nutrition support was beneficial in those without evidence of malnutrition. Further studies in a mixed cohort of patients undergoing laparotomy for gynaecological cancers provided with immuno-nutrition in the post-operative setting demonstrated a reduction in post-operative wound infections (P = 0.049) [21].

There is still a lack of high-quality studies evaluating prehabilitation in GO patients, including the optimal modality of the interventions and set-up of standardised protocols. However, the recognition of sarcopenia as a prognostic indicator supports the development of prehabilitation pathways as treatments for sarcopenia are explored [14] (see Chapter 4).

## OVERVIEW OF SURGICAL PROCEDURES

### Endometrial Cancer

For women with endometrial cancer, hysterectomy, and bilateral salpingo-oophorectomy with staging are considered standard treatment; other treatments include radiotherapy, chemotherapy and immuno-therapy. Historically, surgery for endometrial cancer was performed using laparotomy. Recent evidence suggests that minimally invasive surgical technique is an acceptable alternative to the conventional laparotomy for early-stage disease, with reduction in operative morbidity including wound infection, blood loss, and ileus [22].

### Cervical Cancer

Management of cervical cancer depends on stage, lymph node involvement, and patient comorbidities. Treatment may include surgical resection, radiation, chemotherapy, or a combination. A minimally invasive approach in early-stage, small-volume tumours (<2 cm) is often possible in cervical cancer, with fewer complications and shorter recovery time compared with traditional laparotomy [22].

Treatment of recurrent disease includes medical or surgical options. For women with local recurrence, surgical resection with pelvic exenteration is an option. Exenteration involves en bloc removal of female reproductive organs, the lower urinary tract, and a portion of the involved rectosigmoid. Exenteration is generally used for women who have had previous unsuccessful radiation treatment and it has a 50% cure rate [23].

### Ovarian Cancer

The standard treatment for advanced ovarian carcinoma consists of primary debulking surgery associated with an adjuvant chemotherapy. Neo-adjuvant chemotherapy and interval debulking surgery have been proposed in the management of advanced ovarian carcinoma to increase the rate of complete cytoreductive surgery and to reduce morbidity and mortality in patients with poor performance status at presentation.

### Primary Debulking Surgery

During primary surgery all attempts should be made to achieve complete cytoreduction. When this is not achievable, the surgical goal should be optimal (<1 cm) residual disease. Better understanding of the disease pathology with implementation of radical surgery to achieve no visible residual tumour, alongside chemotherapy, has led to longer survival. Primary debulking surgery consists of hysterectomy, bilateral salpingo-oophorectomy, and total omentectomy, with pelvic and para-aortic lymph node removal followed by platinum-based chemotherapy.

Radical surgery includes the additional steps of bowel resection, appendicectomy, peritoneal or diaphragmatic resection, splenectomy, partial pancreatectomy, partial gastrectomy, and resection of liver disease (both serosal and parenchymal). Overall, prognosis is related to tumour variables such as stage of disease, histology, and grade. Patient and other variables include age, performance status, nutritional status, pre-operative laboratory values, surgical expertise, and achieving nil macroscopic residual disease following surgery. Primary debulking surgery achieves the ideal oncological outcome, but may be at the expense of surgical morbidity and mortality. On the other hand, patients can be treated with alternative, less morbid approaches by neo-adjuvant chemotherapy, but sacrificing the survival benefits of low or no residual disease at outset by surgical cytoreduction and potentially increasing the incidence of resistant clonal disease.

### Interval Debulking Surgery

Interval debulking surgery is considered in poor surgical candidates with poor nutritional status, poor performance status (American Society of Anesthesiologists [ASA] score ≥3), and advanced stage with unresectable disease burden at initial presentation.

These factors may be modifiable by treating the underlying cancer. These patients should be treated with neo-adjuvant chemotherapy and reassessed for surgical debulking. Patients with improvement in their nutritional or performance status and adequate disease response can undergo interval debulking with the goal of resecting all visible disease [24].

## Primary or Interval Debulking Surgery with Bowel Resection and Stoma Formation

Bowel resection is often required for optimal cytoreduction, in selected cases of advanced carcinoma ovary. Of patients with International Federation of Gynaecological Oncologists (FIGO) stage III ovarian cancer, 72% had visible tumour spread in the small and/or large bowel [25] and 87% of these patients undergoing primary debulking surgery were planned for bowel surgery [26]. Depending on spread of the disease, stomas may be either temporary or permanent. It carries a reasonable peri-operative mortality and morbidity risk and improves overall survival. (For stoma management advice, see Chapter 17.)

## Bowel Obstruction and Palliative Resection

Malignant bowel obstruction is common in women with advanced gynaecological cancer, predominantly in ovarian cancer, and it is a clinical challenge as it presents with constitutional symptoms such as the inability to maintain oral intake, vomiting, and abdominal pain. Treatment targets are resolution of obstruction, symptom, and nutritional management (see Chapter 19). Conservative management should be the management of choice in the absence of acute abdomen or intestinal perforation. A venting percutaneous endoscopic gastrostomy tube may effectively palliate women with non-operable bowel obstruction in advanced/recurrent cancer of the ovary [27]. Salvage palliative surgeries should ideally be performed only in a multidisciplinary setting with adequate infrastructure and possibility of home-care support, as it may result in short

bowel syndrome and the need for lifelong parenteral nutrition (PN).

The surgical approach to large bowel obstruction consists of diverting stoma or primary resection and anastomosis, depending on the disease volume, and small bowel obstruction without strangulation is usually treated with conservative measures, as it often relates to multifocal small bowel involvement secondary to peritoneal disease. Some patients could be considered for small bowel resection with anastomosis or internal bypass. Non-operative management of bowel obstruction can also be considered (Chapter 20).

Successful palliation with surgery is achieved in patients without multiple sites of bowel obstruction and widespread recurrence and malignant ascites. Pre-operative poor nutrition and performance status make surgery challenging and contribute to surgical morbidity [28]. It remains unclear how to select patients who derive benefit from continued PN. Balanced in-depth discussions with realistic expectations must be held with patients and family members early on to emphasise the limitations of PN use and situations when PN should be discontinued.

## POST-OPERATIVE COMPLICATIONS AND IMPACT ON NUTRITION

Digestive complications are common after GO surgery, with one study reporting an incidence of 46% [29]. Post-operative nausea, vomiting, and delayed return of bowel function adversely affect recovery after laparotomy (see Chapter 20). Nausea and vomiting are associated with prolonged length of stay, wound dehiscence, electrolyte imbalances, bleeding, and in extreme cases oesophageal perforation. Likewise, delayed return of bowel function can lead to greater catabolism, decreased mobilisation, poorer wound healing, increased risk of infection, and suboptimal nutrition [30].

Enhanced recovery after surgery (ERAS) guidelines support early initiation of oral diet after GO surgery, but are poorly adhered to [31].

## Chyle Leak

Extensive lymph node dissection can result in chyle leak after pelvic clearance. Data is available predominantly in the form of case reports and small case series, demonstrating a progression from conservative management with very low-fat diets, octreotide infusions, PN, and if unsuccessful corrective surgery [32–35].

## Short Bowel Syndrome

Extensive bowel surgery can occur in cases of pelvic clearance, and may result in the formation of a high-output ileostomy (see Chapter 17) or short bowel syndrome (see Chapter 21).

## CONCLUSION

GO surgery presents a variety of nutritional challenges and requires careful consideration of nutritional status in the pre-operative setting and prompt intervention in the patient who is unable to tolerate post-operative nutrition. Long-term considerations in those who have undergone radical surgery should not only focus on the management of any short bowel syndrome, but also consider the impact of resection of stomach and pancreas (see Chapters 11 and 14). More data is required on the role of immuno-nutrition and prehabilitation to strengthen recommendations for pre-operative management.

---

### Routine Case Study

A 68-year-old female was referred on the two-week rule pathway with an eight-month history of worsening abdominal pain and discomfort. She had abdominal bloating and loss of appetite, but she did not report any loss of weight. She was generally fit and well. A transabdominal ultrasound showed large suspicious mass filling abdomen and pelvis with serum cancer antigen 125 (CA 125) of 260 U/ml (reference range [RR] 0–35). A computed tomography (CT) scan revealed a very large mass arising from the pelvis, with cystic and solid components in the periphery of the mass that was occupying most of the abdominal cavity.

On examination, her BMI was 22.5 kg/m² with a body weight of 54 kg, and her abdomen was grossly distended with a mass up to the xiphisternum. Vaginal examination was unremarkable. This large tumour mass had likely masked pre-operative weight loss.

Pre-operatively, she was assessed for fitness for surgery and she underwent an uncomplicated midline laparotomy, extra-fascial total abdominal hysterectomy, bilateral salpingo-oophorectomy, supracolic omentectomy, appendicectomy, and pelvic lymph node sampling.

Post-operatively she was monitored in the intensive care unit for the first 24 h, and she was started with an early oral diet in line with the ERAS pathway. Pain was managed with epidural for the first two days and then with oral analgesics. She was prescribed laxatives, anti-emetics, and a proton pump inhibitor. She mobilised from day 1, opened her bowel on day 4, and was discharged home on day 5. She had uncomplicated recovery from the surgery without significant weight loss or nutritional imbalance. Her iron, magnesium, calcium, and electrolyte levels were normal.

Her histology revealed stage 1c grade 3 endometrioid adenocarcinoma confined to the ovaries. She went on to have adjuvant chemotherapy.

## Complex Case Study

A 75-year-old female presented with a two-month history of abdominal distension, abdominal pain, and mild early satiety. She was diagnosed with high-grade serous carcinoma of ovarian origin after image-guided biopsy. Neo-adjuvant chemotherapy and interval debulking surgery were planned in the multidisciplinary meeting due to her poor performance status and advanced stage of disease.

She was para 4 having had 2 children via vaginal delivery and 2 via caesarean section. She went through the menopause in her early 40s and took hormone replacement therapy (HRT) for 13 years. She had a history of angina, fast atrial fibrillation, type 2 diabetes, hypertension, moderate asthma, and kidney stones. She was an ex-smoker of 20/d having stopped smoking 15 years ago. She had several drug allergies.

Pre-operative preparation was performed with optimisation of medical ailments, assessment of electrolytes: Mg 0.63 mmol/l (RR 0.7–1.0 mmol/l), phosphate 0.7 mmol/l (RR 0.8–1.4 mmol/l), calcium 2.02 mmol/l (RR 2.2–2.6 mmol/l), and carbohydrate loading. Her weight was 73.2 kg and height 156 cm, giving her a BMI of 30.1 kg/m$^2$ pre-operatively. She underwent extra-fascial total abdominal hysterectomy, bilateral salpingo-oophorectomy, supracolic omentectomy, high anterior resection, colorectal anastomosis, excision of tumour deposit from sigmoid colon, and excision of lesion from small bowel serosa.

She was managed in the intensive care unit, and subsequently developed ileus on post-operative day 2. She was managed with anti-emetics, nasogastric tube suction, nil by mouth, and fluid management. The dietitian reviewed her every other day. There was significant weight loss of 4 kg excluding tumour weight on day 8 and this was secondary to reduced appetite and vomiting. She was prescribed intravenous vitamin B in line with the Trust refeeding syndrome guidelines. Nutritional supplementation consisted of Prosource® jelly (90 kcal, 20 g protein, Nutrinovo, Chippenham, UK), Fortijuce BD (200 kcal, 8 g protein each, Nutricia Clinical Care, Trowbridge, UK), and Vitasavoury soups (300 kcal, 6 g protein, Vitaflo, Liverpool, UK), as she did not tolerate milk based products. This was continued until she was able to tolerate solids, after which she was weaned back onto an oral diet.

She unfortunately developed wound infection and superficial dehiscence on day 9, which was managed with antibiotics, reviewed by the wound-care team, and allowed to heal by secondary intention. She stayed in the hospital for 40 days for wound care, requiring input from occupational therapy and physiotherapy. It is likely that her poor nutritional status contributed to her wound infection and prolonged length of stay.

Her weight stabilised after post-operative day 14. The dietitian reviewed her weekly, and nutritional supplements were weaned down as her oral intake improved. Micronutrient supplementation continued until her wounds had healed and she achieved a normal dietary intake. This case demonstrates a difficult post-operative recovery and a missed opportunity (during neo-adjuvant treatment) for prehabilitation.

## REFERENCES

1. Gadducci, A., Cosio, S., Fanucchi, A., and Genazzani, A.R. (2001). Malnutrition and cachexia in ovarian cancer patients: pathophysiology and management. *Anticancer Res* 21 (4B): 2941–2947.

2. Fearon, K., Strasser, F., Anker, S.D. et al. (2011). Definition and classification of cancer cachexia: an international consensus. *Lancet Oncol.* 12 (5): 489–495.

3. Chih, H.J., Lee, A.H., Colville, L. et al. (2013). A review of dietary prevention of human papillomavirus-related infection of the cervix and cervical intraepithelial neoplasia. *Nutr. Cancer* 65 (3): 317–328.

4. Vahedpoor, Z., Jamilian, M., Bahmani, F. et al. (2017). Effects of long-term vitamin D supplementation on regression and metabolic status of cervical intraepithelial neoplasia: a randomized, double-blind. *Placebo-Controlled Trial. Horm Cancer* 8 (1): 58–67.

5. Shao, Y., Cheng, S., Hou, J. et al. (2016). Insulin is an important risk factor of endometrial cancer among premenopausal women: a case-control study in China. *Tumour Biol.* 37 (4): 4721–4726.

6. Bouwman, F., Smits, A., Lopes, A. et al. (2015). The impact of BMI on surgical complications and outcomes in endometrial cancer surgery – an institutional study and systematic review of the literature. *Gynecol. Oncol.* 139 (2): 369–376.

7. Wilkinson, M., Murphy, S., Sinclair, P. et al. (2020). Patient perceptions and understanding of obesity related endometrial cancer. *Gynecol. Oncol. Rep.* 32: 100545.

8. Laky, B., Janda, M., Bauer, J. et al. (2007). Malnutrition among gynaecological cancer patients. *Eur. J. Clin. Nutr.* 61 (5): 642–646.

9. Billson, H.A., Holland, C., Curwell, J. et al. (2013). Perioperative nutrition interventions for women with ovarian cancer. *Cochrane Database Syst. Rev.* (9): CD009884.

10. Laky, B., Janda, M., Cleghorn, G., and Obermair, A. (2008). Comparison of different nutritional assessments and body-composition measurements in detecting malnutrition among gynecologic cancer patients. *Am. J. Clin. Nutr.* 87 (6): 1678–1685.

11. Gillis, C., Gill, M., Marlett, N. et al. (2017). Patients as partners in enhanced recovery after surgery: a qualitative patient-led study. *BMJ Open* 7 (6): e017002.

12. Bisch, S., Nelson, G., and Altman, A. (2019). Impact of nutrition on enhanced recovery after surgery (ERAS) in gynecologic oncology. *Nutrients* 11 (5): 1088.

13. Hogan, S., Steffens, D., Vuong, K. et al. (2022). Preoperative nutritional status impacts clinical outcome and hospital length of stay in pelvic exenteration patients – a retrospective study. *Nutr. Health* 28 (1): 41–48.

14. McSharry, V., Glennon, K., Mullee, A., and Brennan, D. (2021). The impact of body composition on treatment in ovarian cancer: a current insight. *Expert Rev. Clin. Pharmacol.* 14 (9): 1065–1074.

15. Matsuo, K., Moeini, A., Cahoon, S.S. et al. (2016). Weight change pattern and survival outcome of women with endometrial cancer. *Ann. Surg. Oncol.* 23 (9): 2988–2997.

16. McSharry, V., Mullee, A., McCann, L. et al. (2020). The impact of sarcopenia and low muscle attenuation on overall survival in epithelial ovarian cancer: a systematic review and meta-analysis. *Ann. Surg. Oncol.* 27 (9): 3553–3564.

17. Huang, C.Y., Sun, F.J., and Lee, J. (2020). Prognostic value of muscle measurement using the standardized phase of computed tomography in patients with advanced ovarian cancer. *Nutrition* 72: 110642.

18. Huang, C.Y., Yang, Y.C., Chen, T.C. et al. (2020). Muscle loss during primary debulking surgery and chemotherapy predicts poor survival in advanced-stage ovarian cancer. *J. Cachexia. Sarcopenia Muscle* 11 (2): 534–546.

19. Den, E., Steer, B., Quinn, P., and Kiss, N. (2021). Effect of an evidence-based nutrition care pathway for cancer patients undergoing gastrointestinal and pelvic surgery. *Nutr. Cancer* 73 (11–12): 2546–2553.

20. Hogan, S., Solomon, M., Rangan, A. et al. (2020). The impact of preoperative immunonutrition and standard polymeric supplements on patient outcomes after pelvic exenteration surgery, taking compliance into consideration: a randomized controlled trial. *JPEN.* 44 (5): 806–814.

21. Chapman, J.S., Roddy, E., Westhoff, G. et al. (2015). Post-operative enteral immunonutrition for gynecologic oncology patients undergoing laparotomy decreases wound complications. *Gynecol. Oncol.* 137 (3): 523–528.

22. Wang, J., Li, X., Wu, H. et al. (2020). A meta-analysis of robotic surgery in endometrial cancer: comparison with laparoscopy and laparotomy. *Dis. Markers* 2020: 2503753.

23. Berek, J.S., Howe, C., Lagasse, L.D., and Hacker, N.F. (2005). Pelvic exenteration for recurrent gynecologic malignancy: survival and morbidity analysis of the 45-year experience at UCLA. *Gynecol. Oncol.* 99 (1): 153–159.

24. Langstraat, C. and Cliby, W.A. (2013). Considerations in the surgical management of ovarian cancer in the elderly. *Curr. Treat. Options Oncol.* 14 (1): 12–21.

25. Jaeger, W., Ackermann, S., Kessler, H. et al. (2001). The effect of bowel resection on survival in advanced epithelial ovarian cancer. *Gynecol. Oncol.* 83 (2): 286–291.

26. Tamussino, K.F., Lim, P.C., Webb, M.J. et al. (2001). Gastrointestinal surgery in patients with ovarian cancer. *Gynecol. Oncol.* 80 (1): 79–84.

27. Jolicoeur, L. and Faught, W. (2003). Managing bowel obstruction in ovarian cancer using a percutaneous endoscopic gastrostomy (PEG) tube. *Can. Oncol. Nurs. J.* 13 (4): 212–219.

28. Jong, P., Sturgeon, J., and Jamieson, C.G. (1995). Benefit of palliative surgery for bowel obstruction in advanced ovarian cancer. *Can. J. Surg.* 38 (5): 454–457.

29. Spitz, D., Chaves, G.V., and Peres, W.A.F. (2017). Impact of perioperative care on the post-operative recovery of women undergoing surgery for gynaecological tumours. *Eur. J. Cancer Care (Engl.)* 26 (6): doi: 10.1111/ecc.12512.

30. Doorly, M.G. and Senagore, A.J. (2012). Pathogenesis and clinical and economic consequences of postoperative ileus. *Surg. Clin. North Am.* 92 (2): 259–272.

31. Bhandoria, G.P., Bhandarkar, P., Ahuja, V. et al. (2020). Enhanced recovery after surgery (ERAS) in gynecologic oncology: an international survey of peri-operative practice. *Int. J. Gynecol. Cancer* 30 (10): 1471–1478.

32. Baiocchi, G., Faloppa, C.C., Araujo, R.L. et al. (2010). Chylous ascites in gynecologic malignancies: cases report and literature review. *Arch. Gynecol. Obstet.* 281 (4): 677–681.

33. Boran, N., Cil, A.P., Tulunay, G. et al. (2004). Chylous ascites following Para-aortic lymphadenectomy: a case report. *Gynecol. Oncol.* 93 (3): 711–714.

34. Var, T., Gungor, T., Tonguc, E. et al. (2012). The conservative treatment of postoperative chylous ascites in gynecologic cancers: four case reports. *Arch. Gynecol. Obstet.* 285 (3): 849–851.

35. Kim, E.A., Park, H., Jeong, S.G. et al. (2014). Octreotide therapy for the management of refractory chylous ascites after a staging operation for endometrial adenocarcinoma. *J. Obstet. Gynaecol. Res.* 40 (2): 622–626.

# CHAPTER 19

# Major Trauma and Surgery

Jennifer Wetherden[1] and Evanna Leavy[2]

[1] Major Trauma & Critical Care, St George's University Hospitals NHS Foundation Trust, London, UK
[2] Intestinal Failure & Gastrointestinal Surgery, St George's University Hospitals NHS Foundation Trust, London, UK

---

**KEY POINTS**

- Major trauma remains the leading cause of death for people aged 15–44 years and is a significant cause of long-term disability.
- Traumatic injury generally causes a hypermetabolic state in critically ill surgical or medical patients and repeated surgical procedures can prolong this.
- Injury location can dictate specific nutritional considerations, from micronutrients in wound healing to macronutrient losses from wounds, drains, and faeces.
- Dietitians play a key role in overcoming these barriers and ensuring that patients' increased nutritional requirements are met.
- Major trauma patients experience chronic barriers to obtaining adequate nutritional intake, and close liaison is required with the multidisciplinary team to overcome these.

---

Trauma encompasses unintentional and intentional injuries caused by the sudden application of external force to the tissues. It is the leading cause of death for people aged 15–44 years, and the National Audit Office estimates that there are 20 000 major trauma cases a year in the UK, with 5400 deaths [1].

The English Major Trauma system was introduced in 2012 as part of an initiative to improve the care of trauma patients. It consists of 23 Major Trauma regional networks (a major trauma centre or MTC) determined by geographical location, population, and the availability of specialist services, including within the emergency department, surgical specialties, and rehabilitation.

They manage injury care across the region, hosting a network of trauma units (TUs). These are local hospitals with the capability to care for moderately injured patients, or to stabilise them and transfer to

*Nutritional Management of the Surgical Patient*, First Edition. Edited by Mary E. Phillips.
© 2023 John Wiley & Sons Ltd. Published 2023 by John Wiley & Sons Ltd.

the MTC for ongoing care. TUs also receive these injured patients back for further rehabilitation services and local social care.

Since the inception of the Major Trauma system, there has been a 20% reduction in mortality rates [1]. However, trauma remains a significant cause of moderate or severe disability, causing the loss of over 250 million disability-adjusted life years worldwide per year [2].

In 2019, 40% of patients admitted to an MTC required some kind of surgical intervention for their injuries during their admission [3].

Dietitians, and the nutritional therapy they provide, are a key figure in the trauma care spectrum and patient outcomes, from critical care to rehabilitation and discharge.

## PHYSIOLOGICAL RESPONSE TO INJURY

Trauma is defined as physical damage to the body. The major trauma (MT)-induced stress response is similar to that of the surgical-induced stress response that triggers a cascade of physiological processes involving cardiovascular, endocrine, and inflammatory changes. This adaptive response to surviving injury results in a hypermetabolic state affecting nutritional requirements [4, 5].

A quantifiable two-stage response to major trauma was first defined in 1942. The initial stage, called the 'ebb phase', occurs in minutes and hours after injury, where metabolism is reduced to prevent energy depletion. This is followed by the 'flow phase', which is the subsequent increase in metabolism that can last for days to weeks depending on injury severity [6, 7]. Following severe and multiple injuries, the hypercatabolic state can be prolonged by repeated trips to theatre for grafts, revisions, and definitive management of injuries, with the overall effect being catabolism of stored body fuels. The magnitude and duration of stress response are proportional to the surgical injury and the development of complications [6, 8].

Following trauma, the nervous system stimulates increased production and release of catabolic hormones including cortisol, glucagon, and catecholamines and stimulates the release of pro-inflammatory cytokines and the activation of the complement system. These changes mediate the metabolic response, promoting proteolysis of skeletal muscle and lipolysis, providing substrates for gluconeogenesis in the liver that results in increased blood glucose levels. Hyperglycaemia is associated with reduced wound healing, increased infections, inflammation and ventilator dependence, length of hospital stays, and mortality [9].

The final phase of the stress response occurs when there is a transition from catabolism to anabolism, which can take weeks or even months following severe trauma. Fat and protein stores are rendered replete in this anabolic phase [5].

Although initially protective, a prolonged hypercatabolic and metabolic state contributes to complications including muscle wasting, impaired immune function, and reduced wound healing [6]. Exogenous nutrition is important to counteract cumulative nutritional deficits caused by the catabolic phase, and reduce these complications [7]. In addition, the implementation of early enteral nutrition (EN) is known to preserve gut mucosa integrity, reducing the risk of mucosal atrophy, bacterial overproliferation and translocation, and subsequent sepsis. Early EN (defined as <48 h from admission) has been shown to improve outcomes in trauma patients in critical care [8, 10, 11].

## ROUTES OF NUTRITION

EN is the preferred route of nutrition for trauma patients as it maintains the functional and structural integrity of the gastrointestinal tract (GIT), providing immune modulation and attenuation of inflammatory responses [4, 12, 13].

In this heterogeneous patient group, there can be various barriers to achieving adequate nutrition from EN, including mechanical obstruction of the GIT, gut ischaemia, open abdomen, bowel discontinuity following damage-control laparotomy, and paralytic ileus [14]. It is a well-cited concern that EN will contribute to bowel dilatation and increase pressure on the GIT, leading to a higher risk of anastomotic breakdown following surgery; however, it has been shown that initiating EN post anastomoses or in an open abdomen was not associated with worse outcomes [15].

If EN is contraindicated or insufficient to meet requirements, then parenteral nutrition (PN) should be considered. Studies exploring PN versus EN in trauma patients specifically are limited, but studies carried out in critical care (including MT patients) have found varying results, with meta-analyses demonstrating either no difference in infective complications, or mortality [16, 17], or a significant reduction in infectious complications and length of stay in critical care in patients receiving EN compared with PN [18]. It must be considered that these studies varied in nutritional delivery, in both quantity and feed type (see Chapter 8). These studies vary in sample size and in 'standard care' to which the intervention groups are compared [19]. Due to the complexity and diversity of surgeries required for trauma, the post-operative feeding route should be decided on an individual basis.

## NUTRITIONAL REQUIREMENTS

Trauma is generally considered to cause a more severe hypermetabolic state than is seen in medical patients, indicating higher energy requirements. The degree of hypermetabolism varies and appears to relate to systemic inflammation rather than severity or anatomical location of injury. Determining energy requirements is therefore challenging and the use of predictive equations to estimate energy expenditure is the most common practice, and is recommended in the absence of indirect calorimetry [20, 21].

Protein requirements among major trauma patients are still unclear, with research showing varying results. Dickerson et al. [22] concluded that protein provision of 2 g/kg/d or greater was more successful in achieving nitrogen equilibrium than lower-dosage intakes. This, of course, needs to be tailored to appropriate patient groups. Lower provision should be considered for those with renal or hepatic failure, and higher provision for those with poor feed delivery or increased losses (i.e. from wound exudate, drains, or losses from faecal matter). The effects of short-term administration of higher protein doses (i.e. >2.0 g/kg of body weight) are unlikely to cause serious adverse effects in the absence of liver or renal failure.

## OVERVIEW OF TRAUMA INJURIES AND SURGERIES

### Patient and Injury Characteristics

Major trauma admissions used to be predominantly male (just over two-thirds) and under 30 years of age; however, these demographics have changed in recent years [23].

A 2017 report by the Trauma Audit and Research Network (TARN) demonstrated that the typical major trauma patient has changed from being young and male, to older adults with a lower degree of male predominance – 53% of UK TARN-eligible patients admitted in 2019 were male [3]. A fall of less than 2 m is the most common mechanism of injury in older patients, in contrast to the prevalence of road traffic collisions in younger patients. In 2019, the age bracket 80–89 years made up the highest percentage of admissions (24%). This increases the likelihood of pre-existing comorbidities on admission, in addition to frailty and the development of sarcopenia – an independent risk factor for falls and fractures in the elderly [23, 24].

A 2019 review by Dijkink et al. found that within the elderly trauma population, up to 62.5% were malnourished on admission to hospital and up to 60% were at risk of malnutrition. Malnutrition was found to be an independent risk factor for mortality, complications, increased length of stay, and decreased quality of life [25].

### Types of Injury

The energy of the force causing the trauma can be divided in to mechanical, gravitational, thermal, chemical, electrical, and radiant – the latter four of which are related to burns (a complex topic that is not covered in this chapter). The vast majority of traumatic injuries are caused by mechanical or gravitational forces.

Injury mechanisms include blunt trauma (e.g. road traffic collisions, falls), penetrating trauma (stab, impalement, firearm injuries), crush injuries (from machinery or structure collapse), or burn and blast injuries.

The type of tissue involved can also predict subsequent injuries. Solid structures will crack under force – the most obvious example being fractured bones, but solid organs (i.e. spleen, liver, pancreas, and kidneys) also crack and shatter.

Hollow structures tend to pop; that is, air-filled hollow organs (lungs), fluid-filled structures (bladder, eye, or heart), and those filled with both (stomach, intestines, and the abdominal cavity). Fixed points within the body tear from external forces – vessels, tubes, ligaments and tendons, nerves and skin.

Each injury, be it isolated or a combination of these types, presents specific challenges in terms of surgical management and the subsequent effect on nutritional demands and delivery.

## Types of Surgery

### Abdominal Trauma

Abdominal trauma, both blunt and penetrating, can range hugely in severity. Early imaging and assessment are integral to identifying patients with potentially catastrophic injuries. These types of injuries can lead to the previously described shattering of solid organs within the highly vascular abdominal cavity. Also known as lacerations or haematomas, these are graded by severity and can be managed conservatively (with regular monitoring and strict bed rest), by interventional radiology, or surgically.

Pancreatic injuries are relatively rare (reported as 0.32% pancreato-duodenal injuries detected among over 356 000 injured patients in a recent systematic review [12]); however, they can carry significant morbidity and mortality, especially if penetrating (more common in North America). Pancreatic injuries can often be managed conservatively and, if required,

ductal disruption can be handled by early stenting with or without drainage in many cases, although distal resection may be an alternative. If the pancreatic duct is disrupted with an uncontrolled leak, then pancreatic secretory mechanisms can be bypassed with PN or very distal jejunal feeding (see Chapter 14).

Damage-control laparotomies are indicated in trauma patients who present with deranged physiology, for instance those who are actively haemorrhaging or require contamination control and stabilisation before definitive reconstruction [26].

After the initial intervention to stop bleeding, restore perfusion, and limit contamination, patients are often left with an open abdominal wall – rather than run the risk of closure, which can lead to abdominal compartment syndrome from tissue inflammation. The patient is returned to the intensive care unit (ICU) for ongoing resuscitation and restoration of normal physiology, until they are stable for definitive surgery and closure.

If a bowel resection is indicated at this stage, it is likely that the bowel will not be anastomosed, leaving it out of continuity until an anastomosis or stoma is formed in a relook surgery. In this instance, nutrition is not possible via the enteral route and PN may be considered. The length of time until the bowel is back in continuity will help inform the indication for PN.

Early enteral feeding in patients following abdominal trauma with an open abdomen is safe and supported by current guidelines [27], and is associated with a reduction in complications and mortality [28]. However, the case remains less clear in those trauma patients with an open abdomen in addition to bowel injury. EN is not contraindicated in this cohort, but the benefits described have not yet been proven and require further research [13]. These patients should be assessed on an individual basis.

In the patient with an open abdomen, postoperative ileus or reduced gut motility, coupled with increased protein losses from the exposed viscera, can quickly lead to protein and energy malnutrition. Supplementary PN should be considered if nutritional targets cannot be met [4]. MT patients, especially those who have undergone abdominal surgery, are at increased risk of developing abdominal compartment syndrome – where the abdominal organs are subjected to increasing pressures, leading to vascular compromise and ischaemia, and consequently significant morbidity and mortality [29]. Intra-abdominal pressures (IAP) can be monitored via the urinary catheter, and values of <10 mmHg are considered 'normal' in the mechanically ventilated paralysed patient. Intra-abdominal hypertension (IAH) is generally defined as the presence of an IAP (in paralysed patients) higher than 12 mmHg [29].

These increased pressures can affect cardiovascular, respiratory, and renal function, the latter of which is often the first to be compromised. The gut and liver are also sensitive to IAH. Raised pressures can reduce mesenteric blood flow leading to the loss of intestinal barrier function, bacterial translocation, bowel necrosis, and multiple organ failure [30].

## Maxillofacial Trauma

Maxillofacial trauma directly affects the nutritional status of patients by limiting or preventing normal functions such as mouth opening, mastication, and breathing. It is relatively common, with 26% of patients admitted in 2019 undergoing otolaryngology or maxillofacial surgery [3].

The route of feeding can be challenging; associated base-of-skull fractures with trauma to the head and neck mean that blind placement of nasogastric tubes (NGT) is contraindicated. Facial fractures and nasal bone trauma can often mean that the insertion of NGTs is prevented by packing or splinting. Feeding can be undertaken using orogastric tubes (OGTs) while the patient is still ventilated, and following extubation rapid instigation of oral nutritional supplements, with the option for enteral tubes placed under direct visualisation if needed.

Injuries to structures resulting in dysphagia (facial nerve injuries, vocal cord injuries) require multidisciplinary team (MDT) management, especially liaison with the speech and language therapist, regarding swallow rehabilitation, prognosis, and the need for gastrostomy placement to facilitate long-term feeding. Malnutrition, as with most surgical procedures, leads to increased morbidity and mortality rates in maxillofacial patients, especially the elderly, the critically ill, and those who are already malnourished [31].

Patients with isolated maxillofacial trauma are often discharged home rapidly, and the role of the trauma dietitian is crucial in identifying the need for support and education regarding a nutritionally optimal diet if, for instance, dentition is affected, or the jaw is fixed for a period of time to allow for healing.

## Chest Trauma and Thoracic Surgery

Thoracic surgery, while relatively rare (only 2% of major trauma admissions in the UK in 2019 had thoracic surgery [3]), does indicate a significant injury severity score. Rib fractures and fixation bring about significant post-operative pain issues and respiratory compromise, presenting a substantial barrier to starting or increasing oral intake to ensure that requirements are met.

There is still much variation nationally among MTCs in the management of chest wall trauma, with rib fixation growing in popularity, and only approximately 2.4% of patients being managed surgically [32].

Chylothoraxes are also a fairly uncommon but serious condition, where blunt or penetrating traumas to the chest or neck can cause chyle to leak from the lymphatic system into the pleural space, usually on the left side (see Chapter 9).

## Orthopaedic Surgery

Pelvic fractures are relatively common among major trauma admissions, especially the elderly. While most are conservatively managed, those that are surgically repaired, with associated retroperitoneal haematomas, or those that are more severe can develop paralytic ileus [33]. The reason for this remains unclear; it could be due to the severity or mechanism of the trauma itself, manipulation or handling of the gut during surgery, or related to surgical fixation procedures (internal and external) [33].

External fixators (ex-fix) can be placed to immobilise fractured bones – to allow them to heal, or until more definitive management, such as an open reduction internal fixation (ORIF). Ex-fixes can be placed on limbs (typically lower limbs) but also the pelvis. Prior to elective orthopaedic surgeries, enhanced recovery after surgery (ERAS) pathways can be utilised to reduce length of hospital stay and readmission rate, and improve functional recovery [34] (see Chapter 5).

## COMMON POST-OPERATIVE COMPLICATIONS AND THEIR NUTRITIONAL MANAGEMENT

It has been well established that the critical care patient population is under-fed. An international, multicentre observational study in 2010 found that average nutritional adequacy was 59% of targets for energy, 60% for protein, and enteral feeds took on average 46 hours to be commenced [35]. For the major trauma patient, add in pre-operative fasting, time in surgery, scans, and other diagnostic procedures, and the higher energy and protein demands of this population seem aspirational rather than realistic.

Severely injured patients admitted under major trauma will often have damage control surgery within the first 24 h of admission, then undergo reoperation for revisional surgery (i.e. of stumps post amputation) or definitive management (i.e. replacing an ex-fix for an ORIF). Only 20% of ICUs in the UK have fasting protocols, with wide variation in practice for an assortment of procedures; fasting times were on average shorter if a guideline was present [36]. The stoppage of feed for surgery or diagnostic procedures contributes to the nutritional deficits already described, so ensuring that appropriate fasting times are in place and agreed by the ICU team will aid in nutritional targets being met. Other strategies to help overcome stoppages in feed can include higher-concentration enteral feeds, a catch-up/volume-based feeding protocol (i.e. PEPuP [37]), ERAS protocols, or bolus feeding (see Chapter 8).

### Paralytic Ileus

A paralytic ileus is an interruption to gastrointestinal (GI) motility that is common after abdominal and orthopaedic surgeries. The reduction or absence

**TABLE 19.1**   Nutritional composition of fluid losses.

| Losses | Average volume loss/24 h | Nutritional losses |
|---|---|---|
| Wound losses [14] | Soft tissue wounds: 245 ml | 29 g protein/l |
| | Open abdomen: 1031 ml | |
| Faecal losses [42] | >350 g/d leads to nutritional losses | If stool >350 g/d: 627 kcal/d 16.2 g protein/d |

of GI peristalsis results in the accumulation of intra-luminal secretions and gas that causes nausea, vomiting, abdominal pain, and distension [33]. The aetiology of paralytic ileus is thought to be multifactorial, with inflammatory, hormonal, neurogenic, and pharmacological influences [38, 39]. Ileus occurs in 15% of patients after abdominal surgery and 0.3–5.6% after orthopaedic surgery, with spinal and lower-extremity surgery accounting for most cases [40, 41] (see Chapter 20).

### Nutritional Losses

Increased losses may also present a barrier or further challenge to reaching nutritional targets; these can include losses from wounds, drains, topical negative-pressure dressings, amputations, and GI losses (Table 19.1). Protein deficiency contributes to poor wound healing by prolonging the inflammatory process, impairing collagen synthesis, and increasing the risk of wound dehiscence [43].

## LONG-TERM NUTRITIONAL BARRIERS AND COMPLICATIONS

### Impaired Mobility

Restricted mobility from injuries can present barriers to meeting nutritional requirements on acute and rehabilitation wards. Patients with upper-limb injuries, especially those that are bilateral, can be entirely dependent on nursing staff to ensure that their nutrition and hydration needs are met.

Occupational therapists (OTs) play an integral role within the MT rehabilitation MDT to support independence. This may include the use of adapted cutlery, patient hydration bottles attached to the head of the bed with a mouthpiece on the end of a tube, cognitive/psychosocial support, identifying strategies for reducing anxiety, mealtime distractions, and enhancing communication.

## Weight Management

Long-term body composition of patients following spinal cord injury has been well studied, with an overall deterioration in body composition secondary to neurological impairment, specifically a loss of lean muscle mass and an increase in fat mass. This has long-term implications for cardiovascular health, diabetes mellitus, and other chronic diseases associated with an increased proportion of adipose tissue [44]. The long-term health of those post-traumatic injuries is not, however, well studied, and requires further research into the changing metabolic demands of rehabilitation and the types of subsequent nutritional counselling required.

## Micronutrients and Wound Healing

Micronutrients have long been studied for their potential to enhance wound healing, with pressure ulcer wounds improved with oral vitamin B9,

vitamin C, copper, selenium, and zinc supplementation [45]. Traumatic wounds (aside from burns) were not covered in this chapter, and that is an area where further research is needed. Measured serum status levels should be interpreted with care, as low levels may be a result of the inflammatory process and not reflecting a true deficiency (see Chapter 22).

## AREAS FOR FUTURE RESEARCH

Immune-modulating nutrients such as glutamine, omega-3 fish oils, and arginine are theorised to have clinical benefits including membrane stability, mucosal maintenance, attenuation of the inflammatory response to stress, and alterations in blood flow to poorly vascularised areas. Evidence to support their benefit is limited in the trauma patient population. A reduction in complication rates, length of stay, and infectious complication rates has been seen in the abdominal surgery patient population with nutritional formulas enriched with omega-3 fatty acids, arginine, and glutamines. Glutamine has also been linked to improved glycaemic control in critically ill polytrauma patients [45]. However, it must be noted that these studies are limited to small sample sizes with various routes and timings of nutrition.

More widely, micronutrient status and supplementation specifically in traumatic wound healing are under-researched subjects. However, due to the heterogeneous population and injury type, high-quality evidence may be difficult to obtain.

| Routine Case Study | |
|---|---|
| Patient | Mr A, age 49 yr |
| Presenting complaint | Approx 9 ft fall from ladder, onto right side, onto concrete breeze blocks |
| Past medical history | Type 2 diabetes mellitus – diet controlled<br>No allergies |
| Social history | Employed as a builder<br>Lives at home with partner<br>Drinks 4–5 units/wk<br>Smoker – 20/d |

| | |
|---|---|
| Investigations | Trauma computed tomography (CT) scan indicated:<br>• Extensive right-sided rib fractures, including flail segments<br>• Right clavicle fracture<br>• Right humeral fracture<br>• Significant soft tissue injuries to right side |
| Oral intake | No concerns prior to accident – weight stable |
| Anthropometrics | Admission weight reported as 97 kg (by patient). Height 1.88 m. Body mass index (BMI) 27.4 kg/m²<br>Weight stable. Moderate muscle mass due to occupation |
| Bowel function | No concerns |
| Surgical plan | Theatre on day 1 of admission under cardiothoracics/trauma and orthopaedics for clavicle/humeral ORIF and rib fixation<br>Transferred to high-dependency unit (HDU) bed post-operatively |
| Nutritional plan | Aim to meet 100% of nutritional requirements via NGT until oral intake resumes, maintaining nutritional status. Provide ongoing dietetic support, education, and monitoring regarding energy and protein content of oral diet |
| Admission | Patient remained intubated and ventilated post-operatively for 48 h – failed extubation due to chest infection and poor respiratory function<br>Serratus anterior block placed by pain team for management of pain from rib fractures<br>NGT inserted and feeding commenced as per ICU out-of-hours protocol<br>Dietitian saw patient on day 2 and provided a tailored feeding regime<br>Day 4 of ICU stay – patient was successfully extubated on to high-flow nasal oxygen<br>His blood glucose was measured between 14 and 21 mmol/l, therefore he was started on a variable-rate intravenous insulin infusion and subsequently Humulin twice a day<br>Referred to smoking cessation and commenced nicotine patches<br>Stepped down to ward on day 7 of admission<br>Discharged from hospital on day 15 of admission |
| Nutritional support | Commenced on Nutrison Standard 1.0 (Nutricia Clinical Care, Trowbridge, UK) ICU out-of-hours protocol – target 60 ml/h over 24 h<br>Changed to Nutrison Protein Advance (Nutricia Clinical Care), increasing to target 70 ml/h over 24 h continuously while on ICU. This provided 2150 kcal, 140 g protein in 1680 ml (~25 kcal/kg including calories from propofol, 1.3 g protein/kg)<br>On extubation: increased to 88 ml/h over 24 h. Oral intake negligible post extubation due to pain, nausea, oxygen requirements, and breathlessness, therefore NG feeding continued until step-down to ward |
| Outcome | Slow wean off enteral feed onto high-protein oral nutritional supplements (ONS) – tolerating liquids well over solid foods initially due to breathlessness<br>NGT feed initially changed to overnight to aid daytime intake, then ceased altogether on day 10 of admission when patient meeting ~50% of estimated requirements orally<br>New weight on step-down 94 kg, then 92 kg on discharge (5% weight loss during admission) |
| Long term prescriptions | Nil – patient provided with information leaflet and counselling regarding food-first approach prior to discharge. 2-week supply of ONS provided and letter to GP regarding weight monitoring |
| Follow up | Follow-up in MDT clinic 3/12 after discharge<br>Patient's wounds have healed well<br>Weight remains stable (monitored by GP), and patient is actively engaging in regular physiotherapy to aid in rehabilitation |

## Case Study

| Patient | Mr B, 28 yr |
| --- | --- |
| Presenting complaint | Admitted to A&E by helicopter emergency medical services (HEMs) with shotgun wound to abdomen, stabbing to abdomen and groin |
| Past medical history | Nil |
| Social history | Lives with mother |
| Investigations | CT scan: innumerable shotgun pellets throughout the abdomen<br>Surgery: Damage-control surgery |
| Oral intake | No concerns with eating and drinking prior to admission |
| Anthropometrics | Weight 90 kg (estimate)<br>Height 1.74 m<br>BMI 30 kg/m$^2$ (overweight)<br>Adjusted body weight (AdjBW) 78.8kg |
| Diagnosis | Injuries:<br>• Penetrating left abdominal wound with eviscerated omentum<br>• Innumerable shotgun pellets throughout the abdomen and within the bowel<br>• Large blast injury to transverse colon with visible shotgun shell<br>• Multiple small bowel injuries from pellets: from duodenojejunal flexure these were noted at 15, 50, 60, 160, and 190 cm<br>• At least 5 pellet injuries to stomach at inferior portion of greater curve<br>• At least 2 non-bleeding pellet injuries to liver segments<br>• Fractures of left ribs with bone fragments in peritoneal cavity<br>• Laceration to left groin and to right thigh<br>• Multiorgan failure secondary to trauma |
| Surgical plan | Day 1: Damage-control surgery<br>• Small bowel resection ×3: segments resected at 15, 50, and 160 cm. No anastomoses performed. Approx. 250 cm of small bowel remaining but not in continuity<br>• Transverse colectomy. No anastomoses performed<br>• Gastric repairs: at least 5 pellet injuries to inferior portion of greater curve of the stomach repaired. Herniated omentum reduced and resected<br>• Abdomen left open<br>Day 2: Washout and primary closure of laceration to right thigh<br>Day 3: Second-look surgery<br>• Small bowel anastomosis ×3 performed. 250 cm small bowel now in continuity<br>• Hepatic flexure right-sided colostomy, debridement of left flank wound and closure of laparostomy, and closure of left flank wound wall<br>Day 4: Left thigh washout, debridement, and application of vac dressing to thigh |
| Nutritional plan | Intubated and ventilated, requiring artificial nutrition support from PN<br>Indications to initiate PN:<br>• Bowel not in continuity, enteral route unavailable<br>• Following planned re-anastomosis, EN delivery would be limited due to risk of anastomotic breakdown<br>• Post-op ileus expected due to significant intraoperative bowel handling that would limit EN absorption |

| | |
|---|---|
| Nutrition support | Nutrition support initiated on day 2 of admission<br>Day 2: PN started at 50% of energy requirements<br>Day 4: Increased to target energy and protein in PN:<br>18 g nitrogen, 70 g lipid, 230 g glucose (~2040 kcal)<br>Na 80 mmol, K 80 mmol, PO$_4$ 40 mmol, Ca 8 mmol, Mg 16 mmol<br>Standard micronutrients and trace elements<br>2L over 24 hours<br>Required potassium and phosphate intravenous replacement on days 1 and 2<br>Day 7 (4 days post second-look surgery): Trophic NG feed at 10 ml/h permitted by surgeons and increased to tolerance<br>PN/EN titration regime provided. Delays reaching target EN due to high gastric residual volumes, colostomy not active, suspected ileus<br>Remained on target PN during this time<br>Day 11: NG feed delivery reached target nutrition (providing 30 kcal/kg AdjBW, 1.5 g protein/kg AdjBW). PN discontinued<br>Day 13: Weaned off sedation, extubated<br>Day 14: Speech and language therapist assessment following intubation deemed swallow to be safe. Started to eat and drink. ONS provided. Supplementary NG feed continued<br>Day 18: Meeting 80% of requirements with oral intake. NG feed stopped<br>Day 28: Meals, snacks, and ONS |
| Outcome | Discharged home after 42 days<br>On discharge: weight 76kg, BMI: 25 kg/m². Stable for 1 week. 15% body weight loss during admission. 2.5 m small bowel and ascending colon in continuity to colostomy. No signs of malabsorption or fluid and electrolyte disturbances. |
| Long-term prescription | ONS twice a day |
| Follow-up | Dietitian phone review 3 weeks post discharge. Weight 77 kg. Meeting requirements with oral intake. Discontinue ONS. Discharged from dietetic care back to GP |

# REFERENCES

1. NHS England (2013). Independent review of major trauma networks reveals increase in patient survival rates. https://www.england.nhs.uk/2013/06/incr-pati-survi-rts. Accessed 14 February 2022.

2. Murray, C.J., Vos, T., Lozano, R. et al. (2012). Disability-adjusted life years (DALYs) for 291diseases and injuries in 21 regions, 1990–2010: a systematic analysis for the global burden of disease study 2010. *Lancet* 380: 2197–2223.

3. Trauma Audit and Research Network. (2021). Management of surgical patients in England and Wales, 2019. Access on request to research@tarn.ac.uk.

4. Singer, P., Blaser, A.R., Berger, M.M. et al. (2019). ESPEN guideline on clinical nutrition in the intensive care unit. *Clin. Nutr.* 38: 48e79.

5. Şimşek, T., Şimşek, H.U., and Cantürk, N.Z. (2014). Response to trauma and metabolic changes: posttraumatic metabolism. *Ulusal cerrahi dergisi* 30 (3): 153–159.

6. Desborough, J.P. (2000). The stress response to trauma and surgery. *Br. J. Anaes.* 85 (1): 109–117.

7. Finnerty, C.C., Mabvuure, N.T., Ali, A. et al. (2013). The surgically induced stress response. *JPEN.* 37 (5 Suppl): 21S–29S.

8. Li, P.F., Wang, Y.L., Fang, Y.L. et al. (2020). Effect of early enteral nutrition on outcomes of trauma patients requiring intensive care. *Chin. J. Traumatol.* 23 (3): 163–167.

9. Brealey, D. and Singer, M. (2009). Hyperglycemia in critical illness: a review. *J. Diabetes Sci. Technol.* 3 (6): 1250–1260.

10. Herbert, G., Perry, R., Andersen, H.K. et al. (2018). Early enteral nutrition within 24 hours of lower gastrointestinal surgery versus later commencement for length of hospital stay and postoperative complications. *Cochrane Database Syst. Rev.* 10 (10): CD004080.

11. Doig, G.S., Heighes, P.T., Simpson, F., and Sweetman, E.A. (2011). Early enteral nutrition reduces mortality in trauma patients requiring intensive care: a meta analysis of randomised controlled trials. *Injury* 42: 50Y56.

12. Søreide, K., Weiser, T.G., and Parks, R.W. (2018). Clinical update on management of pancreatic trauma. *HPB (Oxford)* 20 (12): 1099–1108.

13. Braga, M., Gianotti, L., Gentilini, O. et al. (2001). Early postoperative enteral nutrition improves gut oxygenation and reduces costs compared with total parenteral nutrition. *Crit. Care Med.* 29 (2): 242–248.

14. Hourigan, L.A., Linfoot, J.A., Chung, K.K. et al. (2010). Loss of protein, immunoglobulins, and electrolytes in exudates from negative pressure wound therapy. *Nutr. Clin. Pract.* 25 (5): 510–516.

15. Osland, E., Yunus, R.M., Khan, S., and Memon, M.A. (2011). Early versus traditional postoperative feeding in patients undergoing resectional gastrointestinal surgery: a meta-analysis. *JPEN.* 35: 473–487.

16. Reignier, J., Van Zanten, A.R.H., and Arabi, Y.M. (2018). Optimal timing, dose and route of early nutrition therapy in critical illness and shock: the quest for the Holy Grail. *Intensive Care Med.* 44: 1558–1560.

17. Harvey, S.E., Parrott, F., Harrison, D.A. et al. (2014). Trial of the route of early nutritional support in critically ill adults. *N. Engl. J. Med.* 371 (18): 1673–1684.

18. Elke, G., van Zanten, A.R., Lemieux, M. et al. (2016). Enteral versus parenteral nutrition in critically ill patients: an updated systematic review and meta-analysis of randomized controlled trials. *Crit. Care* 20 (1): 117.

19. Heyland, D.K., Montalvo, M., MacDonald, S. et al. (2001). Total parenteral nutrition in the surgical patient: a meta-analysis. *Can. J. Surg.* 44 (2): 102–111.

20. Frankenfield, D.C. and Ashcraft, C.M. (2011). Estimating energy needs in nutrition support patients. *JPEN.* 35 (5): 563–570.

21. Lambell, K.J., Tatucu-Babet, O.A., Chapple, L. et al. (2020). Nutrition therapy in critical illness: a review of the literature for clinicians. *Crit. Care* 24: 35.

22. Dickerson, R.N., Pitts, S.L., Maish, G.O. 3rd et al. (2012). A reappraisal of nitrogen requirements for patients with critical illness and trauma. *J. Trauma Acute Care Surg.* 73 (3): 549–557.

23. Trauma Audit and Research Network (2017). Major trauma in older people –2017 Report. https://www.tarn.ac.uk/Content.aspx?c=3793. Accessed 14 February 2022.

24. Yeung, S.S.Y., Reijnierse, E.M., Pham, V.K. et al. (2019). Sarcopenia and its association with falls and fractures in older adults: a systematic review and meta-analysis. *J. Cachexia. Sarcopenia Muscle* 10 (3): 485–500.

25. Dijkink, S., Meier, K., Krijnen, P. et al. (2020). Malnutrition and its effects in severely injured trauma patients. *Eur. J. Trauma Emerg. Surg.* 46 (5): 993–1004.

26. Moore, S.M. and Burlew, C.C. (2016). Nutrition support in the open abdomen. *Nutr. Clin. Pract.* 31 (1): 9–13.

27. Reintam Blaser, A., Starkopf, J., Alhazzani, W. et al. (2017). Early enteral nutrition in critically ill patients: ESICM clinical practice guidelines. *Intensive Care Med.* 43 (3): 380–398.

28. Burlew, C.C., Moore, E.E., Cuschieri, J. et al. (2012). Who should we feed? Western trauma association multi-institutional study of enteral nutrition in the open abdomen after injury. *J. Trauma Acute Care Surg.* 73 (6): 1380–1387.

29. Berry, N. and Fletcher, S. (2012). Abdominal compartment syndrome. *Contin. Educ. Anaesth. Crit. Care Pain* 12 (3): 110–117.

30. Aspesi, M., Gamberoni, C., Severgnini, P. et al. (2002). The abdominal compartment syndrome. Clinical relevance. *Minerva Anestesiol.* 68 (4): 138–146.

31. Giridhar, V.U. (2016). Role of nutrition in oral and maxillofacial surgery patients. *Natl. J. Maxillofac. Surg.* 7 (1): 3–9.

32. Ingoe, H.M., Eardley, W., McDaid, C. et al. (2020). Epidemiology of adult rib fracture and factors associated with surgical fixation: analysis of a chest wall injury dataset from England and Wales. *Injury* 51 (2): 218–223.

33. Daniels, A.H., Ritterman, S.A., and Rubin, L.E. (2015). Paralytic ileus in the orthopaedic patient. *J. Am. Acad. Orthop. Surg.* 23 (6): 365–372.

34. Kaye, A.D., Urman, R.D., Cornett, E.M. et al. (2019). Enhanced recovery pathways in orthopedic surgery. *J. Anaesthesiol. Clin. Pharmacol.* 35 (Suppl 1): S35–S39.

35. Cahill, N.E., Dhaliwal, R., Day, A.G. et al. (2010). Nutrition therapy in the critical care setting: what is 'best achievable' practice? An international multicenter observational study. *Crit. Care Med.* 38 (2): 395–401.

36. Segaran, E., Lovejoy, T.D., Proctor, C. et al. (2018). Exploring fasting practices for critical care patients – a web-based survey of UK intensive care units. *J. Intensive Care Soc.* 19 (3): 188–195.

37. Heyland, D.K., Cahill, N.E., Dhaliwal, R. et al. (2010). Enhanced protein-energy provision via the enteral route in critically ill patients: a single center feasibility trial of the PEP uP protocol. *Crit. Care* 14 (2): R78.

38. Vather, R., Josephson, R., Jaung, R. et al. (2015). Development of a risk stratification system for the occurrence of prolonged postoperative ileus after colorectal surgery: a prospective risk factor analysis. *Surgery* 157 (4): 764–773.

39. Bragg, D., El-Sharkawy, A.M., Psaltis, E. et al. (2015). Postoperative ileus: recent developments in pathophysiology and management. *Clin. Nutr.* 34 (3): 367–376.

40. Kumar, V., Vaish, A., and Vaishya, R. (2020). Postoperative ileus after orthopaedic and spine surgery: a critical review. *Apollo Med.* 17 (1): 16–21.

41. Bugaev, N., Bhattacharya, B., Chiu, W.C. et al. (2019). Promotility agents for the treatment of ileus in adult surgical patients: a practice management guideline from the Eastern Association for the Surgery of Trauma. *J. Trauma Acute Care Surg.* 87 (4): 922–934.

42. Wierdsma, N.J., Peters, J.H., Weijs, P.J. et al. (2011). Malabsorption and nutritional balance in the ICU: fecal weight as a biomarker: a prospective observational pilot study. *Crit. Care* 15 (6): R264.

43. Russell, L. (2001). The importance of patients' nutritional status in wound healing. *Br. J. Nurs.* 10 (6 Suppl): S42–S49.

44. Farkas, G.J., Pitot, M.A., Berg, A.S., and Gater, D.R. (2019). Nutritional status in chronic spinal cord injury: a systematic review and meta-analysis. *Spinal Cord* 57 (1): 3–17.

45. Saeg, F., Orazi, R., Bowers, G.M., and Janis, J.E. (2021). Evidence-based nutritional interventions in wound care. *Plast. Reconstr. Surg.* 148 (1): 226–238.

# CONSEQUENCES OF SURGERY

# CHAPTER 20

# Bowel Obstruction and Dysfunction in Benign and Malignant Disease

Lindsey Allan and Naomi Westran

*Department of Nutrition and Dietetics, Royal Surrey NHS Foundation Trust, Guildford, UK*

---

**KEY POINTS**

- Paralytic ileus occurs most commonly post-operatively.
- Enhanced recovery strategies can be used to reduce the risk of ileus post-operatively.
- Bowel obstruction can be benign (predominantly from surgical adhesions) or malignant from a primary tumour or metastatic spread to the peritoneum.
- Malnutrition rates are high in patients presenting with bowel obstruction.
- More research is required to establish evidence-based nutritional interventions for the management of benign and malignant bowel obstruction.

---

## PARALYTIC ILEUS

A paralytic ileus is defined as an intestinal dysmotility that arises as a consequence of inadequate peristalsis [1]. The most common form occurs post-operatively [2]; however, other causes exist including electrolyte disturbance [3], use of opioid medication [4], and trauma [5].

Post-operative paralytic ileus is the transient cessation of bowel motility following a surgical intervention [6]. A lack of peristalsis within the digestive tract results in a build-up of fluid and gas within the intestine, resulting in a functional obstruction.

## DIAGNOSIS AND INCIDENCE

A definitive diagnosis of post-operative ileus is made with the following criteria [6]:

- Absence of a mechanical obstruction.
- Presence of symptoms including nausea, vomiting, intolerance to oral intake, obstipation

(complete absence of bowel function), abdominal distension, and pain.

It is accepted that some degree of gut paralysis is to be expected following a surgical intervention [7]; however, this is expected to last for only 24 h in the small bowel, 24–48 h in the stomach, and 48–72 h in the colon [8, 9]. A patient is deemed to be in postoperative ileus until there has been passage of stool or flatus and they are tolerating oral intake, events that should occur within four days of surgery [6].

If the ileus has not resolved after the fourth postoperative day and the patient has the presence of two of the following five criteria, they can be defined as having a prolonged postoperative ileus and will likely require medical and nutritional intervention:

- Nausea or vomiting.
- Inability to tolerate oral diet over the previous 24 h.
- Absence of flatus over the previous 24 h.
- Abdominal distension.
- Ileus confirmed radiologically.

The incidence of post-operative and prolonged post-operative ileus reported in the literature varies widely in spite of the presence of an agreed definition and criteria. It is thought that a prolonged postoperative ileus occurs in up to 15.9% of patients following surgery to the colon [10], and has been observed in up to 13% of patients following gastric or pancreatic surgery [11].

The symptoms of post-operative ileus are similar to those of mechanical bowel obstruction (BO). Radiological imaging is therefore recommended to obtain a definitive diagnosis that can distinguish between the two [12].

Patients may be at risk of post-operative mechanical obstruction if they have pre-existing adhesions, or a history of previous abdominal surgeries [13].

Although post-operative ileus and BO can each be initially managed conservatively, prolonged or worsening BO ultimately requires surgery, if appropriate, to prevent complications (e.g. ischaemia, necrosis, perforation) [14].

An ileus can be confirmed radiologically with abdominal x-ray (AXR) or computed tomography (CT) scan [12].

An AXR would show dilated loops of bowel with multiple fluid levels indicating distension, with fluids and air in all of the small bowel and often much, or all, of the large bowel [15].

A CT scan confirming ileus would show multiple air-filled levels throughout the abdomen, an elevated diaphragm, dilatation of one or both the large and small intestine would be evident, and there would be no evidence of mechanical obstruction [12].

## CAUSES AND RISK FACTORS

There are several proposed mechanisms for the pathogenesis of postoperative ileus [16]:

- Electrolyte disturbance is one of the most common causes of all paralytic ileus, notably hypokalaemia, hypocalcaemia, and hypomagnesaemia, due to electrolytes' role in smooth muscle contractility.
- Increased adrenergic motor neuronal activity following a skin incision has an inhibitory effect on gut motility and precipitates the initial acute intestinal paralysis.
- An inflammatory response occurs three to four hours after surgery, causing the release of pro-inflammatory mediators that in turn can directly inhibit smooth muscle contractility.
- Direct handling of the gut increases the systemic inflammatory response.
- Fluid overload induces oedema and can cause intestinal oedema and stretch.
- Use of opioid analgesia decreases intestinal motility.

Several risk factors have been identified that may further increase a patient's risk of developing post-operative ileus [16]. These include increasing age, previous abdominal surgery, use of opioid medication, intraoperative blood loss [17], male sex, low pre-operative albumin, history of peripheral vascular disease or respiratory co-morbidities, and long duration of surgery [18]. Ileus is also deemed more likely following emergency surgery and after stoma formation, due to a higher exacerbation of the inflammatory stress response [18].

## MANAGEMENT

Post-operative ileus can have a profound impact on a patient's reported quality of life (QOL) [19]. It can increase the risk of developing aspiration pneumonia if patients aspirate due to vomiting or regurgitation of the accumulated enteric contents [20]. Patients diagnosed with post-operative ileus are placed nil by mouth (NBM) to reduce the risk of perforation; if this is prolonged it can result in nutritional deficits, put patients at high risk of malnutrition, and subsequently worsen their post-operative recovery [16].

Many strategies have been identified that may prevent post-operative ileus, and have been implemented into enhanced recovery after surgery (ERAS) protocols. Examples include the following [21]:

- Considering laparoscopic or robotic surgery over open procedures.
- Avoiding the use of opioid medications intra- and post-operatively.
- Avoiding nasogastric (NG) tubes intra- and post-operatively.
- Use of early oral nutrition.
- Use of early mobilisation.
- Use of prokinetics and laxatives.
- Use of chewing gum.
- Avoiding salt and water overload.
- Use of carbohydrate loading pre-operatively.

The use of early enteral nutrition (EEN) has also been reported to reduce incidence of post-operative ileus following major rectal surgery [22], and following uncomplicated but emergency intestinal surgery, provided that there are no contraindications to enteral feeding [23].

If a prolonged post-operative ileus occurs, management typically revolves around symptom control [20]. Fluid and electrolyte treatment is required to maintain hydration status and prevent electrolyte imbalance, and it is therefore important to have an accurate measurement of fluid input and output [20].

If the patient is without nutrition for five to seven days or deemed unlikely to restore nutritional intake for five to seven days, then parenteral nutrition (PN) should be considered [24, 25]. Decisions regarding initiation of PN should be taken on an individual basis following discussions with the multidisciplinary and nutrition support teams [26].

## BOWEL OBSTRUCTION

BO is a mechanical or functional blockage of the small and large intestines that restricts the normal passage of food, fluid, and faeces through the gastrointestinal tract. It can present as complete obstruction when the lumen of the gut is totally occluded or as partial or subacute obstruction [27].

### Causes and Incidence

Obstructions can be benign or malignant. They occur mostly in the small intestine, as well as the large bowel, sometimes in both [28], and are due to extrinsic, intrinsic, or intraluminal causes.

Benign obstruction occurs predominantly post-operatively secondary to adhesions. It can also occur in the presence of a volvulus, intussusception, hernia, intraluminal foreign body, extrinsic compression from an abscess, or as a result of radiation enteritis, flare-up of diverticulitis, endometriosis, or inflammatory bowel disease, such as Crohn's disease [29]. The incidence of benign obstruction is difficult to calculate due to the variability of causes; however, it has been reported that mechanical obstructions from adhesions can occur in 9% of patients who have undergone abdominal surgery [30] and 49.1% of admissions for small BO are related to adhesions from previous surgery [31].

Malignant BO is common in cancer patients [32]. It is most often diagnosed in ovarian and bowel primaries and can affect 20–50% and 10–28% of patients, respectively [33–36]. Patients can develop malignant obstruction from the primary tumour when the cancer infiltrates the intestinal wall and the degree of obstruction will depend on the staging of disease. In more serious cases it can result from metastatic spread of disease from the primary tumour following several lines of oncological treatment, usually to the peritoneum [37].

Peritoneal carcinomatosis takes place when tumour cells metastasise from the primary source of disease and infiltrate the serosa of the peritoneum (a thin layer of tissue that lines the abdomen and covers most of the abdominal organs). Hepatomegaly, lymphadenopathy, and nodal disease can also result in BO [27].

## Diagnosis

Diagnosis is made following AXR or CT scans. Water-soluble contrast is commonly used to determine if surgical intervention in acute adhesional BO admissions is necessary. It has been shown to reduce the need for surgery and lower length of hospital stay [38], as a result of a hyperosmolar effect that may relieve the obstruction by drawing fluid into the bowel.

Diagnosis is made in conjunction with clinical symptoms, which are varied and depend on the cause of the obstruction as well as whether it is a complete or partial blockage. Patients report abdominal pain, distension, nausea, vomiting, constipation, acid reflux, early satiety, and bloating after eating.

## Surgical Management

Mortality and morbidity rates are high in both small and large BO, particularly if it is left untreated [39]. In 2015–2016, 12 000 patients underwent major emergency surgery in the UK for small BO and 13% died within three months of their procedure [31].

Adhesional BO can resolve conservatively; however, guidance suggests that if non-operative management measures are unsuccessful after three to five days, laparoscopic adhesiolysis is safe and can reduce post-surgical length of stay and complications, compared to laparotomy [40].

There is limited evidence to support a standardised approach to the surgical management of malignant BO in advanced disease. Decision making is dependent on performance and nutritional status, prognosis, and extent of disease spread. Much of the published literature on malignant BO is limited to palliative surgical and medical management. This includes insertion of colonic stents, use of somatostatin analogues (to reduce gastrointestinal secretions), anti-emetics, intravenous hydration, as well as discussions around the validity of placing a venting gastrostomy to improve QOL [41-44]. A multidisciplinary approach is recommended and decisions regarding surgery should be taken on an individual case-by-case basis [34].

## Nutritional Management

BO can affect nutrient and fluid absorption to varying degrees, depending on the location of the blockage. Build-up of gas from the fermentation of food by intestinal bacteria proximal to the obstruction can result in serosal oedema and reduction in nutrient uptake [45].

Persistent vomiting leads to dehydration and weight loss, and if symptoms are prolonged and severe, strategies should be used to limit the risk of refeeding syndrome once patients are admitted and nutritional interventions introduced [24]. (See Chapter 7.) Symptom control should be a priority and NG tube insertion for drainage considered to alleviate vomiting [32].

When symptoms are severe, patients are often limited to sips of clear fluids or placed NBM, which has adverse impacts on nutritional status and may affect fitness for surgery or being able to proceed to palliative chemotherapy. In a national audit, 63% of cancer patients presenting with malignant BO and 34% of patients with adhesional BO were at medium or severe risk of malnutrition [31]. Nutritional status (defined by Nutritional Risk Index calculated using ideal body weight, current body weight, and admission albumin) has also been shown to adversely affect outcomes in BO surgery [31].

It is documented that malignant BO patients with a poorer performance status and cancer cachexia have worse outcomes and are less likely to be offered surgery [46] This supports the literature demonstrating that poorer nutritional status was shown to result in an inability to complete planned oncology treatment regimens and resulted in reduced overall survival [47, 48]. Furthermore, poor nutritional status is associated with impaired response to chemotherapy [49], reduced QOL [50], delays in treatment [51], chemotherapy toxicity [52], and treatment dose reductions [53].

Recommendations on the nutritional management of BO are based on low levels of evidence [25, 54, 55] and interventions are often dependent on local practice. Most BO surgery is carried out as an emergency procedure, and therefore pre-operative nutrition support is not always possible. Oral intake should be reintroduced as soon as possible postoperatively, with consideration given to adapting the type of food and fluids to each individual patient [25].

More attention has been given to studying PN as an alternative means of providing nutrition in BO, but it is not indicated if BO is intermittent or incomplete, gut function is maintained, and oral diet can be continued [54, 56]. Access to PN in the community in the UK is limited and there is evidence to suggest that it does not have a significant impact on overall survival or QOL [56–58]. A recent qualitative study looking at the QOL of patients and families receiving home PN reported a profound sense of loss at the inability to eat orally [59].

There has been limited attention given to patients at risk of benign or malignant BO who may be experiencing symptoms, but are not fully obstructed and are capable of tolerating some oral intake. Surgical intervention is not always appropriate and nutrition support is challenging. Appropriate nutrition assessment and advice needs to be provided to patients admitted with BO to ensure maintenance or improvement of nutritional status, to minimise delays in surgery and increased risk of complications post-operatively [31].

Although there is limited research regarding the role of nutrition in BO, there are studies in Crohn's disease, which can result in stricturing of the small and large intestines [60].

Research in Crohn's has shown that the most effective means of providing nutrition is exclusive EN with tube feeding for 12 weeks. This liquid diet has been shown to achieve remission in 81.4% of patients [61]. The research in this area has led to the development of guidelines, which also advise that a low-fibre diet should be followed [62].

To date there is no evidence to support the use of low-fibre diets in subacute benign or malignant BO; however, the guidelines for Crohn's disease can be applied to patients with stricturing in the gastrointestinal tract and have been shown anecdotally to reduce symptoms of obstruction and enable patients to increase their oral intake. If intake is impaired by symptoms and inability to meet nutritional requirements, oral nutritional supplements are indicated to prevent weight loss and improve nutritional status [25, 54].

Elemental 028 Extra Liquid* (Nutricia Clinical Care, Trowbridge, UK) is a nutritional supplement licensed for use in conditions causing severe impairment of the gastrointestinal tract and has been shown to maintain nutritional status in Crohn's disease [63]. An elemental diet (ED) has been successfully used and reported in the case of a pregnant woman with adhesional BO [64]. The patient was successfully managed and the use of ED allowed for conservative management, avoiding surgery, and resulting in a healthy delivery at full term. A prospective multicentre feasibility study (http://Clinicaltrials.gov, NCT03150992) examined the effects of ED in women with ovarian cancer treated conservatively for malignant BO. Of the cohort of 19 women, 68.4% tolerated the diet. There was a reduction in incidence of vomiting from 72% at baseline to 23.5% at week 2, and reduction in pain from 96% at baseline to 76% at the end of week 2.

Given the high rates of malnutrition in this patient group, early referral to a dietitian is recommended [24, 54]. Depending on the severity of symptoms, risk of recurrence of a blockage, and outcome of surgical intervention, diet advice will differ

**TABLE 20.1**   Royal Surrey four-step bowel obstruction diet.

| Step 1 | Clear fluids only |
| --- | --- |
| Step 2 | All thin liquids |
| Step 3 | Smooth or puréed foods only, low fibre, no bread products |
| Step 4 | Soft, sloppy foods, low fibre, no bread products |

from one patient to another. Some may be able to tolerate only liquids, while others can manage a puréed or soft diet. If stricturing from adhesions or malignancy is still present, a low-fibre diet is recommended to reduce bulking of stools and increased risk of faecal loading, constipation, and recurrence of symptoms of abdominal bloating, pain, and early satiety [65].

In the absence of clinical guidelines for diet and BO, the evidence established for Crohn's disease has been adapted to develop a structured four-step diet (Table 20.1). This novel approach provides advice that is dependent on the severity of symptoms and risk of obstruction. The four steps are all low fibre. Until patients' symptoms resolve and they are able to tolerate solid foods, they are limited to a liquid diet. Patients either increase the consistency of their food by proceeding to the next step if symptoms improve, or return to clear fluids if they remain or become symptomatic. Oral intake is supplemented where required with nutritional supplements. A feasibility study, BOUNCED, is in progress (ISTCRN 10518796) and a definitive multicentre trial is planned.

## AREAS FOR FUTURE RESEARCH

Research in paralytic ileus has focused primarily on prevention. More work is needed to establish how best to manage the nutritional needs of patients with prolonged post-operative ileus.

Further research is also necessary to establish high levels of evidence supporting nutritional intervention in both benign and malignant BO pre- and post-operatively. Current practice varies markedly and a consensus would be beneficial for patients,

and for medical and surgical teams with no access to specialist dietetic support. Robust clinical trials in parenteral, enteral, and oral diets could provide guidance to ensure that patients with complete and subacute BO are able to improve their nutritional status, and subsequently their QOL.

## REFERENCES

1. Venara, A., Neunlist, M., Slim, K. et al. (2016). Postoperative ileus: pathophysiology, incidence, and prevention. *J. Visc. Surg.* 153 (6): 439–446.
2. Summers, R.W. and Lu, C.C. (1999). Approach to the patient with ileus and obstruction. *Textbook Gastroenterol.* 1: 842–858.
3. Brigode, W.M., Jones, C., Vazquez, D.E., and Evans, D.C. (2015). Scrutinizing the evidence linking hypokalemia and ileus: a commentary on fact and dogma. *Int. J. Acad. Med.* 1 (1): 21.
4. Wintery, E.M., Syam, A.F., Simadibrata, M., and Manan, C.E.L. (2003). Management of paralytic ileus. *Indonesian J. Gastroenterol. Hepatol. Digest. Endoscopy* 4: 80–88.
5. Ebert, E. (2012). Gastrointestinal involvement in spinal cord injury: a clinical perspective. *J. Gastrointestin. Liver Dis.* 21 (1): 75–82.
6. Vather, R., Trivedi, S., and Bissett, I. (2013). Defining postoperative ileus: results of a systematic review and global survey. *J. Gastrointest. Surg.* 17 (5): 962–972.
7. Wilson, J. (1975). Postoperative motility of the large intestine in man. *Gut* 16 (9): 689–692.
8. Holte, K. and Kehlet, H. (2000). Postoperative ileus: a preventable event. *J. Br. Surg.* 87 (11): 1480–1493.
9. Livingston, E.H. and Passaro, E.P. (1990). Postoperative ileus. *Dig. Dis. Sci.* 35 (1): 121–132.
10. Wolthuis, A.M., Bislenghi, G., Lambrecht, M. et al. (2017). Preoperative risk factors for prolonged postoperative ileus after colorectal resection. *Int. J. Colorectal Dis.* 32 (6): 883–890.
11. Shah, D.R., Brown, E., Russo, J.E. et al. (2013). Negligible effect of perioperative epidural analgesia among patients undergoing elective gastric and pancreatic resections. *J. Gastrointest. Surg.* 17 (4): 660–667.
12. Frager, D.H., Baer, J.W., Rothpearl, A., and Bossart, P.A. (1995). Distinction between postoperative ileus and mechanical small-bowel obstruction: value of CT compared with clinical and other radiographic findings. *AJR Am. J. Roentgenol.* 164 (4): 891–894.

13. Garibay-González, F., Navarrete-Arellano, M., Moreno-Delgado, F. et al. (2018). Incidence of intestinal obstruction due to post-surgical adhesions in the central military hospital. Associated risk factors. *Rev. Sanid. Milit.* 71 (6): 534–544.

14. ten Broek, R.P.G., Krielen, P., Di Saverio, S. et al. (2018). Bologna guidelines for diagnosis and management of adhesive small bowel obstruction (ASBO): 2017 update of the evidence-based guidelines from the world society of emergency surgery ASBO working group. *World J. Emergency Surg.* 13 (1): 24.

15. James, B. and Kelly, B. (2013). The abdominal radiograph. *Ulster Med. J.* 82 (3): 179.

16. Bragg, D., El-Sharkawy, A.M., Psaltis, E. et al. (2015). Postoperative ileus: recent developments in pathophysiology and management. *Clin. Nutr.* 34 (3): 367–376.

17. Kronberg, U., Kiran, R.P., Soliman, M.S.M. et al. (2011). A characterization of factors determining postoperative ileus after laparoscopic colectomy enables the generation of a novel predictive score. *Ann. Surg.* 253 (1): 78–81.

18. Chapuis, P.H., Bokey, L., Keshava, A. et al. (2013). Risk factors for prolonged ileus after resection of colorectal cancer: an observational study of 2400 consecutive patients. *Ann. Surg.* 257 (5): 909–915.

19. Kehlet, H. and Holte, K. (2001). Review of postoperative ileus. *Am. J. Surg.* 182 (5): S3–S10.

20. Luckey, A., Livingston, E., and Taché, Y. (2003). Mechanisms and treatment of postoperative ileus. *Arch. Surg.* 138 (2): 206–214.

21. Adiamah, A. and Lobo, D.N. (2020). Postoperative Ileus: Prevention and treatment. In: *Enhanced Recovery after Surgery* (ed. O. Ljungqvist, N.K. Francis, and R.D. Urma), 249–257. New York: Springer.

22. Boelens, P.G., Heesakkers, F.F., Luyer, M.D. et al. (2014). Reduction of postoperative ileus by early enteral nutrition in patients undergoing major rectal surgery: prospective, randomized, controlled trial. *Ann. Surg.* 259 (4): 649–655.

23. Wang, H., Zhao, J., Wang, Y. et al. (2017). Early enteral nutrition reduced postoperative ileus and improved the outcomes in patients with emergency intestinal surgery: results from a propensity score analysis. *Int. J. Clin. Exp. Med.* 10 (4): 7040–7048.

24. National Collaborating Centre for Acute Care (2006). Nutrition support for adults: oral nutrition support, enteral tube feeding and parenteral nutrition. https://www.nice.org.uk/guidance/cg32/evidence/full-guideline-194889853. Accessed 7 May 2023.

25. Weimann, A., Braga, M., Carli, F. et al. (2021). ESPEN practical guideline: clinical nutrition in surgery. *Clin. Nutr.* 40: 4745–4761.

26. National Confidential Enquiry into Patient Outcome and Death (2010). Parenteral nutrition: a mixed bag. https://www.ncepod.org.uk/2010pn.html. Accessed 7 May 2023.

27. Cappell, M.S. and Batke, M. (2008). Mechanical obstruction of the small bowel and colon. *Med. Clin. North Am.* 92 (3): 575–597.

28. Ripamonti, C., Twycross, R., Baines, M. et al. (2001). Clinical-practice recommendations for the management of bowel obstruction in patients with end-stage cancer. *Support. Care Cancer* 9 (4): 223–233.

29. Jaffe, T. and Thompson, W.M. (2015). Large-bowel obstruction in the adult: classic radiographic and CT findings, etiology, and mimics. *Radiology* 275 (3): 651–663.

30. Ten Broek, R.P., Issa, Y., van Santbrink, E.J. et al. (2013). Burden of adhesions in abdominal and pelvic surgery: systematic review and met-analysis. *BMJ* 347: f5588.

31. Lee, M.J., Sayers, A.E., Drake, T.M. et al. (2019). Malnutrition, nutritional interventions and clinical outcomes of patients with acute small bowel obstruction: results from a national, multicentre, prospective audit. *BMJ Open* 9 (7): e029235.

32. Dolan, E.A. (2011). Malignant bowel obstruction: a review of current treatment strategies. *Am. J. Hosp. Palliat. Med.* 28 (8): 576–582.

33. Anthony, T., Baron, T., Mercadante, S. et al. (2007). Report of the clinical protocol committee: development of randomized trials for malignant bowel obstruction. *J. Pain Symptom Manage.* 34 (1): S49–S59.

34. Tuca, A., Guell, E., Martinez-Losada, E., and Codorniu, N. (2012). Malignant bowel obstruction in advanced cancer patients: epidemiology, management, and factors influencing spontaneous resolution. *Cancer Manage. Res.* 4: 159.

35. Ripamonti, C.I., Easson, A.M., and Gerdes, H. (2008). Management of malignant bowel obstruction. *Eur. J. Cancer* 44 (8): 1105–1115.

36. Mercadante, S., Casuccio, A., and Mangione, S. (2007). Medical treatment for inoperable malignant bowel obstruction: a qualitative systematic review. *J. Pain Symptom Manage.* 33 (2): 217–223.

37. Daniele, A., Ferrero, A., Fuso, L. et al. (2015). Palliative care in patients with ovarian cancer and bowel obstruction. *Support. Care Cancer* 23 (11): 3157–3163.

38. Long, S., Emigh, B., Wolf, J. Jr. et al. (2019). This too shall pass: standardized Gastrografin protocol for partial small bowel obstruction. *Am. J. Surg.* 217 (6): 1016–1018.

39. Scott, J.W., Olufajo, O.A., Brat, G.A. et al. (2016). Use of national burden to define operative emergency general surgery. *JAMA Surg.* 151 (6): e160480-e.

40. Pei, K.Y., Asuzu, D., and Davis, K.A. (2017). Will laparoscopic lysis of adhesions become the standard of care? Evaluating trends and outcomes in laparoscopic management of small-bowel obstruction using the American College of Surgeons National Surgical Quality Improvement Project Database. *Surg. Endosc.* 31 (5): 2180–2186.

41. Franke, A.J., Iqbal, A., Starr, J.S. et al. (2017). Management of malignant bowel obstruction associated with GI cancers. *J. Oncol. Pract.* 13 (7): 426–434.

42. Pinard, K.-A., Goring, T.N., Egan, B.C., and Koo, D.J. (2017). Drainage percutaneous endoscopic gastrostomy for malignant bowel obstruction in gastrointestinal cancers: prognosis and implications for timing of palliative intervention. *J. Palliat. Med.* 20 (7): 774–778.

43. Pothuri, B., Montemarano, M., Gerardi, M. et al. (2005). Percutaneous endoscopic gastrostomy tube placement in patients with malignant bowel obstruction due to ovarian carcinoma. *Gynecol. Oncol.* 96 (2): 330–334.

44. Young, C.J., De-Loyde, K.J., Young, J.M. et al. (2015). Improving quality of life for people with incurable large-bowel obstruction: randomized control trial of colonic stent insertion. *Diseases Colon Rectum* 58 (9): 838–849.

45. Reddy, S.R.R. and Cappell, M.S. (2017). A systematic review of the clinical presentation, diagnosis, and treatment of small bowel obstruction. *Curr. Gastroenterol. Rep.* 19 (6): 28.

46. Hamaker, M.E., Oosterlaan, F., van Huis, L.H. et al. (2021). Nutritional status and interventions for patients with cancer – a systematic review. *J. Geriatric Oncol.* 12 (1): 6–21.

47. Lin, J., Peng, J., Qdaisat, A. et al. (2016). Severe weight loss during preoperative chemoradiotherapy compromises survival outcome for patients with locally advanced rectal cancer. *J. Cancer Res. Clin. Oncol.* 142 (12): 2551–2560.

48. Dewys, W.D., Begg, C., Lavin, P.T. et al. (1980). Prognostic effect of weight loss prior tochemotherapy in cancer patients. *Am. J. Med.* 69 (4): 491–497.

49. Andreyev, H., Norman, A., Oates, J., and Cunningham, D. (1998). Why do patients with weight loss have a worse outcome when undergoing chemotherapy for gastrointestinal malignancies? *Eur. J. Cancer* 34 (4): 503–509.

50. Norman, K., Pichard, C., Lochs, H., and Pirlich, M. (2008). Prognostic impact of disease-related malnutrition. *Clin. Nutr.* 27 (1): 5–15.

51. Arrieta, O., De la Torre-Vallejo, M., López-Macías, D. et al. (2015). Nutritional status, body surface, and low lean body mass/body mass index are related to dose reduction and severe gastrointestinal toxicity induced by afatinib in patients with non-small cell lung cancer. *Oncologist* 20 (8): 967.

52. Klute, K.A., Brouwer, J., Jhawer, M. et al. (2016). Chemotherapy dose intensity predicted by baseline nutrition assessment in gastrointestinal malignancies: a multicentre analysis. *Eur. J. Cancer* 63: 189–200.

53. Bozzetti, F., Arends, J., Lundholm, K. et al. (2009). ESPEN guidelines on parenteral nutrition: non-surgical oncology. *Clin. Nutr.* 28 (4): 445–454.

54. Arends, J., Bachmann, P., Baracos, V. et al. (2017). ESPEN guidelines on nutrition in cancer care. *Clin. Nutr.* 36 (1): 11–48.

55. Pironi, L., Arends, J., Baxter, J. et al. (2015). ESPEN endorsed recommendations. Definition and classification of intestinal failure in adults. *Clin. Nutr.* 34 (2): 171–180.

56. Naghibi, M., Smith, T., and Elia, M. (2015). A systematic review with meta-analysis of survival, quality of life and cost-effectiveness of home parenteral nutrition in patients with inoperable malignant bowel obstruction. *Clin. Nutr.* 34 (5): 825–837.

57. Sowerbutts, A.M., Lal, S., Sremanakova, J. et al. (2019). Palliative home parenteral nutrition in patients with ovarian cancer and malignant bowel obstruction: experiences of women and family caregivers. *BMC Palliat. Care* 18 (1): 1–10.

58. Sowerbutts, A.M., Jones, D., Lal, S., and Burden, S. (2021). Quality of life in patients and in family members of those receiving home parenteral support with intestinal failure: a systematic review. *Clin. Nutr.* 40 (5): 3210–3220.

59. Sowerbutts, A.M., Lal, S., Sremanakova, J. et al. (2020). Dealing with loss: food and eating in women with ovarian cancer on parenteral nutrition. *J. Hum. Nutr. Diet.* 33 (4): 550–556.

60. Gajendran, M., Loganathan, P., Catinella, A.P., and Hashash, J.G. (2018). A comprehensive review and update on Crohn's disease. *Dis. Mon.* 64 (2): 20–57.

61. Hu, D., Ren, J., Wang, G. et al. (2014). Exclusive enteral nutritional therapy can relieve inflammatory bowel stricture in Crohn's disease. *J. Clin. Gastroenterol.* 48 (9): 790–795.

62. Lee, J., Allen, R., Ashley, S. et al. (2014). British Dietetic Association evidence-based guidelines for the dietary management of Crohn's disease in adults. *J. Hum. Nutr. Diet.* 27 (3): 207–218.

63. Zoli, G., Care, M., Parazza, M. et al. (1997). A randomized controlled study comparing elemental diet and steroid treatment in Crohn's disease. *Aliment. Pharmacol. Ther.* 11 (4): 735–740.

64. Phillips, M., Curtis, P., and Karanjia, N. (2004). An elemental diet for bowel obstruction in pregnancy: a case study. *J. Hum. Nutr. Diet.* 17 (6): 543–545.

65. Andreyev, H.J.N., Davidson, S.E., Gillespie, C. et al. (2012). Practice guidance on the management of acute and chronic gastrointestinal problems arising as a result of treatment for cancer. *Gut* 61 (2): 179–192.

# CHAPTER 21

# Intestinal Failure and Rehabilitation

Alison Culkin

*Department of Nutrition and Dietetics, St Mark's Hospital, London Northwest Healthcare University Trust, London, UK*

---

**KEY POINTS**

- Patients with intestinal failure require parenteral nutrition.
- Determining anatomy will direct appropriate nutrition support.
- The detection and management of sepsis are crucial.
- Fluid and electrolyte requirements need to include losses from the gastrointestinal tract.
- Close monitoring is required to detect complications.

---

Intestinal failure (IF) is defined as the reduction of gastrointestinal (GI) function below the minimum necessary for the absorption of macronutrients and/or water and electrolytes, such that parenteral supplementation is required to maintain health and/or growth. Surgery and surgical complications are a common cause of IF [1].

The European Society of Parenteral and Enteral Nutrition (ESPEN) has classified IF into three types.

Type 1 is acute, short term, and usually self-limiting, occurring post-operatively and resulting in ileus and/or obstruction. Patients may require a period of parenteral nutrition (PN) until GI function returns. Post-operative ileus and management of bowel obstruction are discussed in Chapter 20.

Type 2 is a prolonged acute condition, often in metabolically unstable patients, requiring complex multidisciplinary care and PN over months. Type 2 can occur after massive bowel resection due to mesenteric ischaemia or volvulus, causing a short bowel with a high-output stoma. Complications from abdominal surgery can result in the development of fistulae that act like short bowel with high GI losses.

Type 2 can develop into type 3 and become a chronic condition requiring PN over years. Some patients with type 2, including those with short bowel/fistula, may be unsuitable for restorative surgery due to comorbidities or inability to undergo an anaesthetic and/or prolonged complex surgery. Some patients with benign disease, including Crohn's and

*Nutritional Management of the Surgical Patient*, First Edition. Edited by Mary E. Phillips.
© 2023 John Wiley & Sons Ltd. Published 2023 by John Wiley & Sons Ltd.

radiation enteritis, have extensive adhesions or strictures, and those with malignancy resulting in obstruction may require lifelong PN (Chapter 20). This obstruction may be reversible or irreversible.

It is not known how many patients require PN in hospital due to surgical complications. UK data exists on the number of patients requiring home parenteral nutrition (HPN). Surgical complications were responsible for 28% of patients requiring HPN. The most common indications for HPN were short bowel (34%), intestinal obstruction (18.8%), malabsorption (16%), and fistula (10.5%). Crohn's disease was the principal diagnosis, accounting for 20% of patients. The UK has seen an increase in patients requiring HPN due to malignancy, with ovarian cancer the most common underlying condition causing obstruction [2].

## MANAGEMENT

ESPEN has produced several guidelines on the management of IF. The prevention and treatment of types 1 and 2 (also known as acute IF) emphasise the detection and management of sepsis, as this is the most common cause of death. Other key aspects include fluid and electrolyte resuscitation, optimisation of nutritional status, wound care, appropriate surgery, and active rehabilitation [3].

### Sepsis

It is easy for sepsis to go unrecognised in a malnourished surgical patient, as they are unable to mount an effective immune response. Patients may not demonstrate the usual signs of infection, such as pyrexia or an increase in C-reactive protein concentration. Therefore, healthcare professionals need to be vigilant and monitor for subtle signs of sepsis, including tachycardia, fatigue, oedema, and jaundice. Biochemical and haematological indicators of uncontrolled sepsis include low haemoglobin, plasma albumin, and transferrin concentration. Abnormal liver function tests (LFTs) are very common and often relate to ongoing unrecognised sepsis [4].

The catheter used to deliver PN may also be a source of infection. The British Intestinal Failure

Alliance (BIFA) has produced UK guidelines on the detection and management of catheter-related bloodstream infections (CRBSI) [5]. This is a crucial aspect of IF care, as the safe and effective provision of PN is paramount to improving nutritional status.

A full septic screen is required if sepsis is suspected. Treatment includes radiological and/or surgical drainage of collections and abscesses, targeted antibiotic/antifungal treatment, fluid and electrolyte resuscitation, and maintenance of acid–base balance, followed by the instigation of nutrition support. It is not possible for patients to improve their nutritional status in the presence of ongoing sepsis and the temptation to overfeed patients must be resisted.

### Nutrition Assessment

Malnutrition is common in IF. The cause is multifactorial and can be due to infection, inflammation, GI losses of fluid/electrolytes, inability to tolerate enteral nutrition (EN), anatomical changes, lack of absorptive surface, and/or limited vascular access (due to complications) impeding the ability to infuse PN.

These circumstances may result in malnutrition, with the consequences of impaired wound healing, infections, increased morbidity, and mortality. Dehydration or oedema is common and must be addressed prior to optimising nutritional status. All patients should be individually assessed by healthcare professionals experienced in nutritional support.

A comprehensive nutritional assessment is required at baseline and should be repeated at regular intervals, as patients can rapidly become dehydrated and malnourished. Nutritional screening and assessment are discussed in Chapter 2.

In patients with IF, sudden weight changes reflect fluid balance and therefore the measurement of body composition is helpful to monitor changes in fat-free mass. Repeating anthropometric measurements (e.g. mid-arm muscle circumference, bioimpedance analysis) monthly helps identify if nutrition support is improving nutritional status rather than just contributing to gains in fat mass. A study comparing the Global Leadership Initiative on Malnutrition (GLIM) criteria with the ESPEN malnutrition diagnosis found an incidence of 93.4% versus 80.9%, respectively. The higher incidence was due to differences in fat-free mass index [6]. The prevalence of sarcopenia in patients ranges from 88% using bioimpedance to 84% using computed tomography (CT) [7, 8]. Therefore, reliance on weight and body mass index (BMI) is inadequate.

Handgrip strength measurement should be repeated regularly to detect changes in functional capacity so that amendments to nutrition support and rehabilitation can be initiated. Mobility should be encouraged at all stages of the patient's journey to promote muscle mass and function.

## Nutrition Support

The nutritional management of IF is an active process involving transitions between PN, EN, and oral nutrition. The most important aspect is that patients receive their estimated requirements via the most appropriate route.

Immediately post-operatively patients will require PN due to high GI losses from a stoma/fistula or diarrhoea. Many patients will need intensive care support until they are stable enough to be cared

for on a surgical ward (Chapter 8). Patients will experience difficulties with fluid, electrolyte, and acid–base balance post-operatively unless managed appropriately [9]. Nutritional requirements will be increased due to surgery, sepsis, malabsorption, and high GI losses.

There is limited evidence to support recommendations on nutritional requirements in IF [1]. The use of indirect calorimetry remains the most accurate measure of resting energy expenditure and should be used if available. The Parenteral and Enteral Nutrition specialist Group (PENG) of the British Dietetic Association recently completed a systematic review of requirements. Energy requirements during sepsis were found to be 26–30 kcal/kg and after GI surgery ranged from 22 to 28 kcal/kg, but studies were not conducted in patients with IF [10]. Other guidelines recommend 25–35 kcal/kg and 1.5–2.5 g/kg of protein in those with an enterocutaneous fistula (ECF) [1, 10, 11]. Evidence to support these recommendations was not based on trial data and therefore ongoing monitoring of response to nutrition support is essential (Table 21.1).

**TABLE 21.1**  Clinical monitoring requirements of patients with intestinal failure.

| Parameter | Frequency | Rationale | Consequence |
|---|---|---|---|
| Anthropometry | Monthly | Assess body composition | Loss of muscle mass unrecognised |
| Weight | Daily | Monitor hydration | Risk of overload and dehydration |
| Capillary blood glucose | Every 6 h until stable | Risk of hypo- and hyperglycaemia | ↑ Risk of infection and dehydration |
| Urinalysis | Daily | Ketones, glucose | Refeeding risk, glycosuria |
| Urine sodium | Weekly | Assess hydration | Risk of dehydration |
| Fluid balance | Hourly/daily | Monitor hydration | Risk of dehydration and overload |
| Temperature | Every 4–6 h | Sign of infection | Infection unrecognised |
| Clinical condition | Daily | Requirements | Under- and overfeeding |
| Assessment of catheter | Daily | Risk of infection/ displacement | Interruption in parenteral nutrition (PN) delivery |
| Food chart/enteral nutrition regimen | Daily | Assess oral/enteral intake | Delayed transition to oral diet |
| Handgrip | Weekly | Functional capacity | Effect of PN unknown |
| Medications | Daily | Effects and side effects | Gastrointestinal (GI) side effects, e.g. ↑GI losses, nausea, taste changes, electrolyte disturbances, ↑liver function tests |

## Fluid and Electrolytes

Guidelines on the requirements for fluid and electrolytes are based on clinical expertise as no trial data exists. Fluids should be prescribed to cover baseline requirements plus losses from the GI tract (Table 21.2) to maintain a urine output of at least 1 ml/kg/h (or 25 ml/kg/d) [3]. Urea and creatinine may be low in patients with reduced muscle mass and therefore biochemical dehydration can be easy to miss. Any trends should be noted, especially when results remain within the normal range. A random urine sodium concentration of <20 mmol/l is a useful early warning that patients are becoming sodium deplete and dehydrated. An important aspect of managing IF is that the losses from the GI tract are accounted for when prescribing PN. An assessment of the composition of GI losses is required and the composition of body secretions is shown in Figure 21.1 [12].

## Parenteral Nutrition

PN is required for all patients, but the length of treatment will depend on the type of IF. In types 2 and 3 it is usual practice for patients to receive a

**TABLE 21.2** Recommendations on fluid and electrolyte requirements for patients requiring intravenous support from European Society of Parenteral and Enteral Nutrition (ESPEN) and National Institute for Health and Care Excellence (NICE).

|  | ESPEN [1] | UK [10] |
|---|---|---|
| Fluid (ml/kg) | 25–35 | 25–30 |
| Sodium (mmol/kg) | 1–1.5 | 1 |
| Chloride (mmol/kg) | 1–1.5 | 1 |
| Potassium (mmol/kg) | 1–1.5 | 1 |
| Calcium (mmol/kg) | 0.1–0.15 | 0.1–0.15[a] |
| Magnesium (mmol/kg) | 0.1–0.15 | 0.1–0.2[a] |
| Phosphate (mmol/kg) | 0.3–0.5 | 0.5–0.7 or 10/1000 kcal[a] |

[a] Adapted from [12].

combination of PN and EN to meet requirements. PN is a lifesaving treatment, but is associated with fatal complications if not managed well. There is growing interest in whether the provision of different types of lipid emulsions can influence clinical outcomes. Concerns regarding high omega-6 content due to its pro-inflammatory effects have led to the development of omega-3–containing emulsions including fish oils. A systematic review and meta-analysis of 49 randomised control trials comparing omega-3–enriched PN with standard PN found a reduction in infection, sepsis, length of intensive care unit (ICU) and hospital stay, but no difference in mortality [13]. Ongoing monitoring is essential to minimise the risks associated with PN (Table 21.1).

## Enteral Nutrition

EN can be instigated early in those with IF as it promotes intestinal adaptation. The success depends on the quantity and quality of the remaining bowel after surgery. EN may have limited application in patients with severe mucosal disease, obstruction, or those with <100 cm of small bowel, as previous studies have shown dependence on parenteral support [14]. A study of EN in patients with short bowel demonstrated that the provision of 1000 kcal from a polymeric fibre-free formula significantly increased absorption of energy, protein, and fat without increasing intestinal losses [15]. The study was short term and it is not known whether patients were able to be weaned off parenteral support permanently. The sodium content of available EN is below the recommended 90 mmol/l to optimise sodium and fluid absorption in the jejunum. The addition of 10 ml of 30% sodium chloride can help maximise absorption by reaching the optimum sodium concentration [16].

Initiating EN in a patient with an ECF can be a challenge. It is crucial that EN is not feeding an abdominal cavity, as this will lead to ongoing intra-abdominal sepsis [17]. In fistulas arising from the proximal small bowel, EN is likely to exacerbate GI losses and distal EN may be a more appropriate strategy. Distal EN includes feeding through a distal limb of an ECF (fistuloclysis) or through a

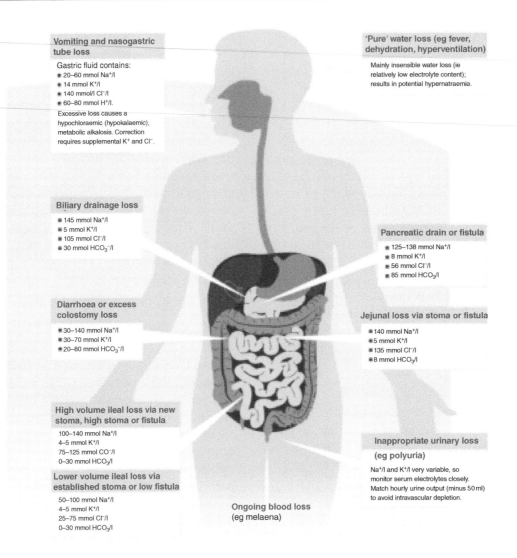

**Vomiting and nasogastric tube loss**

Gastric fluid contains:
- 20–60 mmol Na$^+$/l
- 14 mmol K$^+$/l
- 140 mmol/l Cl$^-$/l
- 60–80 mmol H$^+$/l.

Excessive loss causes a hypochloraemic (hypokalaemic), metabolic alkalosis. Correction requires supplemental K$^+$ and Cl$^-$.

**'Pure' water loss (eg fever, dehydration, hyperventilation)**

Mainly insensible water loss (ie relatively low electrolyte content); results in potential hypernatraemia.

**Biliary drainage loss**
- 145 mmol Na$^+$/l
- 5 mmol K$^+$/l
- 105 mmol Cl$^-$/l
- 30 mmol HCO$_3$$^-$/l

**Pancreatic drain or fistula**
- 125–138 mmol Na$^+$/l
- 8 mmol K$^+$/l
- 56 mmol Cl$^-$/l
- 85 mmol HCO$_3$/l

**Diarrhoea or excess colostomy loss**
- 30–140 mmol Na$^+$/l
- 30–70 mmol K$^+$/l
- 20–80 mmol HCO$_3$$^-$/l

**Jejunal loss via stoma or fistula**
- 140 mmol Na$^+$/l
- 5 mmol K$^+$/l
- 135 mmol Cl$^-$/l
- 8 mmol HCO$_3$/l

**High volume ileal loss via new stoma, high stoma or fistula**
- 100–140 mmol Na$^+$/l
- 4–5 mmol K$^+$/l
- 75–125 mmol CO$^-$/l
- 0–30 mmol HCO$_3$/l

**Inappropriate urinary loss**

**(eg polyuria)**

Na$^+$/l and K$^+$/l very variable, so monitor serum electrolytes closely. Match hourly urine output (minus 50 ml) to avoid intravascular depletion.

**Lower volume ileal loss via established stoma or low fistula**
- 50–100 mmol Na$^+$/l
- 4–5 mmol K$^+$/l
- 25–75 mmol Cl$^-$/l
- 0–30 mmol HCO$_3$/l

**Ongoing blood loss (eg melaena)**

**FIGURE 21.1**   Diagram of ongoing losses. *Source*: Reprinted with permission © NICE [2013]. Intravenous fluid therapy in adults. Available from www.nice.org.uk/Guidance/CG174. All rights reserved. Subject to Notice of rights.

defunctioned distal small bowel stoma/mucus fistula (enteroclysis). Feeding may be complete, where the aim is to administer all nutrition and hydration (+/− chyme), or trophic, where EN is provided to maintain bowel structure and function before reconstructive surgery. Polymeric, semi-elemental, and elemental formulae have all been described in the literature. A systematic review demonstrated effective weaning from PN, and improvements in post-operative ileus, renal, and liver function [18].

## Oral Nutrition

The dietary management of short bowel and that of ECF are similar once an established fistula tract has formed and oral nutrition is safe to administer. The decision to allow patients with a fistula oral nutrition is lacking evidence. There are no prospective studies comparing oral/EN verses PN post fistula formation [11]. A European survey found disparity in practice regarding the management of

ECF, with 50% of units not having a policy on when to allow oral nutrition [19].

Spontaneous fistula closure occurs in about 30% of patients, with 90–95% resolving within four to five weeks. After this time, patients are likely to need surgery. There are situations where recommending the patient remains nil by mouth (NBM) may aid in spontaneous closure (during the acute phase, or if the fistula is very proximal or high output). In all other cases the patient should be allowed to introduce oral nutrition and be encouraged to follow the short bowel regimen [3].

All patients with short bowel require a high-energy, high-protein diet to compensate for the malabsorption experienced due to high GI losses. Patients with a jejunostomy or ECF arising within the small bowel benefit from a high-fat, low-fibre diet. This contrasts with patients with a jejuno-colonic anastomosis, who are recommended a high-carbohydrate, low-fat diet, as the colon can readily absorb carbohydrate. After restorative surgery, patients may require a low-fibre diet until adaptation in the colon has occurred, especially if distal feeding was not possible [16]. Over months patients can increase fibre intake while monitoring bowel function (Table 21.3).

**TABLE 21.3**   Dietary management of short bowel intestinal failure.

| | Jejunostomy/entero-cutaneous fistula | Jejuno-colonic anastomosis |
|---|---|---|
| Energy | High | High |
| Protein | High | High |
| Fat | High | Low to moderate (↑medium-chain triglycerides) |
| Carbohydrate (complex) | High | High |
| Lactose | No restriction | No restriction |
| Salt | High | Moderate |
| Oral fluid restriction | 1 l restriction + oral rehydration solution | Not required long term |
| Oxalate | No restriction | Low |

## Anatomy

It is imperative that the anatomy of the bowel is identified to focus treatment and aid in decision making regarding nutrition support. Short bowel is when <200 cm of small bowel remains, but the requirement for parenteral support usually occurs when <100 cm remains. The exact location within the GI tract of an ECF is important to determine if PN will be required long term (<100 cm proximally) or if the patient has adequate functioning bowel to wean from PN. The underling disease should be managed (i.e. Crohn's disease), as the presence of strictures or obstruction will limit the success of oral nutrition.

## Surgical Management

Surgery should be planned and occur at least 100 days after the initial insult, or not before six months in a patient with an open abdomen or ECF. This is to allow the patient to recover and rehabilitate before undergoing restorative surgery [17].

## Prehabilitation

Patients with types 2 and 3 should be considered for a period of prehabilitation prior to restorative surgery. Patients with type 3 who may be candidates for bowel-lengthening procedures or intestinal transplant will benefit from prehabilitation to ensure they are optimised for surgery. Prehabilitation is discussed in Chapter 4.

## LONG-TERM NUTRITIONAL CONSEQUENCES

### Renal Issues

Prolonged dehydration due to high GI losses can result in acute kidney injury (AKI) and chronic kidney disease. Ongoing education to manage a high-output stoma/fistula is essential [9]. Renal stones occur in 25% of patients with a jejuno-colic anastomosis due to increased absorption of oxalate in the colon. Treatment includes a low-oxalate, low-fat, high-calcium diet, and the prevention of dehydration [17] (Table 21.3).

## Intestinal Failure–Associated Liver Disease

Abnormal LFTs are common, especially during episodes of sepsis. The cause is multifactorial and a study by Baker and Nightingale [20] found that 34% of patients already had pre-existing raised LFTs before PN was started, with the presence of sepsis a significant contributing factor. Other causes include hepatotoxic medications, lack of EN, and the underlying disease, including liver and biliary disease (e.g. hepatitis, gallstones). Treatment should focus on the identification and aggressive management of sepsis. It is paramount that patients are not overfed, as excess glucose and lipid can contribute to intestinal failure–associated liver disease. ESPEN recommends limiting soybean oil–based lipid to <1 g/kg/d [21]. A five-year follow-up study of type 3 patients on HPN demonstrated that the provision of a lipid emulsion containing fish oil resulted in reduced bilirubin compared to other lipids not containing fish oil [22].

## Micronutrient Deficiencies

Micronutrient deficiencies used to be common due to increased requirements, high GI losses, and inadequate provision. The importance of ongoing monitoring to ensure deficiencies are identified and treated appropriately depending on anatomy is a vital aspect of care. A micronutrient screen should be undertaken once C-reactive protein (CRP) is <20 mg/l to avoid the influence of the systemic inflammatory response on concentration [23] (see Chapter 22). Patients on PN should receive a daily intravenous (IV) micronutrient supplement to prevent deficiencies. Patients weaning from PN or on EN/oral diet are at risk of deficiencies and need frequent monitoring [24]. All patients after terminal ileum resection should receive intramuscular (IM) vitamin B12 every three months unless on PN.

## AREAS FOR FUTURE RESEARCH

- What is the best method to assess body composition in IF?
- What are the energy and protein requirements for patients with IF?
- What route of nutrition is optimal for patients with an ECF?
- What is the optimal enteral nutrition for distal feeding/fistuloclysis?
- What is the best lipid emulsion for short- and long-term PN?

Patients with IF should be looked after by experienced healthcare professionals as part of a multidisciplinary team, since management is complex.

| Case Study | |
|---|---|
| Patient transferred to St Mark's Intestinal Rehabilitation Unit. Handover states patient unable to gain weight despite increasing energy provision from PN. Ongoing abnormal LFTs. | |
| **Patient** | **Mrs F, age 67 yr** |
| Presenting complaint | Road traffic collision. Laparotomy for small bowel and mid-ileal injury: small bowel resection with subsequent ECF formation 6 weeks ago. AKI requiring haemofiltration on ICU. High-output fistula >3 l/d despite NBM and anti-secretory and anti-motility drugs. Omeprazole 40 mg twice a day. Loperamide 8 mg qds. Codeine 30 mg qds. PN via peripherally inserted central catheter (PICC) |

| | |
|---|---|
| Past medical history | Depression and headaches |
| Social history | Lives with her son |
| Investigations | Sepsis surveillance:<br>CRBSI: *Staphylococcus epidermidis* (central, peripheral, exit site, and tip) and *Staphylococcus aureus* (central)<br>*Coliform* and *Staphylococcus aureus* urinary tract infection<br>Mapping/imaging:<br>CT abdo and pelvis: increasing calibre of common bile duct compared to previous CT, suggesting biliary obstruction. 60 cm from duodenojejunal flexure to ECF and 40 cm of ileum with no obstruction in colon.<br>Magnetic resonance imaging (MRI) spine lumbar and sacral and pelvis: osteomyelitis |
| Anthropometrics | Height 1.78 m, weight 56 kg, BMI = 17.7 kg/m$^2$<br>Usual weight 70 kg 3–6 months ago, 20% weight loss<br>Mid-arm circumference 5th centile<br>Triceps skinfold thickness <5th centile<br>Mid-arm muscle circumference <5th centile |
| Biochemistry | White cell count (WCC) 9.8, sodium 140, potassium 3.8, urea 3.7, creatinine 35, CRP 16.1↑, bilirubin 4, alkaline phosphatase 700↑, alanine transaminase 169↑, albumin 28↓, corrected calcium 2.60, magnesium 0.6↓, phosphate 1.41, urine sodium <20<br>Dehydrated with normal urea and creatinine due to low muscle mass<br>Ongoing inflammatory response. Patient unable to mount normal response due to malnutrition<br>Vitamin D 18↓, vitamin A 0.55↓, selenium 0.45↓<br>All other micronutrients normal |
| Clinical | Fluid balance:<br>Urine output 800 ml, fistula output 3 l = negative fluid balance<br>National Early Warning Score (NEWS) score 2 (low blood pressure, tachycardic) |
| Diet | Oral: NBM<br>Current PN: 2200 kcal, 15 g nitrogen, 715 kcal lipid (soybean), 2500 ml over 24 h |
| Environmental | Low mood |
| Functional | Handgrip 16 kg (poor functional capacity) |
| Diagnosis | Short bowel–associated IF due to post-surgical ECF formation. CRBSI, urinary tract infection, and osteomyelitis |
| Medical plan | IV antibiotics for CRBSI. PICC removed<br>Plan for central venous catheter placement for HPN and IV antibiotics for osteomyelitis<br>Change omeprazole to IV pantoprazole 40 mg twice a day<br>Increase loperamide to 16 mg qds<br>Increase codeine 60 mg qds<br>Psychological support |
| Nutrition plan | Re-establish PN and start fistuloclysis |
| Surgical plan | Bowel mapping and fistula repair in 6 months |

| | | | |
|---|---|---|---|
| Nutrition support | Oral: Start short bowel protocol (high energy, protein, fat, low fibre) | | |
| | Oral fluid: 1 l oral rehydration solution (St Mark's solution), 1 l all other fluids | | |
| | Requirements: Current weight 56 kg, but as dehydrated likely actual weight 60 kg to be used for estimating requirements. Sepsis treated with IV antibiotics. Aim to meet requirements with combination of oral, EN, and PN | | |
| | Parenteral nutrition | | |

| | Requirement | Requirement | PN prescription |
|---|---|---|---|
| Energy | 20–25 kcal/kg + physical activity level (PAL) 1.2 | 1440–1800 | 1775 kcal |
| Protein | 1.5 g/kg | 90 g = 14 g nitrogen | 11 g |
| Fluid | 25–30 ml/kg + losses | 1.5–1.8 + 3 l = 4.5–4.8 | 3 l |
| Sodium | 1 mmol/kg + losses | 60 + 300 = 360 | 300 mmol |
| Potassium | 1 mmol/kg + losses | 60 + 15 = 75 | 60 mmol |
| Calcium | 0.1–0.15 mmol/kg | 6–9 | 6 mmol |
| Magnesium | 0.1–0.2 mmol/kg | 6–12 | 12 mmol |
| Phosphate | 0.5–0.7 mmol/kg or 10/1000 kcal | 30–42 14–18 | 20 mmol |

| | |
|---|---|
| | Aim to gradually increase rate of PN over 12 h for overnight HPN |
| | Fistuloclysis: 1.5 kcal/ml semi-elemental 100 ml twice a day via balloon gastrostomy placed distal to ECF (300 kcal and 12 g protein) |
| | Micronutrients: Vitamin D 300 000 IU IM, Vitamin A 10 000 IU IM, Selenium 500 µmol 3/7 IV |
| Outcome | Discharged on HPN and fistuloclysis. Once sepsis and dehydration treated, ECF output reduced, patient improved nutritional status, and LFTs normalised. Fistuloclysis resulted in daily bowel movement |
| Follow-up | Review in intestinal rehabilitation clinic Ongoing sepsis surveillance Recheck micronutrients to ensure supplementation successful Repeat body composition and handgrip to monitor fat-free mass, functional capacity, and fitness for surgery |

# REFERENCES

1. Pironi, L., Arends, J., Bozzetti, F. et al. (2016). Home Artificial Nutrition & Chronic Intestinal Failure Special Interest Group of ESPEN. ESPEN guidelines on chronic intestinal failure in adults. *Clin. Nutr.* 35: 247–307.

2. Smith, T. and Naghibi, M. (2016). BANS report 2016: artificial nutrition support in the UK 2005-2015. Adult home parenteral nutrition and home intravenous fluids. https://www.bapen.org.uk/images/pdfs/reports/bans-report-2016.pdf. Accessed 23 March 2023.

3. Klek, S., Forbes, A., Gabe, S. et al. (2016). Management of acute intestinal failure: a position paper from the European Society for Clinical Nutrition and Metabolism (ESPEN) Special Interest Group. *Clin. Nutr.* 35: 1209–1218.

4. Gabe, S.M. and Culkin, A. (2010). Abnormal liver function tests in the parenteral nutrition fed patient. *Frontline Gastroenterol.* 1: 98–104.

5. Bond, A., Chadwick, P., Smith, T.R. et al. (2020). Diagnosis and management of catheter-related bloodstream infections in patients on home parenteral nutrition. *Frontline Gastroenterol.* 11: 48–54.

6. Liu, H., Gao, X., Zhang, L. et al. (2022). Application of the GLIM criteria in patients with intestinal insufficiency and intestinal failure at nutritional risk on admission. *Eur. J. Clin. Nutr.* 76 (7): 1003–1009.

7. Kopczynska, M., Barrett, M.P., Cloutier, A. et al. (2022). Body composition in patients with type 2 intestinal failure. *Nutr. Clin. Pract.* 37: 137–145.

8. Oke, S.M., Rye, B., Malietzis, G. et al. (2020). Survival and CT defined sarcopenia in patients with intestinal failure on home parenteral support. *Clin. Nutr.* 39: 829–836.

9. Nightingale, J.M.D. (2022). How to manage a high-output stoma. *Frontline Gastroenterol.* 13: 140–151.

10. Cope, J., Culkin, A., Judges, D. et al. (2018). Adult requirements. In: *A Pocket Guide to Clinical Nutrition* (ed. V. Todorovik and B. Mafrici). Birmingham: British Dietetic Association.

11. Kumpf, V.J., de Aguilar-Nascimento, J.E., Diaz-Pizarro Graf, J.I. et al. (2017). American Society for Parenteral and Enteral Nutrition. ASPEN-FELANPE clinical guidelines. *J. Parenter. Enteral Nutr.* 41: 104–112.

12. National Institute for Health and Care Excellence, NICE. (2013). Intravenous fluid therapy in adults in hospital. Clinical guideline [CG174]. www.nice.org.uk/guidance/cg174. Accessed 23 March 2023.

13. Pradelli, L., Mayer, K., Klek, S. et al. (2020). ω-3 Fatty-acid enriched parenteral nutrition in hospitalized patients: systematic review with meta-analysis and trial sequential analysis. *J. Parenter. Enteral Nutr.* 44: 44–57.

14. Nightingale, J.M., Lennard-Jones, J.E., Gertner, D.J. et al. (1992). Colonic preservation reduces need for parenteral therapy, increases incidence of renal stones, but does not change high prevalence of gall stones in patients with a short bowel. *Gut* 33: 1493–1497.

15. Joly, F., Dray, X., Corcos, O. et al. (2009). Tube feeding improves intestinal absorption in short bowel syndrome patients. *Gastroenterologia* 136: 824–831.

16. Culkin, A. (2014). Intestinal failure and nutrition. In: *Advanced Nutrition and Dietetics in Gastroenterology* (ed. M. Lomer), 210–217. Chichester: Wiley Blackwell.

17. Lal, S., Teubner, A., and Shaffer, J.L. (2006). Review article: intestinal failure. *Aliment. Pharmacol. Ther.* 24: 19–31.

18. Dilke, S.M., Gould, L., Yao, M. et al. (2020). Distal feeding-bowel stimulation to treat short-term or long-term pathology: a systematic review. *Frontline Gastroenterol.* 12: 677–682.

19. Gabe, S.M., Shaffer, J.L., Forbes, A. et al. (2012). The management of patients with high output enterocutaneous fistulae: a European survey. *Clin. Nutr.* 7 (Suppl 1): 14–15.

20. Baker, M. and Nightingale, J.M.D. (2004). Abnormal liver function tests and parenteral nutrition. *Clin. Nutr. Suppl.* 23: P864.

21. Lal, S., Pironi, L., Wanten, G. et al. (2018). Clinical approach to the management of Intestinal Failure Associated Liver Disease (IFALD) in adults: a position paper from the Home Artificial Nutrition and Chronic Intestinal Failure Special Interest Group of ESPEN. *Clin. Nutr.* 37: 1794–1797.

22. Klek, S., Szczepanek, K., Scislo, L. et al. (2021). Intravenous lipid emulsions and liver function in adult chronic intestinal failure patients: results after 5 y of home parenteral nutrition. *Nutrition* 82: 111029.

23. Duncan, A., Talwar, D., McMillan, D.C. et al. (2012). Quantitative data on the magnitude of the systemic inflammatory response and its effect on micronutrient status based on plasma measurements. *Am. J. Clin. Nutr.* 95: 64–71.

24. Buchman, A.L., Scolapio, J., and Fryer, J. (2003). AGA technical review on short bowel syndrome and intestinal transplantation. *Gastroenterologia* 124: 1111–1134.

# CHAPTER 22

# Nutritional Biochemistry in the Post-operative Patient

Callum Livingstone

*Clinical Biochemistry Department, Royal Surrey NHS Foundation Trust, Guildford, UK*

---

## KEY POINTS

- Consider assessing micronutrient status in any patient who is having major surgery, especially those with a prolonged and complicated post-operative course or who require post-operative nutrition support.
- Measure micronutrients concurrently as a panel of tests along with a serum C-reactive protein concentration to assess the acute-phase response.
- Know the limitations of the available micronutrient tests, which include limited diagnostic sensitivity and specificity, high biological variation, and susceptibility to artefacts.
- Interpret micronutrient results in the clinical context, in particular being aware of risk factors for deficiency, possible consequences of deficiency, and the results of other investigations.
- Keep provision of micronutrients under close review given the uncertainty inherent in assessing their status.

---

The surgical patients most likely to require assessment of micronutrient status are those who require major surgery, especially if there is a complicated post-operative course or under-nutrition. Micronutrient results are a key component in assessing micronutrient status. However, the available tests have numerous limitations, which confound the interpretation of results, especially in the acute setting. Consequently, micronutrient status cannot currently be assessed using these results alone.

All available clinical information should be considered, including possible features of deficiency and the results of other laboratory tests. Many patients requiring post-operative nutrition support have subclinical micronutrient deficiency – a state in which clinical features of deficiency may be absent and serum micronutrient concentrations within reference limits. Nevertheless, these patients are still at risk of an adverse outcome. The only available pointers to this state may be risk factors – that is, possible

---

*Nutritional Management of the Surgical Patient*, First Edition. Edited by Mary E. Phillips.
© 2023 John Wiley & Sons Ltd. Published 2023 by John Wiley & Sons Ltd.

causes – for deficiency. It is good practice therefore to be alert to these risk factors, as their presence implies that the patient may benefit from generous provision of the micronutrient. Even when all the available information is considered, there is often uncertainty about patients' micronutrient status. As the interpretation of micronutrient results is inextricably linked to decisions on provision, this uncertainty necessitates that clinical judgement is applied when making these decisions.

A factor confounding interpretation of many micronutrient results is the acute-phase response (APR). Researchers have sought to establish cut-off levels of APR markers, such as C-reactive protein (CRP), for the purpose of interpreting or adjusting results. However, this has proven difficult to achieve because APR markers have different time courses of change during illness and change to different extents depending on the patient's age [1]. Moreover, APR markers may not be linearly correlated with micronutrient concentrations. Currently, there are no widely accepted methods for adjusting measured micronutrient concentrations to account for the APR. Although cut-off levels for interpreting results have been suggested in the literature, these should be used with caution. Acute illness can in addition compromise micronutrient status directly, resulting in deficiency coexisting with the effects of the APR.

It is appropriate to mention two aspects of test requesting. First, it is advisable to request micronutrient levels concurrently as a panel of tests. This is because micronutrient deficiencies often occur together, when an underlying cause affects multiple micronutrients. Second, many micronutrient tests are costly, in part because specimens may have to be sent to a specialist laboratory for analysis. Before requesting tests, practitioners should ensure that the results are essential to the clinical management of the patient.

This chapter suggests a practical approach to assessing micronutrient status. Discussion is confined to those micronutrients that most commonly give cause for concern in post-operative patients. For convenience the micronutrients are discussed individually, but in practice they should be considered together. Comprehensive lists of causes of abnormal micronutrient results are provided in order to assist practitioners with interpreting results. For advice on interpreting results, practitioners should consult their provider laboratory. Most laboratories offering measurement of micronutrient levels also offer an interpretative service.

## TRACE ELEMENTS

Currently, the biochemical assessment of trace element (TE) status requires measuring the concentration of the TE itself in blood [2]. This approach is limited because blood TE levels do not necessarily correlate well with tissue levels and as such may be diagnostically insensitive. Consequently, results within reference limits do not rule out abnormal status of the TE. The tests also have low diagnostic specificity; that is, results outside the reference range can occur for reasons other than abnormal status of the TE. Finally, practitioners should be aware of the possibility of artefactual results, including TE contamination of specimens. Specimens should be collected into the tube recommended by the provider laboratory. Causes of abnormal TE results are listed in Table 22.1.

### Zinc (Zn)

Serum Zn concentration is the most widely used biomarker of Zn status, but has numerous limitations [3]. It is an insensitive marker for deficiency, tending to remain unchanged even in patients with deficiency severe enough to impair growth. This is because adaptation initially maintains the serum Zn concentration within normal limits. Neither is hypozincaemia specific for Zn deficiency, being present in hypoalbuminaemia of any cause, notably the APR, haemodilution, and pregnancy [4, 5]. Serum Zn is also subject to wide biological

**TABLE 22.1**    Causes of abnormal trace element levels.

| Trace element | Decreased | Increased | Reference range[a] |
|---|---|---|---|
| Zn (serum/plasma) | Insufficient intake:<br>  Dietary deficiency<br>  Insufficient provision in PN<br><br>Redistribution:<br>  APR<br>  Hypoalbuminaemia<br><br>Increased demand:<br>  Growth<br>  Pregnancy<br>  Lactation<br>  Oxidative stress<br><br>Decreased absorption:<br>  Malabsorptive GI disease<br>  Inhibitors of absorption<br>  (phytic acid, Fe)<br>  IBD<br><br>Increased GI loss:<br>  Diarrhoea<br>  Fistula losses<br>  Stomal losses<br>  Nasogastric aspiration<br>  Chyle leak<br><br>Increased urinary loss:<br>  Sepsis<br>  Drugs (thiazides,<br>  angiotensin-converting<br>  enzyme inhibitors, angio-<br>  tensin receptor blockers)<br>  Cysteine infusion<br><br>Dialysate losses:<br>  RRT<br><br>Decreased delivery:<br>  Complexing in PN<br>  Adsorption to lines | Increased provision:<br>  Excessive IV or oral Zn<br><br>Decreased excretion:<br>  Cholestasis<br><br>Increased absorption:<br>  Cu deficiency | 9.6–20.5 µmol/l (F)<br><br>10.1–20.2 µmol/l (M) |

**TABLE 22.1**   (Continued)

| Trace element | Decreased | Increased | Reference range[a] |
|---|---|---|---|
| Cu (serum/plasma) | Insufficient intake:<br>  Dietary deficiency<br>  Insufficient provision in PN<br><br>Decreased absorption:<br>  Gastric surgery<br>  Malabsorptive GI disease<br>  Short bowel syndrome<br>  Bariatric surgery<br>  ZICD<br><br>Increased GI loss:<br>  Diarrhoea<br>  Fistula losses<br>  Stomal losses<br><br>Increased urinary loss:<br>  Chelating agents<br>  Cisplatin<br><br>Dialysate losses:<br>  RRT<br><br>Cutaneous losses:<br>  Extensive skin burns | Increased provision:<br>  Excessive IV or oral Cu<br><br>Increased absorption:<br>  Zn deficiency<br><br>Decreased excretion:<br>  Cholestasis<br><br>Increased Cp synthesis:<br>  APR<br>  Treatment with<br>  oestrogens | 11.0–25.1 µmol/l |
| Se (serum/plasma) | Redistribution:<br>  APR<br><br>Insufficient intake:<br>  Dietary deficiency<br>  Insufficient provision in PN<br><br>Increased demand:<br>  Acute illness<br>  Oxidative stress<br>  Smoking<br><br>Increased GI loss:<br>  Diarrhoea<br>  Fistula losses<br>  Stomal losses<br><br>Dialysate losses:<br>  RRT<br><br>Increased urinary losses:<br>  Diuretics<br>  Alcohol | Increased provision:<br>  Excessive IV or oral Se<br><br>Decreased excretion:<br>  Renal impairment<br><br>Occupational exposure:<br>  Paints, dyes, rubber<br>  and fungicides<br><br>Interference:<br>  Gadolinium (MRI<br>  contrast media) | 0.75–1.46 µmol/l |

(Continued)

**TABLE 22.1**  (Continued)

| Trace element | Decreased | Increased | Reference range[a] |
|---|---|---|---|
| Mn (whole blood) | Decreased provision:<br>  Mn withheld from PN | Increased provision:<br>  Excessive IV or oral Mn | 80–260 nmol/l |
| | | Decreased excretion:<br>  Cholestasis | |
| | | Increased absorption:<br>  Fe deficiency | |
| | | Occupational exposure:<br>  Welders | |
| Fe (serum/plasma) | Insufficient intake:<br>  Low dietary intake<br>  Insufficient IV provision | Excessive provision:<br>  Excessive IV or oral Fe<br>  Frequent blood<br>  transfusions | 9–30 µmol/l (F)<br><br>12–31 µmol/l (M) |
| | Redistribution:<br>  APR | Increased absorption:<br>  Haemochromatosis | |
| | Decreased absorption:<br>  Decreased dietary intake<br>  Insufficient absorptive<br>  surface area<br>  Inhibitors of absorption<br>  (phytate, antacids)<br>  Malabsorptive GI disease<br>  IBD | | |
| | Increased losses:<br>  Blood loss | | |
| | Impaired transport:<br>  Cu deficiency | | |

APR, acute phase response; Cp, caeruloplasmin; F, female; GI, gastrointestinal; IBD, inflammatory bowel disease; IV, intravenous; M, male; MRI, magnetic resonance imaging; PN, parenteral nutrition; RRT, renal replacement therapy; ZICD, Zn-induced Cu deficiency.

[a] Reference ranges are from the author's laboratory. Refer to local reference ranges when interpreting results.

variation (BV), which limits the weight that can be attached to individual results and has the consequence that the difference between consecutive results needs to be large (>30%) before it is likely to reflect a 'real' change as opposed to one attributable to BV [6]. Finally, artefactually high results can be caused by gel separators, rubber, heparin, and haemolysis [2, 3]. If undetected, this could result either in failure to diagnose Zn deficiency or in misdiagnosis of Zn toxicity.

These limitations demand that factors other than serum Zn concentration are considered when assessing Zn status. Seek the characteristic skin rash of overt Zn deficiency, and non-specific clinical features such as delayed wound healing, recurrent infections, alopecia, poor growth, and cognitive impairment. Identify possible causes of Zn deficiency, the most important of which, in the post-operative patient, is persistent gastrointestinal (GI) losses. The gold standard for diagnosing Zn deficiency is observation of the clinical response to supplementation [3]. In practice, however, this approach is limited because the clinical features are usually non-specific and, as such, not necessarily attributable to Zn deficiency. In addition, resolution of these features cannot necessarily be attributed to Zn provision.

Other biochemical tests may provide useful information. CRP should be measured to assess the APR. Researchers have reported that serum Zn can be reliably interpreted only when CRP is <20 mg/l (reference range [RR] <10 mg/l) [7]. In Zn deficiency serum copper (Cu) increases because of increased absorption. Consequently, a diagnosis of Zn deficiency is supported by the observation of hypercupraemia and a serum Cu : Zn ratio >1.5. In addition, serum insulin-like growth factor-I (IGF-I) decreases during Zn deficiency. Both Cu and IGF-I results are themselves affected by the APR, however, and as such may be limited in the acute setting. Zn toxicity is unusual in post-operative patients. If it is suspected seek hyperzincaemia, the presence of which should suggest the possibility of toxicity, irrespective of whether there is an APR. Zn toxicity is also characteristically accompanied by Zn-induced Cu deficiency (ZICD) [8].

Difficulty in assessing Zn status in the acute setting often results in uncertainty about how much to provide. A common dilemma is whether to give additional Zn to hypozincaemic hospitalised patients. While these patients will likely have an APR, there may be concurrent Zn deficiency that, if unsupplemented, may lead to clinical consequences. On the other hand, excessive Zn supplementation in the absence of deficiency may lead to toxicity. Given that most hospitalised patients referred for nutrition support have multiple risk factors for deficiency, it is appropriate in the short term to err on the side of over-provision. The presence of large and persistent GI losses implies that Zn requirements are considerably increased. In these patients, the American Society for Parenteral and Enteral Nutrition (ASPEN) recommends that Zn provision should be guided by the volume of GI losses [9].

## Copper (Cu)

Serum Cu has limitations as a biomarker of Cu status [10]. It is an insensitive test of deficiency, a result within the RR not ruling out deficiency [11]. It is also an insensitive biomarker of Cu overload, tending to remain within normal limits despite hepatic accumulation of Cu [12–14]. Various factors cause serum Cu to increase in the absence of Cu overload, especially the APR. This is because the Cu-binding protein caeruloplasmin (Cp), to which most of the serum Cu is bound, is a positive APR reactant [15]. Increased Cp synthesis also occurs in response to oestrogens, resulting in misleadingly high serum Cu results in women who are pregnant or treated with hormone replacement therapy (HRT). This hypercupraemia is of no pathological significance, but could result in Cu deficiency being overlooked or inadequately treated.

When assessing Cu status, seek possible causes and features of deficiency [8, 16]. The main features are anaemia, which is usually normocytic or microcytic, neutropenia, secondary iron (Fe) deficiency, and neurological abnormalities resembling those occurring in deficiency of vitamin B12. Note that while hypocupraemia usually suggests Cu deficiency, it can also occur in Wilson's disease (WD), an inherited disorder of Cu metabolism [17]. WD can be ruled out by 24 h urinary Cu ≤0.6 mmol [18]. Once WD has been ruled out, hypocupraemia suggests Cu deficiency whether or not there is an APR. Always request a CRP to quantitate the APR, Zn to rule out Zn excess, and a full blood count (FBC) to rule out haematological features of Cu deficiency. Resolution of haematological features in response to Cu supplementation suggests a diagnosis of Cu deficiency [19, 20]. It is also advisable to measure an Fe profile and other micronutrients, especially vitamin B12, deficiency of which can coexist with or mimic that of Cu. If the cause of Cu deficiency is unclear, consider a diagnosis of ZICD. ZICD can be ruled out by a 24 h urine Zn <19 mmol [21]. Patients are at risk of Cu overload if they have cholestasis or have received excessive provision. If overload is suspected, seek stigmata of liver disease and deranged liver function tests (LFTs) and consider measuring Cu on a liver biopsy specimen.

Where there is uncertainty about Cu status, the priority during nutrition support in the acute setting is to avoid deficiency. Over-provision is unlikely to be harmful in the short term, but can result in Cu overload if it continues long term.

## Selenium (Se)

The serum Se concentration is the test most commonly used to assess Se status in clinical practice and, in the non-acute setting, is simpler to interpret than serum Cu or Zn. It changes in parallel with selenoproteins, which in turn parallel the patient's recent intake of Se. This is because about 90% of serum Se is bound to selenoproteins. The serum Se concentration therefore tends to decrease in unsupplemented patients and increase in response to supplementation. As such, it has utility in assessing recent intake and the response to supplementation [22]. The test also has relatively high diagnostic sensitivity, which in practice means that Se deficiency is unlikely if results are within the RR [23]. The serum concentration also has prognostic value, correlating with mortality in the critically ill [24]. However, serum Se is an unreliable biomarker of Se status in the acute setting [25]. This is because during the APR Se is taken up by tissues for use by the immune and antioxidant systems, resulting in a decrease in its serum concentration, irrespective of Se status. Se results can be reliably interpreted only when the serum CRP is <20 mg/l [7]. A serum CRP should therefore be measured concurrently to assess the APR. Serum Se is also an unreliable test for ruling out toxicity, because its concentration tends to reach a plateau once requirements are met [26].

Patients with a prolonged post-operative course are likely to have some degree of Se deficiency. Usually this is subclinical, but be aware of the clinical features, which are muscle weakness, predisposition to infection, anaemia, macrocytosis, hair loss, and poor growth. Severe deficiency can result in cardiomyopathy and organ failure. Se toxicity is unlikely in patients requiring post-operative nutrition support,

but has been observed in patients with regular daily intakes >800 µg [27]. It presents with garlic breath and GI symptoms such as nausea, vomiting, diarrhoea, and abdominal pain. Note that Se results can be artefactually high after magnetic resonance imaging (MRI) because of interference from gadolinium present in the contrast medium. To avoid this problem, postpone Se measurement until five days post MRI.

Although Se results may be difficult to interpret in sick post-operative patients, decisions on Se provision are typically straightforward. It is usually appropriate to provide additional Se given the likelihood that some degree of deficiency will have resulted from the various risk factors. Se supplementation is unlikely to cause harm at daily provision <800 µg.

## Manganese (Mn)

In patients treated with parenteral nutrition (PN) for longer than one month, Mn status should be assessed, the aim being to avoid Mn excess. The test of choice is a whole-blood Mn concentration [28]. This correlates with Mn deposition in the basal ganglia, as measured by MRI, and changes in a dose-dependent manner, increasing with increased provision and normalising when supplementation is withheld. Whole-blood Mn is relatively unaffected by the APR because most Mn in the blood is inside red blood cells (RBCs). Consequently, the finding of hypermanganesaemia is consistent with Mn excess whether or not there is an APR. Hypermanganesaemia is a risk factor for Mn toxicity, but most hypermanganesaemic patients do not develop toxicity. Mn should not be measured on serum because, unlike whole-blood Mn, serum Mn correlates poorly with tissue deposition and decreases during the APR, both of which could cause a false-negative result. Mn deficiency is rare and highly unlikely to occur in the post-operative patient. Although hypomanganesaemia has occasionally been reported in patients in whom supplemental Mn has been withheld, it has not been associated with clinical features of deficiency [28].

Practitioners should have a high index of suspicion for Mn toxicity in patients with hypermanaganesaemia. To assess Mn status, identify risk factors for toxicity [9]. These include cholestatic liver disease, Fe deficiency, and prolonged high doses of Mn. Request LFTs and an Fe profile. If Parkinsonian-like features of Mn toxicity are present, supplemental Mn should be withheld and a neurological opinion sought. Consider MRI of the basal ganglia. An important limitation of Mn measurement is artefactually high results caused by contamination of specimen tubes [29]. When there is uncertainty about whether hypermanganesaemia is artefactual or genuine, the safest approach is to withhold supplemental Mn. In artefactual hypermanganesaemia this approach is unlikely to cause harm, whereas continuing to supplement Mn in the presence of genuine hypermanganesaemia risks toxicity.

## Iron (Fe)

When assessing Fe status, a full Fe profile should be requested along with an FBC and concurrent CRP concentration. Fe profiles usually include serum Fe, transferrin (Tf), Tf saturation, and ferritin concentration, although some laboratories report total iron-binding capacity (TIBC) and saturation of TIBC instead of Tf and Tf saturation, respectively. Table 22.2 shows the typical changes in the Fe profile during deficiency and overload.

While assessment of Fe status is likely to be straightforward in patients who are clinically well, it may be problematic in post-operative patients with an APR. During the APR, ferritin increases by 30–1400% depending on the severity of the insult, Fe and Tf decrease by 30–50%, and Tf saturation decreases to about 20% [1]. In this situation, Fe deficiency cannot therefore be ruled out by the finding of a ferritin result within the RR. Another common condition causing serum ferritin to increase in the absence of Fe overload is non-alcoholic fatty liver disease (NAFLD). Note also that Tf concentrations can be misleadingly low in patients with protein-energy nutrition. Because of these limitations, an iron profile should be interpreted in the light of all available findings. Clinical features of Fe deficiency include tiredness, pallor, and koilonychia (spoon-shaped nails), and an FBC typically shows a decreased haemoglobin (Hb) concentration and a decreased mean cell volume (MCV) of RBCs.

## VITAMINS

With the exception of vitamin B12 and folate, it is rarely necessary to measure water-soluble vitamins in post-operative patients. This is because these vitamins, which have low toxicity potential, can be safely supplemented at high doses. Indeed, most post-operative patients requiring nutrition support will receive generous supplementation of vitamins B1, B2, B6, and C in addition to the standard provision contained in the nutrition support. Measuring

**TABLE 22.2**   Interpreting serum Fe profile results.

| Test | Fe deficiency | Fe overload | Inflammation | Reference range[a] |
|---|---|---|---|---|
| Fe | ↓ | ↑ | ↓ | 9–30 µmol/l (F) |
| | | | | 12–31 µmol/l (M) |
| Ferritin | ↓ | ↑ | ↑ | 15–250 µg/l (F) |
| | | | | 15–300 µg/l (M) |
| Tf | ↑ | ↓ | ↓ | 2.50–3.80 g/l (F) |
| | | | | 2.15–3.05 g/l (M) |
| Tf saturation | ↓ | ↑ | ↓ | 15–50% (F) |
| | | | | 20–50% (M) |

**Key:** F, female; M, male; Tf, transferrin; ↓, decreased; ↑, increased.
[a] Reference ranges are from the author's laboratory. Refer to local reference ranges when interpreting results.

the levels of these vitamins is therefore unlikely to influence clinical management. Deficiency of fat-soluble vitamins tends to occur later in the course of disease because these vitamins have dedicated stores. Clinical deficiency of fat-soluble vitamins is uncommon in post-operative patients, but subclinical deficiency is relatively common and can adversely affect outcome. Vitamins A and D, unlike the water-soluble vitamins, have potential for toxicity and as such cannot be routinely supplemented in megadoses. Causes of abnormal vitamin results are listed in Table 22.3.

**TABLE 22.3**   Causes of abnormal vitamin levels.

| Vitamin | Decreased | Increased | Reference range[a] |
|---|---|---|---|
| Thiamine (serum/ whole blood) | Decreased intake:<br>  Dietary deficiency<br>  Chronic alcohol misuse<br>  Chronic illness<br>  Malignancy<br>  WE<br><br>Decreased absorption:<br>  GI surgery<br>  Enteropathy<br><br>Increased requirement:<br>  Critical illness<br>  Congestive cardiac failure<br>  APR<br><br>Increased renal losses:<br>  Prolonged diuretic use<br>  RRT | Haematological disease<br>  Leukaemia<br>  Hodgkin's disease<br>  Polycythaemia vera | 66.5–200.0 nmol/l |
| Vitamin B12 (serum) | Decreased intake:<br>  Vegetarian diet<br>  Alcohol excess<br><br>Decreased absorption:<br>  Pernicious anaemia<br>  Gastrectomy<br>  Gastric atrophy<br>  Pancreatic insufficiency<br>  Ileal resection<br>  IBD affecting small bowel<br>  Vitamin B6 deficiency<br>  Tropical sprue<br>  Tapeworms<br>  Congenital malabsorption (infants)<br><br>Increased utilisation:<br>  Colonic bacterial overgrowth | Supplementation:<br>  Oral or parenteral<br>  delivery of vitamin B12<br><br>Liver disease:<br>  Hepatitis<br>  Cirrhosis<br>  Liver cancer (primary or<br>  secondary)<br><br>Haematological disease:<br>  Leukaemias<br>  Myeloma<br>  Polycythaemia vera | 200–900 ng/l |

**TABLE 22.3**    (Continued)

| Vitamin | Decreased | Increased | Reference range[a] |
|---|---|---|---|
| | Drugs:<br>  Phenytoin<br>  Metformin<br>  Proton pump inhibitors<br>  H2 blockers<br><br>Plasma expansion:<br>  Pregnancy | | |
| Folate (serum) | Decreased intake:<br>  Dietary deficiency (low intake of<br>  green leafy vegetables)<br>  Decreased absorption<br><br>Decreased absorption:<br>  Intestinal disease<br>  Antacids<br><br>Increased losses:<br>  Haemodialysis<br><br>Increased demand:<br>  Pregnancy<br>  Exfoliative skin disease<br>  Malignancy<br><br>Drugs:<br>  Alcohol<br>  Azathioprine<br>  Trimethoprim<br>  Methotrexate<br>  Phenytoin | Increased intake:<br>  Oral supplementation<br>  PN | 4–26 µg/l |
| Vitamin A (serum retinol) | Decreased intake:<br>  Dietary deficiency<br>  Insufficient supplementation of PN<br>  Pre-term infants<br><br>Decreased absorption:<br>  Fat malabsorption<br>  Pancreatic exocrine insufficiency<br>  Intestinal disease<br>  Bile acid sequestrants<br><br>Decreased RBP synthesis:<br>  Liver disease<br>  Zn deficiency<br>  APR | Excessive intake:<br>  Excessive oral or<br>  parenteral intake | 0.99–3.35 µmol/l (F)<br><br>0.77–3.95 µmol/l (M) |

(Continued)

**TABLE 22.3**  (Continued)

| Vitamin | Decreased | Increased | Reference range[a] |
|---|---|---|---|
| | Increased demand:<br>  APR<br>  Pregnancy | | |
| Vitamin D (serum 25OHD) | Decreased intake:<br>  Dietary deficiency<br>  Lack of sun exposure<br><br>Increased demand:<br>  Pregnancy<br>  Breastfeeding<br><br>Decreased absorption:<br>  Elderly<br>  Fat malabsorption<br>  Pancreatic exocrine insufficiency<br>  IBD<br>  Coeliac disease<br>  Liver disease<br>  Bile acid–binding resins<br><br>Increased metabolism:<br>  Drugs: phenytoin, carbamazepine, phenobarbital, rifampicin, corticosteroids, HAART<br><br>Decreased binding proteins:<br>  Critical illness<br>  APR | Excessive intake:<br>  Excessive oral or parenteral intake | 76–250 nmol/l |
| Vitamin E (serum alpha-tocopherol : cholesterol ratio) | Decreased intake:<br>  Dietary deficiency<br>  Insufficient supplementation of PN<br>  Pre-term infants<br><br>Decreased absorption:<br>  Cholestasis<br>  Pancreatic exocrine insufficiency<br>  Intestinal disease<br><br>Impaired mobilisation:<br>  Abetalipoproteinaemia<br><br>Increased utilisation:<br>  Metabolic syndrome | Excessive intake:<br>  Excessive oral or parenteral intake | 9.5–41.5 |

APR, acute-phase response; F, female; GI, gastrointestinal; HAART, highly active antiretroviral treatment; IBD, inflammatory bowel disease; M, male; PN, parenteral nutrition; RBP, retinol-binding protein; RRT, renal replacement therapy; WE, Wernicke's encephalopathy.

[a] Reference ranges are from the author's laboratory. Refer to local reference ranges when interpreting results.

## Thiamine (Vitamin B1)

Thiamine should be supplemented promptly if there is clinical suspicion of deficiency. For this reason, thiamine results are unlikely to inform the clinical management of most patients. However, in patients with clinical features of severe deficiency, it is appropriate to measure thiamine for retrospective confirmation of the diagnosis in the event that the patient fails to respond to supplementation [30]. Severe deficiency usually presents with Wernicke's encephalopathy (WE), a triad of confusion, ataxia, and ophthalmoplegia. Other possible features of thiamine deficiency include peripheral neuropathy, cardiac failure, and Korsakoff's psychosis (that is, severe memory loss). Tests of thiamine status include total serum thiamine, RBC thiamine, or thiamine diphosphate, and RBC transketolase and transketolase activation. Practitioners should consult their local laboratory for advice on the choice of test and specimen requirement.

## Vitamin B12 (Cyanocobalamin)

The need to assess vitamin B12 status may arise in those who have undergone gastric surgery, post-operative patients requiring long-term nutrition support, patients on treatment for known vitamin B12 deficiency, and those in whom new features arise that are consistent with deficiency. Clinical features tend to occur late following the causal insult, the interval to deficiency depending on the status of hepatic stores at the time of the insult. Deficiency leads to impaired formation of RBCs resulting in megaloblastic anaemia, and later compromises growth and repair of nerve cells, leading to neurological features such as weakness, paraesthesia, and sensory loss. Awareness of these clinical features is important because there is no gold-standard test for diagnosis of vitamin B12 deficiency [31]. In established deficiency, the Hb concentration is decreased, MCV increased, and a blood film shows macrocytes. Note however that Hb has poor sensitivity and specificity for the diagnosis and MCV has poor specificity, also increasing in alcohol excess and hypothyroidism.

The first-line biochemical test of choice is serum vitamin B12. It generally has good sensitivity for diagnosis of deficiency, decreasing pre-symptomatically and likely to be significantly decreased in patients with clinical features of deficiency. However, its sensitivity is poor in patients who have liver disease or myeloproliferative disorders, both of which cause misleadingly high results [32]. In the event of an unexpectedly normal result in a patient with clinical features of deficiency, secondary biomarkers of vitamin B12 status may be useful. Methylmalonic acid (MMA) is a sensitive and specific biomarker, the serum concentration of which increases in deficiency. However, it is a costly test and not readily available. Plasma homocysteine is another sensitive biomarker, increasing in vitamin B12 deficiency, but it is non-specific, also increasing in deficiencies of folate and vitamin B6. Serum vitamin B12 has relatively poor specificity for diagnosis of deficiency because low results can occur in non-anaemic patients and in patients with non-specific symptoms. Low results, not necessarily requiring treatment, can occur in vegetarians, and patients on a strict vegan diet are at increased risk of deficiency.

Following a diagnosis of vitamin B12 deficiency, the cause should be sought by a combination of dietetic assessment, drug history, endoscopy, and measurement of anti-intrinsic factor antibodies, which if positive suggest pernicious anaemia. If vitamin B12 levels are increased rule out recent supplementation, and check LFTs and an FBC to investigate the possibility of haematological or liver disease. Note that in patients treated with PN, serum vitamin B12 concentrations are likely to reflect what has been infused rather than the status of stores. In this situation, monitor the FBC and MCV.

## Folate

Folate deficiency presents with haematological features similar to those of vitamin B12 deficiency. This is because both micronutrients are required for blood cell formation in the bone marrow. There will be megaloblastic anaemia and possibly leucopaenia and thrombocytopaenia as well.

The main biochemical tests of folate status are serum folate and RBC folate. Serum folate is sensitive to recent changes in folate intake, but has high BV, limiting the use of single measurements. RBC folate reflects longer-term body status [32], but has the limitation of giving misleadingly low results in concurrent vitamin B12 deficiency. In established deficiency, both serum and RBC folate concentrations decrease, whereas recent poor intake results in decreased serum folate and normal RBC folate concentrations. Serum folate concentrations above the RR are not pathological, but can occur in patients treated with PN.

It is recommended that serum folate alone is measured initially, a concentration $<3\,\mu g/l$ suggesting deficiency [31]. It is unnecessary to measure RBC folate routinely. It should however be measured in patients treated with PN and if serum folate is normal in the presence of strong clinical suspicion of deficiency. In the former group of patients, serum folate is likely to reflect recently infused folate rather than the status of the vitamin. Plasma homocysteine is a secondary biomarker of folate status increasing in deficiency, but is non-specific, also increasing in deficiencies of vitamins B6 and B12. When assessing folate status it is advisable to assess vitamin B12 status concurrently. This is because high-dose folic acid supplementation in a patient with undetected vitamin B12 deficiency can result in irreversible neurological symptoms.

## Vitamin A

Vitamin A deficiency can occur in post-operative patients, particularly those who have multiple predisposing causes or are critically ill. Critical illness can compromise vitamin A status by decreasing dietary intake, decreasing intestinal absorption, and increasing urinary excretion [1]. If illness is prolonged, demands on the antioxidant system also cause a deficit in retinol resulting from increased utilisation [33, 34]. In patients with characteristic clinical features of vitamin A deficiency, the underlying cause is usually readily identifiable. Clinical vitamin A deficiency usually presents with night blindness that, untreated, may lead to xerophthalmia and

ultimately blindness. Other consequences of vitamin A deficiency relevant in the post-operative patient are poor wound healing [9], pressure ulcers, and increased susceptibility to infection [35, 36].

Vitamin A status is usually assessed by measuring the serum retinol concentration, but this test has two major limitations. First, it decreases late in deficiency [37]. This is because homeostasis tends to maintain its serum concentration within narrow limits until hepatic stores are depleted. As such, serum retinol has low diagnostic sensitivity, potentially resulting in failure to diagnose mild deficiency. Second, its specificity is poor in the acute setting. Falsely low results can occur because the APR decreases serum retinol-binding protein (RBP) levels irrespective of vitamin A status. In subjects without acute illness, serum retinol $<1.0\,\mu mol/l$ suggests deficiency [37].

Vitamin A toxicity is unusual post-operatively, but patients with acute renal impairment are at greater risk because there is reduced renal clearance of RBP [38]. It presents with bone pain, hepatomegaly, and higher liver enzymes [39, 40]. To confirm vitamin A toxicity, the test of choice is serum retinyl esters. These increase in toxicity from the normal concentration of $<0.2\,\mu mol/l$ [9].

## Vitamin D

Vitamin D deficiency and insufficiency are common in the UK because of lack of sun exposure. In addition, deficiency is commoner in elderly patients because of an age-related decrease in hepatic and renal activation of vitamin D. Consequently, many surgical patients will have suboptimal vitamin D status long before they become unwell, and will be at considerably increased risk of developing vitamin D deficiency if they suffer post-operative complications.

When assessing vitamin D status, be aware of the clinical features of deficiency, which include muscle weakness, myalgia, and bone pain, and seek possible causes of vitamin D deficiency [41]. The biochemical test of choice is serum 25-hydroxyvitamin D (25OHD), deficiency being defined as 25OHD $<25\,nmol/l$ and insufficiency as $25–50\,nmol/l$ [42]. In addition, it is useful to measure parathyroid hormone (PTH) and serum calcium. PTH increases in response to vitamin D deficiency. This secondary hyperparathyroidism tends to maintain serum calcium concentrations within normal limits until the deficiency is severe. At this point hypocalcaemia develops, possibly accompanied by symptoms of paraesthesia and muscle spasm. Serum 25OHD levels >250 nmol/l may be associated with toxicity. Practitioners should be aware that there is ongoing debate about cut-off levels and that different assays may give different results.

While serum 25OHD results are usually straightforward to interpret in patients who are clinically well, they are difficult to interpret in many postoperative patients, especially the critically ill. Serum 25OHD is bound to albumin and vitamin D–binding protein (DBP), both of which leave the circulation during the APR. There is also decreased synthesis of these binding proteins and increased renal wasting of vitamin D [43]. Results may also decrease because of haemodilution from the administration of intravenous fluids. Up to 90% of critically ill patients have 25OHD <50 nmol/l [44]. This is associated with increased mortality and higher risk of respiratory infection, but it is unknown whether the decreased 25OHD levels truly reflect vitamin D status in these patients [45]. In future, it may be possible to measure bioavailable vitamin D, but at present it is not possible to assess vitamin D status reliably in the critically ill. Note also that BV is wide in these patients, making single measurements unreliable [45].

Avoid routinely measuring the active form of vitamin D, 1,25-dihydroxyvitamin D (1,25OHD), the level of which paradoxically increases in vitamin D deficiency. Its measurement should be confined to assessment of patients with chronic kidney disease, who may have features of vitamin D deficiency as a result of impaired renal activation of 25OHD. Its measurement is also useful in the investigation of some hypercalcaemic patients.

## Vitamin E

Severe vitamin E deficiency is uncommon, but is more likely to occur in patients with severe intestinal, liver, and pancreatic disease, especially if the illness is prolonged. The presenting features are neuropathy, myopathy, and haemolytic anaemia [46, 47]. Mild vitamin E deficiency is commoner and is implicated in the development of pressure ulcers [48]. Vitamin E toxicity has not been described in patients treated with nutrition support, but could in principle be caused by excessive supplementation. Its main feature is bleeding resulting from impaired blood clotting [49].

Current laboratory assessment of vitamin E status is unreliable and there is a need for new biomarkers of deficiency. Alpha-tocopherol is the most abundant and most commonly measured form of vitamin E in serum, but interpretation of results is complicated by its association with lipoproteins. The serum alpha-tocopherol concentration tends to decrease as the serum cholesterol decreases. To account for this, laboratories report the alpha-tocopherol : cholesterol ratio along with serum alpha-tocopherol results. However, evidence suggests that use of the ratio may not always be appropriate. In undernourished or acutely ill patients, in whom both alpha-tocopherol and cholesterol are abnormally low, the ratio may be misleadingly normal, resulting in failure to diagnose vitamin E deficiency. Consequently, some authors have advised against correction for lipids, instead relying on serum total alpha-tocopherol concentrations [50]. In obese patients, on the other hand, who tend to have mild vitamin E deficiency resulting from the oxidative stress associated with chronic inflammation, the ratio is likely to be a more reliable measure of status. This is because these patients often have hyperlipidaemia, resulting in the alpha-tocopherol being misleadingly normal but a ratio below that of non-obese subjects, reflecting mild vitamin E deficiency [51]. The US Institute of Medicine defines vitamin E deficiency in adults as a serum alpha-tocopherol concentration <12 μmol/l [52].

These difficulties emphasise the importance of assessing clinical features and seeking possible causes of deficiency rather than relying solely on laboratory results. Where clinical features are consistent with vitamin E deficiency, consider a trial of treatment, because the features usually respond promptly to supplementation.

## CONCLUSION

There is an urgent need to develop new tests of micronutrient status that are reliable in the acute setting. It is likely that such tests will consist of panels of biomarkers, identified using the '-omics' technologies, rather than single biomarkers. Hopefully, as better tests become available, the assessment of micronutrient status will become more accurate, thereby removing some of the uncertainty from decisions on provision.

---

### Case Study:   Manganese Toxicity

A 62 year-old male patient with acute pancreatitis was admitted to the intensive care unit (ICU). He was critically ill, requiring multiorgan support. Because of intestinal failure, he also required PN, which was infused continuously over 24 h to meet nutritional requirements. From early in the admission the patient's serum alkaline phosphatase level was noted to be increased, ranging from 347 to 674 U/l (RR 30–130 U/l), but alanine transaminase (ALT) and total bilirubin concentrations remained within normal limits.

Ten weeks after admission to ICU, the patient started experiencing episodic tremor that became increasingly severe, affecting all limbs. A standard neurological examination showed some limb weakness, but was otherwise normal and a cerebral computed tomographic (CT) scan showed no abnormalities. A micronutrient profile indicated that whole-blood Mn was increased at 429 nmol/l (RR 80–260). This finding, in combination with the Parkinsonian-like symptoms, suggested Mn toxicity. Ideally, the diagnosis would have been made definitively by MRI of the basal ganglia, but this was technically not possible because of the amount of ferrous equipment attached to the patient.

The toxicity was thought to be caused by the combination of relatively high doses of Mn and prolonged, albeit mild, cholestasis. TEs had been provided as a standard multi-TE (MTE) product added to the PN bag. This delivered a daily Mn dose of 270 µg in line with 2009 ESPEN recommendations [53], but higher than the 55 µg daily dose recommended by ASPEN in 2012 [9]. Staff were aware of the ASPEN guidance, but no MTE product delivering a 55 µg dose was available at the time. The patient was managed by withholding the MTE product and providing Cu, Zn, and Se in the PN as individual micronutrient supplements. The symptoms started to improve after four months and resolved after nine months.

This case study emphasises the importance of being alert to risk factors for Mn toxicity. It also illustrates that this micronutrient disorder can occur after a relatively short duration of PN in susceptible patients.

---

### Case Study:   Vitamin A Deficiency Night Blindness

A 37 year-old female patient presented with night blindness at 33 weeks of gestation. She also complained of persistent diarrhoea, but was otherwise well. Serum retinol was significantly decreased at 0.20 µmol/l (RR 0.92–2.76), confirming vitamin A deficiency. Hb was low at 97 g/l (RR 115–165) and an Fe profile confirmed Fe deficiency with serum Fe 15 µmol/l (RR 9–30), ferritin 12 µg/l (RR 15–250), TIBC 95 µmol/l (RR 45–70), and saturation of TIBC 16% (RR 15–50).

The cause of the deficiency was pancreatic exocrine insufficiency. Six years previously the patient had required pancreatico-duodenectomy for a benign pancreatic tumour. Thereafter she was commenced on a multivitamin supplement and pancreatic enzyme replacement therapy (PERT). However, 4½ years post-operatively she discontinued these treatments because of concerns about possible side effects. The vitamin A deficiency presented late, presumably because of the length of time taken for hepatic stores to become depleted. In addition, prior to the pregnancy the patient had regularly eaten liver, an abundant source of vitamin A, but had avoided it during pregnancy. The deficiency was likely precipitated by the extra demands incurred during the third trimester of pregnancy.

The patient was given a vitamin infusion containing 3300 IU (415 µg) of retinol, 200 IU (5 µg) ergocalciferol, 10 IU of alpha-tocopherol, and 150 µg of phytomenadione (vitamin K), after which the night blindness resolved. She was also treated by blood transfusion and was discharged from hospital on a daily oral micronutrient supplement providing 1250 IU retinol along with other vitamins and minerals. She later agreed to restart PERT.

This case study illustrates how clinical deficiency of different micronutrients can coincide. It also emphasises the importance of adhering to micronutrient supplements and PERT if micronutrient deficiency is to be avoided. Because of the teratogenicity of vitamin A, supplementation should not exceed a daily dose of 10 000 IU in women of child-bearing age [54].

# REFERENCES

1. Bresnahan, K.A. and Tanumihardjo, S.A. (2014). Undernutrition, the acute phase response to infection and its effects on micronutrient status markers. *Adv. Nutr.* 5: 702–711.

2. Taylor, A. (1996). Detection and monitoring of disorders of essential trace elements. *Ann. Clin. Biochem.* 33: 486–510.

3. Livingstone, C. (2015). Zinc: physiology, deficiency and parenteral nutrition. *Nutr. Clin. Pract.* 30: 371–382.

4. Solomans, N.W. (1979). On the assessment of zinc and copper nutriture in man. *Am. J. Clin. Nutr.* 32: 856–871.

5. Hobisch-Hagen, P., Mortl, M., and Schobersberger, W. (1997). Hemostatic disorders in pregnancy and the peripartum period. *Acta Anaesthesiol. Scand. Suppl.* 111: 216–217.

6. Lux, O. and Naidoo, D. (1995). The assessment of biological variation components of copper, zinc and selenium. *J. Nutr. Biochem.* 6: 43–47.

7. Duncan, A., Talwar, D., McMillan, D.C. et al. (2012). Quantitative data on the magnitude of the systemic inflammatory response and its effect on micronutrient status based on plasma measurements. *Am. J. Clin. Nutr.* 95: 64–71.

8. Livingstone, C. (2017). A review of copper provision in the parenteral nutrition of adults. *Nutr. Clin. Pract.* 32: 153–165.

9. Vanek, V.W., Borum, P., Buchman, A. et al. (2012). ASPEN position paper: recommendations for changes in commercially available parenteral multi-vitamin and multi-trace element products. *Nutr. Clin. Pract.* 27: 440–491.

10. Harvey, L.J., Ashton, K., Hopper, L. et al. (2009). Methods of assessment of copper status in humans: a systematic review. *Am. J. Clin. Nutr.* 89: 2009S–2024S.

11. Frankel, D.A. (1993). Supplementation of trace elements in parenteral nutrition: rationale and recommendations. *Nutr. Res.* 13: 583–596.

12. Food and Nutrition Board (2001). *Institute of Medicine. Dietary Reference Intakes for Vitamin a, Vitamin K, Arsenic, Boron, Chromium, Copper, Iodine, Iron, Manganese, Molybdenum, Nickel, Silicon, Vanadium, and Zinc.* Washington, DC: National Academies Press.

13. Blaszyk, H., Wild, P.J., Oliveira, A. et al. (2005). Hepatic copper in patients receiving long-term total parenteral nutrition. *J. Clin. Gastroenterol.* 39: 318–320.

14. Howard, L., Ashley, C., Lyon, D., and Shenkin, A. (2007). Autopsy tissue trace elements in eight long term parenteral nutrition patients who received the current US FDA formulation. *J. Parenter. Enteral Nutr.* 31: 388–396.

15. McKay, M., Mulroy, C.W., Street, J. et al. (2015). Assessing copper status in pediatric patients receiving parenteral nutrition. *Nutr. Clin. Pract.* 30: 117–121.

16. Osland, E.J., Ali, A., Isenring, E. et al. (2014). Australasian Society for Parenteral and Enteral Nutrition guidelines for supplementation of trace elements during parenteral nutrition. *Asia Pac. J. Clin. Nutr.* 23: 545–554.

17. Steinlieb, L. and Scheinberg, I.H. (1994). Wilson disease. In: *Current Therapy in Gastroenterology and Liver Disease*, 4e (ed. T.M. Bayliss), 578. Maryland Heights, MO: Mosby.

18. Roberts, E.A. and Schilsky, M.L. (2008). AASLD practice guidelines. Diagnosis and treatment of Wilson disease: an update. *Hepatology* 47: 2089–2111.

19. Fuhrman, M.P., Herrmann, V., Masidonski, P., and Eby, C. (2000). Pancytopenia after removal of copper from total parenteral nutrition. *J. Parenter. Enteral Nutr.* 24: 361–366.

20. Huff, J.D., Keung, Y.K., Thakuri, M. et al. (2007). Copper deficiency causes reversible myelodysplasia. *Am. J. Hematol.* 82: 625–630.

21. Duncan, A., Gallacher, G., and Willox, L. (2016). The role of the clinical biochemist in detection of zinc-induced copper deficiency. *Ann. Clin. Biochem.* 53: 298–301.

22. Hardy, G., Menendez, A.M., and Manzanares, W. (2009). Trace element supplementation in parenteral nutrition: pharmacy, posology, and monitoring guidance. *Nutrition* 25: 1073–1084.

23. Hatanaka, N., Nakaden, H., Yamamoto, Y. et al. (2000). Selenium kinetics and changes in glutathione peroxidase activities in patients receiving long-term parenteral nutrition and effects of supplementation with selenite. *Nutrition* 16: 22–26.

24. Manzanares, W., Biestro, A., Galusso, F. et al. (2009). Serum selenium and glutathione peroxidase-3 activity: biomarkers of systemic inflammation in the critically ill? *Intensive Care Med.* 35: 882–889.

25. Stefanowicz, F., Gashut, R.A., Talwar, D. et al. (2014). Assessment of plasma and red cell trace element concentrations, disease severity and outcome in patients with critical illness. *J. Crit. Care* 29: 214–218.

26. Food and Nutrition Board (2000). Institute of Medicine–National Academy of Sciences. Selenium. In: *Dietary Reference Intakes for Vitamin C, Vitamin E, Selenium, and Carotenoids.* (ed. Institute of Medicine Panel on Dietary Antioxidants and Related Compounds), 284–324. Washington, DC: National Academies Press.

27. Shenkin, A. (2009). Selenium in intravenous nutrition. *Gastroenterologia* 37: S61–S69.

28. Livingstone, C. (2018). Manganese provision in parenteral nutrition: an update. *Nutr. Clin. Pract.* 33: 404–418.

29. Santos, D., Batoreu, C., Mateus, L. et al. (2014). Manganese in human parenteral nutrition: considerations for toxicity and biomonitoring. *Neurotoxicology* 43: 36–45.

30. Galvin, R., Brathen, G., Ivashynka, A. et al. (2010). EFNS guidelines for diagnosis, therapy and prevention of Wernicke's encephalopthy. *Eur. J. Neurol.* 17: 1408–1418.

31. Devalia, V., Hamilton, M.S., and Molloy, A.M. (2014). Guidelines for the diagnosis and treatment of cobalamin and folate disorders. *Br. J. Haematol.* 166: 496–513.

32. Green, R. (2011). Indicators for assessing folate and vitamin $B_{12}$ status and for monitoring the efficacy of intervention strategies. *Am. J. Clin. Nutr.* 94 (Suppl): 666S–672S.

33. Goode, H.F., Cowley, H.C., Walker, B.E. et al. (1995). Decreased antioxidant status and increased lipid peroxidation in patients with septic shock and secondary organ dysfunction. *Crit. Care Med.* 23: 646–651.

34. Stephenson, D., Alvarez, J.O., and Kohatsu, J. (1994). Vitamin a is excreted in the urine during acute infection. *Am. J. Clin. Nutr.* 60: 388–392.

35. World Health Organization (1996). Indicators for assessing vitamin A deficiency and their application in monitoring and evaluating intervention programmes. Geneva: WHO. https://apps.who.int/iris/handle/10665/63064. Accessed February 2021.

36. Field, C.J., Johnson, I.R., and Scley, P.D. (2002). Nutrients and their role in host resistance to infection. *J. Leukoc. Biol.* 71: 16–32.

37. Tanumihardjo, S.A., Russell, R.M., Stephenson, C.B. et al. (2016). Biomarkers of nutrition for development: vitamin A review. *J. Nutr.* 146 (Suppl): 1816S–1848S.

38. Lipkin, A.C. and Lenssen, P. (2008). Hypervitaminosis A in pediatric hematopoietic stem cell patients requiring renal replacement therapy. *Nutr. Clin. Pract.* 23: 621–629.

39. Rohde, C.M., Manatt, M., Clagett-Dame, M., and DeLuca, H.F. (1999). Vitamin a antagonizes the action of vitamin D in rats. *J. Nutr.* 129: 2246–2250.

40. Ramanathan, V.S., Hensley, G., French, S. et al. (2010). Hypervitaminosis a inducing intra-hepatic cholestasis: a rare case report. *Exp. Mol. Pathol.* 88: 324–325.

41. Rosenberg, I.H. and Miller, J.W. (1992). Nutritional factors in physical and cognitive functions of elderly people. *Am. J. Clin. Nutr.* 55: 1237S–1243S.

42. National Institute for Health and Care Excellence (2020). Vitamin D deficiency in adults – treatment and prevention. https://cks.nice.org.uk/topics/vitamin-d-deficiency-in-adults. Accessed February 2021.

43. Schulman, R.C. and Mechanick, J.I. (2012). Metabolic and nutrition support in the chronic ctitical illness syndrome. *Respir. Care* 57: 958–978.

44. Nierman, D.M. and Mechanick, J.I. (1998). Bone hyperresorption is prevalent in chronically critically ill patients. *Chest* 114: 1122–1128.

45. Quraishi, S.A. and Camargo, C.A. (2012). Vitamin D in acute stress and critical illness. *Curr. Opin. Clin. Nutr. Metab. Care* 15: 625–364.

46. Kumar, N. (2007). Nutritional neuropathies. *Neurol. Clin.* 25: 209–255.

47. Oski, F.A. and Barness, L.A. (1967). Vitamin E deficiency: a previously unrecognised cause of haemolytic anaemia in the premature infant. *J. Pediatr.* 70: 211–220.

48. Rojas, A.I. and Phillips, T.J. (1999). Patients with chronic leg ulcers show diminished levels of vitamins A and E, carotenes and zinc. *Dermatol. Surg.* 25: 601–604.

49. Owen, K.N. and Dewald, O. (2020). Vitamin E toxicity. In: *StatPearls [Internet]*. Treasure Island, FL: StatPearls Publishing.

50. Traber, M.G. (2014). Vitamin E inadequacy in humans: causes and consequences. *Adv. Nutr.* 5: 503–514.

51. Strauss, R.S. (1999). Comparison of serum concentrations of alpha-tocopherol and beta-caroten in a cross-sectional sample of obese and non-obese children (NHANES III). *J. Pediatr.* 134: 160–165.

52. Food and Nutrition Board (2000). *Institute of Medicine. Dietary Reference Intakes for Vitamin C, Vitamin E, Selenium, and Carotenoids.* Washington, DC: National Academic Press.

53. Braga, M., Ljungqvist, O., Soeters, P. et al. (2009). ESPEN guidelines on parenteral nutrition: surgery. *Clin. Nutr.* 28: 378–386.

54. World Health Organization (1998). *Safe Vitamin A Dosage during Pregnancy and Lactation: Recommendations and Report from a Consultation.* Geneva: WHO.

# CONSOLIDATE YOUR LEARNING

# CHAPTER 23

# Test Yourself

This chapter is designed to consolidate your knowledge by utilising the content of this book to plan the nutritional management of patients in different clinical situations. For each case consider the questions posed. The answers can all be found in one or more of the chapters in this book.

| Case 1 |
| --- |

Mr A (age 65 yr, weight 87 kg, BMI 32 kg/m², normal weight 94 kg) is referred following a total laryngectomy.

1. What factors would you consider in your initial assessment and management?
2. What should the surgeon have considered prior to surgery?
3. What nutritional management would you recommend in the immediate post-operative period?
4. What long-term considerations are there?
5. Unfortunately, Mr A was assessed as dysphagic. What feeding option might you consider now?

*Nutritional Management of the Surgical Patient*, First Edition. Edited by Mary E. Phillips.
© 2023 John Wiley & Sons Ltd. Published 2023 by John Wiley & Sons Ltd.

| Case 2 |
| --- |

Mrs B (age 47 yr, weight 98 kg, height 156 cm) is admitted following a road traffic collision. She is day 1 following orthopaedic surgery during which an external fixation device was inserted to pin her left femur. She has five rib fractures (flail segment), a radial fracture in her dominant arm, and a spinal injury (C4) requiring immobilisation with a cervical collar. She is on 0.45 μg/kg/min noradrenaline and is currently intubated and ventilated. She is awaiting further imaging to determine the management of her cervical spine injury.

1. What would you consider in your initial assessment?
2. How would you initially feed this patient?
3. As she becomes more haemodynamically stable, how might your management change?
4. What would you calculate her nutritional requirements as initially, and again five days later?
5. Mrs B is extubated and weaned off inotropes, she has no obvious sensory defect, but needs to remain in a cervical collar. What might you need to put in place to support her nutritionally now?

| Case 3 |
| --- |

Mr C (aged 74 yr, weight 124 kg, height 172 cm) has just had an emergency coronary artery bypass graft (CABG) and is recovering well. He is day 4 post-op and is mobilising gently.

1. What initial social and lifestyle factors should be considered before any advice is given?

2. What long-term options should be recommended for this patient?
3. Mr C develops a significant wound infection on day 5 requiring intravenous antibiotics. How does this affect your nutritional management?

| Case 4 |
| --- |

Mr D (aged 27 yr, weight 54 kg, height 168 cm) was referred into a gastrointestinal surgery clinic with chronic abdominal pain, weight loss, and constipation. A CT scan revealed extensive calcification throughout the pancreas with a dilated pancreatic duct but no obvious masses. Tumour markers were normal, and a subsequent EUS did not detect any signs of malignancy. A blood test revealed low levels of vitamin A, D, and zinc.

1. What lifestyle advice should be provided?
2. What factors should be considered within his nutritional assessment?
3. What do you need to interpret the blood tests?
4. What medications might you consider?
5. What impact does pain management have on nutritional management?
6. What long-term screening would you put in place?

## Case 5

Mrs E (aged 72 yr, weight 78 kg, height 158 cm) is day 6 post pancreatico-duodenectomy and has developed a pancreatic leak, her abdomen is distended, and she has not passed flatus. Her drain amylase is 65 450 and her CRP is elevated at 250 mg/l; she is nauseated.

1. How does a pancreatic leak affect the digestive function?

2. What would you consider when determining how to feed her?
3. When would you consider parenteral nutrition?
4. Assuming the leak resolves with conservative management, what medication should she be started on and what else should she be screened for?

## Case 6

Mr F (aged 78 yr, weight 134 kg, height 169 cm) is undergoing chemotherapy prior to an extended right liver resection for colorectal liver metastases. He has had his primary removed (right hemi-colectomy), he has been weight stable throughout his chemotherapy, but has bloating and watery diarrhoea that has not settled since his first operation.

1. What could be the cause of the diarrhoea?
2. What might you consider during the chemotherapy to try to reduce the risk of his liver surgery?
3. What long-term health advice should you provide this patient with?

## Case 7

Miss G (aged 42 yr, weight 92 kg, height 172 cm) underwent a total pelvic clearance for ovarian cancer. Day 3 post-op she starts vomiting. Her ileal conduit produces very little urine and an NGT is sited that drains 2800 mls in the first 12 h. After 2 more days her symptoms are no better.

1. What management would you consider now you are at day 5?
2. What does her ileal conduit render her more susceptible to?
3. When might you consider allowing her to eat?

## Case 8

Mr H (age 19 yr, weight 84 kg, height 178 cm) was admitted to intensive care after a damage-control laparotomy for multiple abdominal sharp-force injuries following a stabbing incident. He underwent a total colectomy, nephrectomy, left hepatectomy, extended distal pancreatectomy, splenectomy, and extensive small bowel resection. The operating surgeon thought there was approximately 80 cm of jejunum left, three drains were left in situ, and a loop ileostomy was formed. The laparotomy wound was packed, with a further laparotomy planned in two days.

1. What factors would determine which route of feeding you considered?
2. What would your initial nutritional management be?
3. Once he has stabilised, an NGT is placed and feeding commences.
4. What type of feed would you choose and what else what might you use?
5. What are the long-term implications of his surgery?

## Case 9

Miss J (age 35 yr, weight 98 kg, height 154 cm) was admitted to ICU with type two respiratory failure on day 3 of her admission with gallstone pancreatitis. Her CRP was 457 and she was commenced on CPAP. An NGT is sited and left on free drainage while she is on CPAP.

1. What would you recommend on her initial admission to ICU?
2. What factors may determine your choice of feeding route?

3. At week 1, her CT scan shows extensive fluid collections and her abdomen is distended. She is intubated and paralysed. Her intra-abdominal pressures are recorded at 24 and she is started on haemofiltration. How would this change your management?
4. At week 3, her CT scan shows 90% necrosis of the pancreas. What additional factors might you consider now?

## Case 10

Mr K (aged 68 yr, weight 67 kg, height 170 cm) is due to be admitted for elective oesophagectomy for adenocarcinoma. He has a history of hypertension, hypercholesterolaemia, and his pre-assessment blood tests revealed significant iron-deficiency anaemia. He is weight stable and aside of fatigue reported to be feeling well pre-operatively.

1. What pre-operative nutritional management would you recommend?

2. On day 4 post oesophagectomy and insertion of feeding jejunostomy, he develops a new abdominal distension, his CRP increases, and his lactate rises. A CT scan shows intestinal pneumatosis. What would your feeding options consist of now? What medical management might be implemented?
3. Once recovered, Mr K continued to struggle with weight loss and loose bowel motions. What else might you consider?

# Index

*Nutritional Management of the Surgical Patient*, First Edition. Edited by Mary E. Phillips.
© 2023 John Wiley & Sons Ltd. Published 2023 by John Wiley & Sons Ltd.